The Fragmented Personality

The Fragmented Personality

An Integrative, Dynamic, and Personalized Approach to Personality Disorder

Dragan M. Svrakic, MD, PhD

Professor of Psychiatry
Washington University School of Medicine;
VA Medical Center
St. Louis, Missouri

and

Mirjana Divac-Jovanovic, PhD

Associate Professor of Clinical Psychology
Faculty of Media and Communications
Department of Psychology
Singidunum University
Belgrade, Serbia

OXFORD
UNIVERSITY PRESS

OXFORD
UNIVERSITY PRESS

Oxford University Press is a department of the University of Oxford. It furthers the University's objective of excellence in research, scholarship, and education by publishing worldwide. Oxford is a registered trade mark of Oxford University Press in the UK and certain other countries.

Published in the United States of America by Oxford University Press
198 Madison Avenue, New York, NY 10016, United States of America.

CIP data is on file at the Library of Congress
ISBN 978-0-19-088457-4

9 8 7 6 5 4 3 2 1

Printed by WebCom, Inc., Canada

Gratitude
To my wife Sanja and my daughter Neda for
their love and continuing support
Dr. D. Svrakic

I dedicate this book to my patients, whose desire and courage
to change crucially advanced my understanding of mental
processes in the background of their problems
Dr. M. Divac-Jovanovic

CONTENTS

PREFACE

In this book we present our understanding of the concepts of personality and personality disorder, forged over a cumulative of 60 years of clinical practice and research between the two of us. We also review the contributions of other authors, with a focus on those works that have passed the test of time to become an integral part of the knowledge base in the field. The book is primarily intended to be a guide for mental health professionals, notably psychiatrists, psychologists, social workers, and psychotherapists of any orientation, for those already in practice and equally for those in training. The book may also prove informative to a selected subsection of the educated general public who may find it stimulating, as it covers a number of topics of wide interest (e.g., from the biosocial evolution of morality to the impact of postmodern "accelerated" time on psychological concepts, among many others). Last but not least, we trust that the book may inspire our patients[1] and all of us who are, in a very figurative sense, someone's patient, to reflect on own emotions, thoughts, motivations, and behaviors. If nothing else, the very act of introspection may help people grow mentally and we dare say even become happier. We are profoundly grateful to all those individuals whose desire, determination, and courage to change helped us formulate our understanding of the processes underlying their problems. In fact, with their intuition and keen self-observation they were often the first to grasp the operating patterns underlying their mental struggles. In many cases we simply connected the dots while following their lead.

We also have learned a great deal from our colleagues, Otto F. Kernberg and Robert C. Cloninger, two of the most influential contemporary authors in the field of personality. Kernberg's book *Borderline Conditions*

1. The term "patient"—even though less politically correct—better captures the essence of the notion of a suffering person than the term "client," which, in our view, seems better suited for a business relationship than for the therapeutic relationship.

and Pathological Narcissism published in 1975 has defined our professional choices, as both of us, inspired by the book, chose the field of personality and its disorders. At the time, at the beginning of our careers, we were open to Kernberg's leadership to move the field forward, and thus away from the authoritarian dogma that pervaded classical psychoanalysis. Now, 40 years later, we are still inspired by Kernberg's talent for synthesis, his powerful insights, and his eloquence in describing them. One of us (DMS) was also greatly influenced by a longstanding close and continuing collaboration with Cloninger whose pioneering work on the psychobiology of personality, particularly the visionary idea to connect human temperament with the underlying neurobiological mechanisms, has not only scientifically demystified the hitherto esoteric concept of personality traits but has also set a new standard in theory and research in the field. We incorporate Kernberg's and Cloninger's work as the foundation upon which we build our original contributions and formulations.

The position of clinical psychology and psychiatry in contemporary society is somewhat paradoxical. They are expected to not only explain all sorts of mental and social phenomena in the general population but also to diagnose (classify, evaluate) these phenomena and in, many cases, to correct (treat, change) them. At the same time, these allocated powers are being closely scrutinized due to fear of abuse of these roles given the not unreasonable concern that our private mental experiences may gradually become less so over time. In this book we systematically uphold the scientific approach to the assessment of personality and psychopathology (*the principle of objectivity*) along with our genuine respect of these persons who turn to us for help (*the principle of respect*). In formulating our ideas, we followed the descriptive-analytical approach (qualitative analysis) while taking great care to avoid labels of any kind, particularly any sort of moral qualifications (*the principle of non-labeling*). We are aware that this may not always be possible when describing individuals who are socially maladapted, because the descriptors themselves in many cases may already carry labels with derogatory connotations. Contrary to widespread prejudice, a person's weakness lies not in him or her seeking psychological help but rather in him or her not addressing his or her problems. People who seek help for psychological problems demonstrate a high level of awareness, mental strength, and, above all, courage to face their weaknesses, fears, confusion, or insecurity. It is our professional responsibility to employ all available knowledge and the most effective methods to help these courageous individuals overcome their mental struggles. It is our professional obligation not just to keep up to date with scientific advances in the field but also to share insights and ideas with other colleagues. It is in this spirit that we undertook the considerable expenditure of energy involved in writing a book, which we wish in time will be commensurate with whatever benefit may accrue to the reader.

ACKNOWLEDGMENTS

Charles F. Zorumski, MD, Washington University School of Medicine in St. Louis, provided helpful guidance and insightful suggestions.

Patrick J. Lustman, PhD, Washington University School of Medicine in St. Louis, provided useful comments.

Tamara Džamonja- Ignjatović, PhD, University of Belgrade, School of Philosophy, Department of Psychology, Serbia, provided useful suggestions and is the coauthor of the Inventory of Defense Mechanisms presented in this book.

Aaron Mofsen, MD, Washington University School of Medicine in St. Louis, provided useful comments and helped with editing the manuscript.

Introduction

When we consult colleagues about patients with personality disorder, the discussion typically centers on how the patient in question functions psychologically or interpersonally rather than whether he or she conforms to a specific diagnosis. To us as therapists and even more so to the patient who is expecting help, a traditional diagnosis of personality disorder is of secondary importance. Behind a variable behavior façade, individuals with personality disorder are more alike than not with respect to their underlying personality organization and symptom dynamics. Despite chronic interpersonal problems, they persist in social deviance, as if their behaviors were primarily subserving some vital internal needs, at the expense of adaptability. Over the years we have searched for a deeper understanding of the mechanisms underlying manifest symptoms and the dynamics that maintain them. The search has resulted in our understanding that personality disorder reflects the mind's pursuit of organization and survival through fantasy, excess, and deviance, akin to a lump of callus that heals the bone. Our efforts to solve the "so different yet so similar" gestalt have helped us create a dynamic, dimensional, time- and context-sensitive personalized model and therapy of personality disorder that is the centerpiece of this book.

Moving beyond static structures, typology, and population averages, modern psychology conceptualizes mental health and disorder through the prism of mental function, which it defines dynamically, in time and context. The current digital era has increasingly fragmentated society in the real world and fostered its abstracted organization in the cyberspace, thus redefining many fundamental concepts related to personality. Almost all aspects of self, identity, socialization, intimacy, and community are perceived, experienced, and validated in a qualitatively new way. In this book, we revisit the concept of personality disorder. As one's mental potentials are expanded by the technologies, fragmentation of personality into multiplicity of self-images that would have been diagnosed as personality disorder only 30 years ago today are viewed as a normal "multiphrenia" (Gergen, 1991) or adaptive fragmentation of the self. The antithetical but no less relativizing proposal of the World Health Organization (WHO) includes a vague category of "personality problems that may emerge in interpersonal relations," which, if accepted, would be likely to affect no less than 80% of the earth's population, a grave and unrealistic pathologization of everyday human life. We support diagnostic flexibility in assessing mental phenomena but caution against wanton efforts to expand the catchment area of psychopathology, perhaps acceptable to philosophical anthropology, but not to the applied sciences of psychology and clinical psychiatry.

Diagnostic aspects pivotal to the analysis of personality and its disorders are twofold. One aspect examines the level of mental functioning (a qualitative aspect of personality integration) while the second aspect is concerned with that individual's style of adaptation in relation to the environment (habitual behavior patterns). These aspects can be thought of as "vertical diagnosis" and "horizontal diagnosis," respectively. The former captures in-depth features, like defense mechanisms or identity coherence; the latter describes the adaptive façade with typical patterns of behavior, thought, and emotion. These two aspects are the pillars of the assessment of personality in health and personality disorder. They provide answers to the three most important questions concerning the diagnosis: *what* (adaptive style, patterns of behavior and relationships), *how* (characteristics of mental functioning), and *why* (factors in the development and maintenance of the observed patterns). Cross-matching one's specific adaptive style with one's level of personality integration, in the given context and a unit of time, defines the unique position for that individual in the tridimensional diagnostic cylinder (Chapter 3). Our dynamic nosology allows for a personalized diagnosis, time and context sensitive, and a personalized (patient-specific) method of help.

As an official diagnosis, personality disorder first appeared in 1952, in the first edition of *Diagnostic and Statistical Manual of Mental Disorders* (DSM) developed by the American Psychiatric Association (APA, 1952). The new diagnosis polarized clinicians as soon as it was conceived. Some welcomed it with enthusiasm, primarily due to the fact that it finally made official an important mental syndrome hitherto overshadowed by other, clinically more impressive affective or psychotic disorders. Others reacted with skepticism, voicing concerns of potential abuse whereby any variant of uncommon behavior could be now formally diagnosed as psychopathological, leading to what some feared could become a "psychiatrization of life." Incidentally, the anticipated misuse has not materialized, perhaps because the profound implications of being the arbiters of "amorality" forced clinicians to reserve the diagnosis for carefully analyzed and well documented outpatients.[1] Another milestone was the introduction of explicit, operationalized criteria for personality disorder in the third edition of the DSM (APA, 1980). The descriptive criteria were expected to increase the reliability and the specificity of the diagnosis. This expectation has not been met due to overlapping and heterogeneous criteria, which fail to reliably separate individual subtypes and do not account for mixed and atypical forms. The latter are more frequent than prototypical cases, because individual differences are as great in illness as they are in health. On the positive side, the new diagnosis provided clinicians with the ability to correctly diagnose individuals who were misdiagnosed as having other mental disorders, most commonly atypical depression, anxiety disorder, bipolar disorder, dysthymia, or incipient Schizophrenia, which in many instances led to better outcomes. Practicing clinicians expected that the new diagnosis would stimulate the development of specific therapies. The expectation has been met to an extent, especially with regard to psychotherapy (new psychotherapies for this category of patients are discussed in Chapter 4) but also with regard to pharmacotherapy (discussed in Chapter 5), which has moved from symptom centered to mechanism-based (targeting underlying temperament vulnerabilities) and symptom domain based (targeting domains of symptoms shared by most individual variants of personality disorder). In any case, the new diagnosis rekindled the old public debate surrounding normalcy. Critics in the second half of the 20th century derided the field's tendency to pathologize behavior it presumably found unpalatable and tended to regard diagnosis as little more than another institutional decree of what constituted acceptable social behavior.

The ineluctable controversies surrounding what constitutes a personality disorder continue to inspire clinicians efforts to explore, understand, and, perhaps even resolve them. This interest is by no means limited to clinicians as it continues to provide fodder for artistic creation. Artists have been long been intrigued by the coexistence of polarized extremes in the same personality: flexible and rigid, cold and compassionate, scared and fearless, brilliant and limited, permissive and strict. Marcel Proust (1871–1922) in the opus *In Search of Lost Time*, through the character of Baron

1. The diagnosis is used more freely with psychiatric inpatients and ER agitated patients

de Charlus, brilliantly captures the essence of narcissistic personality disorder based in part on the life of Robert de Montesquiou (1855–1921), a contemporary French aesthete, symbolist poet, art collector, and dandy. More recently, Jonathan Frentzen (1959–) provided another great literary portrayal of fragmented personality in his novel *Purity* through the character of Anabel. Captivated by the same general interest, the media, with varying degrees of responsibility, continues to opine on deviant behaviors of politicians, celebrities, and notorious transgressors, among others.

When psychotherapists say "personality disorder," they mean "borderline" or, as we refer to it, "fragmented" personality. Indeed, we have shown that fragmentation appears as a common characteristic of all bona fide variants of personality disorder (Divac et al., 1993). Because of the misuse, overuse, stigma, and therapeutic nihilism associated with the term "borderline," we prefer the term "fragmented personality." The term "borderline" refers to differences between persons with neurosis and psychosis, has become a negative prototype for mental instability, rather than providing more specific information about the person. The term "fragmented" evokes the psychological essence of personality disorder consistent with our personalized approach (i.e., suboptimal brain and mind integration within a person that secondarily leads to social maladaptation, together known as a personality disorder).

The term and the concept of "adaptation" are used with multiple meanings in the literature. We understand it as a long-term yet dynamic balance within and between one's internal and external environments, resulting in mental flexibility and functional adaptation to the society. By internal environment we mean one's unique biogenetic heritage (e.g., inherited emotional biases associated with temperament, cognitive capabilities [IQ]), personalized mental functions [emotions, motivations, cognition] derived from internalized object relations [we refer to the latter as the elementary particles of the mind], and one's autobiographical chronicle and mental prospection of possible futures [mediated by the subsystem of identity]. External environment refers to sociocultural and interpersonal context which are adaptively "handled" by character and moral values. In contrast, periodical coping with changing internal or external conditions constitutes adjustment. "Fragmented personality" should not be confused with the "postmodern fragmented self," a healthy adaptation to the postmodern world.

In our opinion, assessment of personality disorder is paradigmatic for differential diagnosis in general concerned as it is with a specific level of mental functioning, which overlaps with normalcy, neuroses, and psychoses. As such, all must be ruled out. In the process of diagnosing personality disorder one always finds indices of normalcy and psychopathology, including elements of psychoses: once we understand personality disorder, we begin to understand the majority of nonpsychotic and psychotic phenomena. As personality disorder increases susceptibility to many other psychiatric and medical problems, the diagnosis and treatment planning of any psychological, psychosomatic, or psychosocial syndrome is incomplete without a systematic assessment of personality that "carries" the syndrome.

In this book we present our understanding of personality (Chapter 1) and personality disorder (Chapter 2). In Chapter 3, we introduce our model of dynamic dimensional nosology and specify differential diagnostic parameters of personality disorder, including a detailed differentiation from neuroses. We outline the basic principles of reconstructive interpersonal psychotherapy in Chapter 4 and discuss mechanism- and symptom domain–based pharmacotherapy as it applies to personality disorder in Chapter 5. We conclude the book by sharing our vision as to "what lies ahead for human personality."

CHAPTER 1

What Is Personality?

In this section, we describe the neural and psychological processes that transform units of sensory information about internal and external environment into complex faculties of the mind, notably cognition, emotion, and motivation, or "mental triology" as LeDoux (2003) calls them. We also hypothesize how the mind self-organizes into semi-stable configurations of these faculties (the "subsystems" of the mind),[1] with highly complex functional outcomes, such as the sense of self, identity, character, or moral values, among others. To this end, we borrow from cognitive, molecular, and computational neuroscientists (Joseph LeDoux, Charles Zorumski, Olaf Sporns, Susumu Tonegawa) and cite other work as indicated.

THE HUMAN BRAIN: THE MATTER UNDER MIND

Neuroscience understands the human brain, its structural organization and neurophysiological function, to be the physical substrate, the matter of the mind. The brain, a collection of about 80 billion neurons, and the mind, the brain's adaptive agency subserved by mental faculties, are structural and functional analogues. Mental faculties and behavior are associated with neuronal activity in distributed networks of neuronal populations and brain regions. The mind and its matter are involved in a bidirectional, modifying influences (positive feedback), where increasingly complex neural organization of the brain promotes the increased complexity of the

1. As modern psychology has moved away from structures to functions, we use the term "systems" instead of "structures" to capture the dynamic nature of the mind.

mind and vice versa. Both processes are observed in the psychosocial development of a child, that is, his or her increasing motoric, cognitive, behavioral, and social capacities achieved via bidirectional interacting neural and mental plasticity that continues throughout the lifetime.

Brain organization: a modular design cobbled during evolution. In all biology, more complex systems are built upon the older more primitive structures; in other words, the latter are not replaced but incorporated into and controlled by higher complexity. Applied to the human brain, more complex brain networks (a set of nodes[2] and edges forming a network) are not built *de novo* but through combinations and/or extension of existing networks, the latter referring to the addition of network elements in positions where they maximize the overall processing power of the neural organization (Sporns and Kotter, 2004) or, simply, attaching new nodes to highly connected existing nodes. Such cobbling of the brain creates redundancy ("back-up" functions) and inefficiency (error-prone, gap-filling) that nevertheless works to produce the mind when things are normal and resulting in varying degrees of mental disorder when the system malfunctions.

Two types of networks characterize brain organization: structural and functional. Structural networks correspond to a pattern of anatomical connections, summarizing synaptic links between neurons or projections among brain regions. These are exemplified by large-scale networks that link cortical and subcortical gray matter regions (aka "human connectome"). In contrast, functional networks are deduced from estimates of statistical dependencies between neuronal or regional time series data (reviewed in Sporns and Betzel, 2016). These are exemplified by large-scale functional networks (aka "intrinsic connectivity networks" [ICNs]), believed to be the mechanism of the mind, from basic mental faculties to self-awareness. There is solid evidence that brain networks, structural and functional, are modular. Modules are defined as subcomponents of a network, clusters of nodes strongly internally and weakly externally connected that work together to achieve a relatively specialized function (e.g., to process specific information). From the standpoint of evolution, modular organization of a system is adaptively advantageous as it promotes the system's evolvability (capability of quickly adapting to new environments) through stability (compartmentalization increases resilience in the context of continuous changes), flexibility (rearranging suboptimal modules is less costly than redesigning the entire system), conserving wiring length (most brain modules

2. Nodes are highly connected points within a network.

are spatially compact), complex neuronal dynamics (promotes specialization), and robustness (the effects of local perturbations are mainly confined to the module provided that a vital node is not involved).

In his discussion of the oceanic feeling, Freud (1930) used the city of Rome in Italy as a metaphor for the psyche in which "nothing that has once come into existence will have passed away and all the earlier phases of development continue to exist alongside the latest one. . . . The earlier phases of development are in no sense still preserved; they have been absorbed into the later phases for which they have supplied the material" (p. 5). Freud was using the metaphor to explain the adult residuals of the early, all-embracing "oceanic" ego. We use the city of Rome as a metaphor for the process of brain and mind development. The city has been developing over thousands of years, many times structurally modified to fit the evolving social models, the growing needs of its growing population, and the likings of the Roman emperor de jour. In the process, some worn-out structures were replaced, some were demolished to free the space for new construction, and some were modified and integrated into the new plan of the city. Clay-brick arches and iron-fortified concrete columns side by side supporting buildings and bridges testify to such cobbling of the city. No brick arch or concrete beam is superior in function: they co-support the structures which, altogether, make the city of Rome. A walk through the center (Il Centro) vividly illustrates the city's developmental history, here used to metaphorize the sequential and progressive development leading to a largely nonhierarchical and canonical brain and mind organization.

The brain networks cross-talk through shared motifs. The concepts of structural and functional motifs are important to understand the organization of brain networks of information processing. Modules and motifs differ in that the former (modules) are specialized subcomponents of a network, and the latter (motifs) are smaller building blocks of a biological network, defined as frequently repeated patterns that occur in the real network significantly more often than in randomized networks. Motifs are shared among interacting networks as "points of contacts" for a specific communicated event. The term "motif" is used as an analogy for driving elements that are elaborated in a musical composition. To explain the basics of functional and structural motifs we borrow from Sporns and Kotter (2004). Structural motifs are smaller network building blocks defined as a set of brain areas and pathways that can potentially engage in different patterns of interactions. Functional motifs are different combinations of selectively activated nodes and connections within the constraints of the underlying structural motif in the course of particular information processing. One structural motif may contain many instances of functional motifs. The real brain networks maximize the number and diversity of functional motifs to ensure a large repertoire of functional circuits, and minimize the number and diversity of structural motifs, to allow for efficient assembly and encoding. The resulting networks are of the small world attributes that lie between regular and random and promote functional cooperation, recurrent processing, and efficient information exchange (Sporns and Kotter, 2004, p. 1915). The highly connected nodes (hubs) and modularity (physical or functional isolation of subsystems) may give rise to "scale-free"[3] properties of information processing in the brain. A scale-free connectivity involves a few highly connected hubs ("power centers"), many scarcely connected nodes (about 20% of nodes have 80% of the "power"), and long-range connections. The power centers in the human brain or vital hubs are the hippocampus (the "super hub"), amygdala, prefrontal cortex (PFCx), among others. Scale-free systems have the ability to incorporate biogenetic and mental imperfections and still fall within the range of physiological variation. This type of connectivity enhances the robustness of the system and resists system failures, provided that a sufficient number of highly connected hubs are not all compromised at the same time, which can lead to a cascade failure.

Complex biological systems: toward ever more efficient information processing and output complexity. The increasingly complex forms of biological systems have been proposed to have evolved following "non-zero" sumness or "win-win" sumness in game theory, that is, the prospect of creating new interactions that are not zero-sum (do not have the loser and the winner, but all participants win) (Wright, 1999). The thesis is that both natural selection and cultural evolution promote better information processing. Competing organisms mutually promote each other's complexity: the increasing ability of a prey to defend itself promotes increasing abilities on the part of the predator.

The brain is organized into multiple parallel processing systems, each specialized to process a specific modality of the *same* information (e.g., visual, emotional, rewarding). This provides "pieces" to be unified into a mental portrait of reality (Zorumski and Rubin, 2011). The parallel processing systems are not independent, as the simplest perceptions are instantly made more complex by the input from other systems, for example, by integrating memories and affects into unified memory-and-affect experience. Such coordinated activity is achieved in part by activity-dependent

3. In scale-free networks, the distribution of connections that nodes have is a rapidly decreasing function of the number of nodes in the network, with no true average number of connections, making the network difficult to measure or scale ("scale free") (Zorumski and Rubin, 2011).

Hebbian-type synaptic plasticity within and between the parallel systems whereby synapses that connect neurons involved in timed co-activity tend to strengthen and those not involved tend to weaken. This leads to circuit forming where the type of "cells that fire together wire together" and vice versa.[4]

The described lower level information processing is integrated by several highly connected neocortical regions called "convergence zones" (LeDoux, 2003), for example, parietal or PFCx, among others. The high connectivity makes the convergence zones optimal for synthesizing multimodal information complexes. At these "meeting points," lower level processing outcomes are integrated into multimodal information complexes embedded within a higher order cognitive frame of reference. The convergence zones likely represent highly connected nodes ("hubs") within scale-free networks. The zones may be the point of neural-mental interface, where the neurophysiology of the brain (percepts) gives rise to the abstractions of the mind (concepts). For example, working memory involves the ability of the PFCx (one of the convergence zones) to temporarily hold relevant perceptions in a "cognitive buffer," a form of rudimentary abstraction crossing from the realm of the brain into that of the mind, where internal representations of the external world are reliable and readily available to inform active reasoning, decision-making, and behavior (Nestler et al., 2015).

The human connectome refers to large-scale structural networks anatomically linking cortical and subcortical gray matter regions. However, it is the functional connectivity among distributed brain regions that appears to be the mechanism of the mind. The complex functions of the mind (e.g., decision-making, language, motivation, conscious emotion among others) are believed to result from activity in large-scale functional networks (ICNs). Unlike structural networks, which are thought to be relatively stable, functional networks are variable, with spontaneous dynamic changes during rest as well as characteristic modulations in different task conditions—basically variations of the resting state architecture (reviewed in Sporns and Betzel, 2016). In other words, the brain's functional network architecture during task performance appears to be shaped primarily by an intrinsic network architecture that is also present during rest and secondarily by evoked task-general and task-specific network changes (Cole et al., 2014).

The ICNs are functionally connected distributed brain regions that resonate or "hum" together in slow activity (<0.1 Hz). Such resonant activity

4. Another mechanism facilitating flexible coordination within and across the parallel processing systems is via neuromodulators and neurotransmitters, whether inhibitory or excitatory, slow or fast acting.

and its associated functional connectivity, perhaps reflecting co-active functional motifs, have been postulated to underlie higher order processing of information (Zorumski and Rubin, 2011). Recent work in animals (Mitra et al., 2018) documents a high correspondence of spatiotemporal trajectories and infra-slow frequency of <0.1 Hz between the resting state BOLD[5] signals and wide-field optical calcium imaging of neuronal activity. In other words, the same resting state network is identified by two different methodologies, indicating that spontaneous infra-slow BOLD signals reflect reality (i.e., spontaneous infra-slow neuronal activity [ISA] in the identified regions). Moreover, by measuring time delays (dubbed "lag threads") in the BOLD signal in resting awake humans, the same group (Mitra et al., 2015) demonstrated multiple, highly reproducible, temporal sequences of propagated activity unidirectional within conventionally understood resting-state networks. The finding is suggestive of a sequential process of dynamic and unidirectional propagated activation, rather than static co-occurrence.[6] Modeling experiments showed that resting state networks *naturally emerge as a consequence of this shared patterns of propagation*. The ISA wave-like propagation is highly stereotypical, shows laminar specificity and traveling direction (bottom to top layers of cortex) and reverses the direction along the same trajectories with a change in brain states, notably consciousness vs anesthesia. The authors postulate that such spatiotemporal organization of ISA might have emergent, system-level organizational properties, such as governing or marking functional brain rather than itself reflecting information flow. The exact origins of the slow resonant synchrony is not fully understood. Subthreshold activity, neuromodulators from neurons and the glia, or metabolic glia signaling may play a role as these mediate more widespread, diverse, volumetric transmission than relatively precise synaptic transmission and can alter the function of local or distant neuronal partners (Mitra et al., 2018; Zorumski and Rubin, 2011). Functional connectivity among brain regions often follows anatomical connectivity but may also include functional co-occurrences (perhaps even coincidences?) without hard connection.

5. Functional magnetic resonance imaging (fMRI) uses blood oxygen-level dependent (BOLD) signal, presumed to reflect an increased blood flow due to increased neuronal activity of the neurons in question, to measure behavior-related neural activity in the human brain; its relationship with underlying neural activity has been questioned, and the Mitra (2018) study offers some insights on the subject.

6. The term "chronnectome" has been coined to capture such time-varying levels of correlated or mutually informed activity between brain regions whose spatial properties may also be temporally evolving.

Several ICNs have been identified thus far, for example default mode network mediating spontaneous internal mentation, working memory network, prefrontal executive network, emotional salience network, among a number of others. Some "super-hubs" are involved in multiple ICNs (e.g., the hippocampus, amygdala). The shared hubs help coordinate the flow of information within and between the ICNs. Activity in some functional systems is specifically decreased ("anti-correlated") when another system is active.

Physiological variations in the organization of ICNs likely underlie individual differences, perhaps even uniqueness, in the mind's function and adaptive effectiveness. Recently, nine scientists from Washington University in St. Louis scanned own brains for more than 10 hours of functional connectivity (fcMRI) at rest with eyes open and while performing different tasks (visual, semantic, memory, motor) (Gratton et al., 2018). The brain networks were dominated by common organizational principles (i.e., stable general structure) and stable individual differences, the latter to the point that the individual could be identified by his or her brain networks with a glance (record@wustl.edu, April 4, 2018). The brain networks of the participants were remarkably stable from day to day and while undertaking different tasks. Due to the organizational stability and sensitivity to individual differences of the networks, Gratton et al. (2108) suggest that fcMRI scans may hold promise as diagnostic biomarkers to identify individuals with mental health vs disorder. To this end, some distinguishing brain markers of dysfunction would have to show specificity for specific mental disorders. We expect brain networks to be as individually distinctive in mental disorder as they are in health, and thus might be of more benefit to precision or personalized medicine than to evidence based medicine. In other words, personality can be thought of as "personalized mind", a unique ontogenetic outcome of the general phylogenetic capacity of our species; although BOLD neuroimaging captures only a fraction of the mind's function, the task and time stability of unique individual features justifies the metaphor.

The dynamic functional interaction among the large scale ICNs allows for integration of processing outcomes in diverse neural circuits. The interaction is believed to create the complex faculties of the mind, aka "mental trilogy". As Zorumski and Rubin (2011) note, cognition (thought) may involve co-activity of the working memory network, attention/reorienting network, executive functioning network, and face recognition network, among others. Emotion (meaning) may involve the extended amygdala processing network, emotional-salience network, and explicit memory network. Motivation (goals) may involve the reward processing network and the ventral tegmentum—ventral striatum network (Zorumski and Rubin, 2011, p. 48). The exact mechanism underlying the formation of complex mental faculties is unknown, but the mentioned spontaneous regulatory ISA and cross-regional talk through shared motifs could provide some answers.

How do the mental faculties of emotion, motivation, and thought become organized into one's personality? Although the exact mechanism has not been demonstrated, it can be outlined as a rather straightforward speculation. At the highest level of cognitive integration, driven by self-organizing multidirectional optimization processes to meet the increasing adaptive demands before the mind, the ICNs involved in thought, emotion, and motivation self-organize into semi-stable emerging configurations which we refer to as the subsystems of the mind, such as the sense of self, character, moral standards, and identity, each providing a unique adaptive function to the system of the mind as a whole. If homeostatic optimization is the driving force behind such self-organization, the operative force is the increasingly capable general network of cognition, with crucial inputs from emotional and motivational networks. The general network of cognition is an interactive composite in its own right (involving the lateral and medial PFCx, posterior parietal cortex, and insular cortex), through the works of cognitive functions (attention, working memory, and metacognition[7]) (LeDoux and Brown, 2017). The network has been implicated in the phenomena of self-awareness and emotional consciousness (LeDoux and Brown, 2017). In addition, it interacts with other brain regions to give rise to a number of related phenomena, nonconscious, actively or passively conscious, such as theory of mind of others, autobiographical memory, spontaneous mentation, prospection, empathy and related social emotions, moral evaluations of right or wrong, among others. Together, such highest-order cognitive processes and the respective emerging subsystems contribute to the unified and personalized experience of mental and physical reality, as we discuss later.

Prefrontal cortices and cognitive feedback control: the executives of human mind. One of the most frequently cited neurobiological deficits in personality disorder are hypofunctional PFCx with suboptimal top-down control of subcortical processes, which are frequently overreactive in the first place. The mismatch may explain the majority of symptoms of personality disorder: mood instability, defective mentalization and theory of mind of others (defined as ability to appreciate the independent mental processes and states of oneself and others, respectively), lack of empathy, difficulties in self-related episodic memory[8] and future

7. Metacognition refers to the awareness and the understanding of one's own thought processes.

8. Memory of autobiographical events (times, places, associated emotions, and other contextual who, what, when, where, why knowledge) that can be explicitly stated or conjured. It is the collection of past personal experiences that occurred at a particular time and place or interaction.

planning, polarization of experience into cognitive-affective extremes, among others. The hypofrontality appears to result from the interplay of heritable neurobiology (inborn reactivity to stress) and environment (stressogenic), singly or in concert interfering with the early organization of large-scale brain networks, even fracturing the already formed ones. This in turn interferes with the integrative processes of the early mind, which remains polarized into contradictory units of memories and affects and is adaptively suboptimal. In a vicious circle, hypoactive brain networks and mental fragmentation perpetuate each other, in the process perpetuating the psychopathology of personality disorder. Here we describe the organization and function of the PFCx as well as the executive function (EF) and working memory, which are all important to understanding the neurobiology of personality disorder.

Functional organization of the PFCx. The PFCx is the brain region that subserves EF, perhaps the most "human" of its many other functions, which encompasses a set of cognitive processes, such as reasoning, problem solving, planning and decision-making, drawing inferences, cognitive flexibility, making predictions based on recognized patterns and regularities, among others (Nestler et al., 2015; Zorumski and Rubin, 2011). Other PFCx functions, more or less overlapping with EF, include working memory (instrumental in conscious thinking), attention shifting, resolving ambiguities and handling uncertainties, anticipation of reward and punishment, the experience of empathy and other complex and prosocial (secondary) emotions, and a close involvement with ICNs for language, the latter important for abstractions and complex concepts. Here we focus on EF, which is defined as top-down control of decision-making and behavior, sometimes called "supervisory attentional system" (D Norman and T Shallice). The PFCx is a multimodal association cortex, one of the highly connected regions called "convergence zones," that draws information form stored memories in other areas of neocortex, primary sensory areas, and other convergence zones such as parietal cortex and the hippocampus. Such connectivity enables information from various processed sensory modalities to be integrated here in a multimodal fashion within a higher order cognitive frame of reference to form the complex constructs of memory, perception, and diverse cognitive processes, such as mentation (that is spontaneous or deliberate mental activity), theory of mind of others, and mentalization, among others (reviewed in Siddiqui et al., 2008). The PFCx communicates via extensive feedback and feedforward reciprocal connections with subcortical structures, notably the amygdala, hypothalamus, midbrain, and pons (the thalamus is the traffic controller of this "extended prefrontal neural system"), not only to integrate these subcortical affects and motivations into higher cognitive functions but also to "top-down" regulate the more instinctive subcortical processes. Keeping in mind that functional subdivisions of the PFCx are a simplification, are still somewhat vague, and vary in the literature, we list the most recent understanding as reported in Nestler et al. (2015): the *anterior cingulate* is involved in processes requiring correct decision-making (e.g., in conflicts) or cortical stopping of activity to switch to another task; the *medial PFCx* is involved in supervisory attentional functions ("action-outcome" rules) and behavioral flexibility (ability to switch strategies); the *dorsolateral PFCx* is implicated in matching sensory inputs with planned motor responses (many associate this region with judgment of responsibility for actions, top-down regulation of attention, reasoning and dealing with ambiguity, planning, and working memory); *the ventromedial PFCx* regulates empathy and social cognition, regulation of emotion, and perhaps also self-reflection, moral emotions and cognition; the *orbitofrontal PFCx* is involved in social decision-making and representing affective valuation assigned to different experiences and impulse control. In some other works, the *ventrolateral PFCx* or, alternatively, inferior PFCx, was implicated in mediation of cognitive control of behavior (inhibitory control, interference control, and cognitive flexibility). The PFCx also has extensive connections specialized for each processing domain with the cerebellar cortex via the pontine nuclei, with parallel projections through the basal ganglia. With these connectivity and functional effects, the PFCx is positioned to orchestrate all aspects of behavior in accordance with short- and long-term goals, prior experience, and environmental context (Zorumski and Rubin, 2011).

The executive top-down control of affects, motivation, and behavior by the PFCx depends on its fundamental ability to represent information not currently in the environment. This representational knowledge is known as working memory. Goldman-Rakic (1996) referred to it as a "mental sketch pad" and Nestler et al. (2015) as a short-lived, capacity-limited cognitive buffer that maintains a representation of sensory information "on line" and permits the integration of this information to guide thought, emotion, and behavior. In this way, working memory can be seen as fundamental to an adaptively effective mind and behavior. As noted, working memory represents a form of rudimentary abstraction crossing from the realm of the brain into that of the mind and from percepts to concepts. As Zorumski and Rubin (2011) noted working memory is not a "storage device" but a series of operations that pulls information from multiple sources and keeps track of that information while it is being used (p. 57).

The neurochemical environment of the PFCx: it has to be just right. The regulatory functions of the PFCx are based on local microcircuits that consist of glutamatergic pyramidal neurons and gamma-aminobutyric acid (GABA)-ergic inhibitory interneurons (Goldman-Rakic, 1995). The activity of these circuits is modulated by the brain's neurotransmitters and neuromodulators, for example, dopamine, norepinephrine, serotonin, acetylcholine, and orexin, among others. The PFCx is very sensitive to its neurochemical environment, and small variabilities in the available neuroactive molecules can produce large effects on mediated functions. The brain systems regulating the level of arousal (the midbrain norepinephrine and hypothalamic orexin, among others) or those involved in stress reactions (the midbrain dopamine and hypothalamic corticotropin releasing factor, among others) can functionally strengthen or weaken microcircuit cortical connections to coordinate cognition with arousal state or stress level (Arnsten and Rubia, 2012). Mild arousal or stress improves performance on various cognitive tasks, but if it becomes too great, performance declines (reflecting an inverted-U-shaped relationship between arousal/stress and performance [the Yerkes-Dodson principle]). The role of dopamine and norepinephrine, associated with stress and arousal, is discussed in more detail later.

The mesocorticolimbic dopaminergic system modulates a number of fundamental aspects of motivation, reward-related behaviors, and attention, as well as multiple forms of memory, all of which are coordinated in response to potent rewards. The neocortical arm of the dopaminergic system modulates multiple functions of the PFCx, most notably the EF. The dopaminergic role in EF involves working memory, suppression of prepotent behaviors that compete with goal-directed actions, and control of attention in order to overcome distractions (Nestler et al., 2015). Optimal levels of DA and NE are needed for proper PFCx executive control of behavior and diverse aspects of attention. Moderate levels of dopaminergic D1 receptor stimulation are essential for normal functioning of PFCx (D1 receptors are abundant there). As a cellular correlate, moderate D1-receptor stimulation suppresses neuronal processing of irrelevant information (i.e., reduces "noise") rendering PFCx firing more selective. High levels of D1 stimulation in PFCx (during high stress or negative affects) impair working memory. Similar patterns are observed for noradrenergic modulation of PFCx functions. In an inverted-U dose response pattern, norepinephrine improves PFCx function through actions at postsynaptic alpha (α) 2A receptors. Cognitive effects include improved working memory, attention regulation, and behavioral inhibition and/or planning in humans (Hunt et al., 1995). Cellular correlates of the cognitive effects include increased delay-related neuronal firing, a cellular correlate of working memory, and behavioral inhibition. The increased delay-related firing is observed for the preferred spatial direction, indicating that α2A receptor stimulation increases "signal strength" in PFCx. However, high levels of norepinephrine release (e.g., high stress) impair PFCx function through action at α1 receptors, both at the cellular level (decreased delay-related firing) and the cognitive level (impaired working memory; reviewed in Arnsten, 2006). In a simplified summary, Arnsten pointed out that norepinephrine enhances "signals" through postsynaptic α2A adrenoceptors, while dopamine decreases the "noise" through modest levels of D1 stimulation in PFCx. The inverted-U dose response pattern for dopamine and norepinephrine may help explain impressive clinical similarities between two neuropathologically different entities, the attention deficit hyperactivity disorder (ADHD) at the low end of the inverted U (deficient dopamine and norpeinpehrine) and the excessive temperament trait of novelty seeking at the high end of the inverted U (surplus dopamine and norpeinephrine). The respective treatments also fundamentally differ as discussed in Chapter 5.

Monoaminergic modulatory effects on PFCx overlap and are complementary. For example, noradrenergic projections from the locus coeruleus (hereafter referred to as LC-NA) to the PFCx interact with dopaminergic projections from the ventral tegmental area (VTA) to co-regulate cognitive, top-down control of behavior and working memory. Second, norepinephrine has high affinity for the D4 dopaminergic receptors (Van Tol et al., 1991), thus D4 receptors are able to respond to either dopamine or norepinephrine. Finally, serotonin, dopamine, and norepinephrine receptors in PFCx anatomically overlap and are frequently complementary (Goldman-Rakic et al., 1990).

GENOME, EPIGENOME, BRAIN/MIND, AND ENVIRONMENT: INTERACTIVE FORCES IN MENTAL DEVELOPMENT

DNA sequence (genotype) is not the final blueprint for physical and behavioral features. Rather, DNA outlines overall physical and neuropsychological capabilities of an organism ("what is possible") which then funnel into specific adaptive features (phenotype) in an interactive response to specific environmental stimuli. Such gene (G) × environment (E) interaction (G × E) is mediated by epigenetic mechanisms which reversibly "program" the genes (by chromatin remodeling, promoter methylation, etc.) to modulate their expression and activity as well as time and tissue specificity, in response to changing environmental conditions. Incidentally, epigenetic programming does not only refer to G × E interaction but also to programs of embryonic development that specify activity and expression of genes at different times and in different tissues, thus enabling one gene to serve multiple functions (aka "pleiotropy"). Back to G × E interaction, epigenetic programming can be thought of as the DNA response to signals from the environment that is *fast* (occurs within one generation, while mutations take many generations to spread in a population), *effective* (as effective as a mutation), stable but *reversible*, cell and tissue *specific* (affect only cells relevant to the environmental factor, whereas mutations affect all cells in the body), and allows *nongenomic inheritance* (whereby features acquired by the parents and/or their experience with the environment can be transmitted to offspring without changing the DNA sequence). The nongenomic inheritance occurs either through incomplete removal of epigenetic programs during meiosis or by behavioral inheritance: epigenetic effects of maternal behavior (high level of care) lead to an increased expression of glucocorticoid receptors in the brains of offspring, who are hence resistant to stress and themselves tend to be caring for their offspring (Champagne, 2008).

Basic structural features of the human brain, its general cytoarchitecture and neurophysiological characteristics, are encoded in the genome. Ontogenetically, the brain and the mind finalize structural and functional organization through G × E interaction, which cross-matches the specific genetic architecture and specific environmental factors. The "nature *and* nurture" paradigm posits that environmental factors, internal and external, modulate gene activity in the neurons and the related physiological processes as well as the structural and functional organization of brain networks and their dynamic output, the mind. The brain's ability to reorganize synaptic connections and remodel its networks in response to environmental conditions, learning, or experience is known as neuroplasticity. The latter is, we believe, the force behind psychoplasticity, that is, dynamic and reversible configurations of the mind and its subsystems as a function of adapting to the changing environment. Both neural and mental plasticity are lifelong; although they both tend to saturate with advancing age, they are rarely completely lost. Together the genome, the brain/mind, and the environment form a complex interactive triad in the brain-mind system development: at every point in the process, the development is influenced by the phase-specific gene activity and phase-relevant environmental factors[9] and the characteristics of the brain/mind system at the previous point. In a multidirectional feedback–feedforward interaction among the three variables, genes × brain/mind × environment, each new phase is

9. Epigenetic programming defines tissue and time specificity of gene activity; environmental stimuli also change relevance with the phase of life and cognitive abilities.

influenced by the degree of success at the previous phase and indirectly by the degree of success at all previous phases.

To summarize, the effects of the environment and genes are powerful enough to modify brain, mind, and behavior in any direction. A good environment can compensate for the effects of bad genes, while a bad environment can sabotage the effects of good genes. Fortunately, the epigenetic effects of a bad early environment, even though relatively stable, are open to correction in healthier, enriched, or therapeutic environments, known as environment × environment (E × E) interaction. The concept of E × E interaction refers to corrective powers of healthy environments in which the epigenetic influences of early experiences interact with environmental conditions experienced later in development (Champagne, 2008). Simply put, a healthy environment can epigenetically reverse brain structure, function, and maladaptive behaviors developed in earlier pathogenic environments in animals, much like what happens in psychotherapy. Neuroimaging reports (Hirvonen et al., 2011; Karlsson et al., 2010) provide evidence for the long-held belief that psychotherapy can modify not just the function (the mind) but also the neural structure of the brain (dubbed "molecular psychodynamics"). One can think of psychotherapy as both E x E and E x G effect: it is powerful enough to reach the nuclei of neurons, modify the activity of their genes, change the brain structurally and functionally, and impact personality traits in a lasting way, correcting in the process the impact of previous bad environments and/or heritable trait vulnerabilities.

THE HUMAN MIND: THE BRAIN'S ADAPTIVE AGENCY INDIVIDUALIZED INTO PERSONALITY

The human mind is best conceptualized as a progressively differentiated agency that mediates the brain's dynamic and interactive communication with the environment (Proust, 2009). The mind enables the brain to achieve its main adaptation tasks: to perceive environment, learn about it, remember it, analyze it using pre-existing knowledge, predict it, act toward it in a goal-oriented way, modify it toward one's own needs, and itself adjust to it. The concepts of mind, mental function, and personality can be thought of as equivalents. The first two derive from the Latin *mens* for "mind," whereas personality refers to the unique configuration of the mind in a given individual. Recent neuroimaging results, which show that functional brain networks are dominated both by common organizational principles (i.e., stable general structure) and stable individual differences (Gratton et al, 2018), appear to support the concept of personality as a unique configuration of the mind for any given individual. In other words, personality can be thought of as "personalized mind".

The default of the human brain is aimless mind-wandering ("day-dreaming"). ICNs can be roughly classified into task negative and task positive. The task-negative network, known as the default mode, is active when the brain is at wakeful rest and engages in spontaneous internal mentation (mind-wandering or daydreaming), also called the intrinsic attention system or self-generated cognition. If working memory is necessary for conscious thinking, the content of thinking involves the default network and the ICN involved in attention (Zorumski and Rubin, 2011). The task-positive networks are active during attention-demanding tasks involving the external environment (the extrinsic attention system). The two main groups of networks, task and non-task, are anticorrelated but not completely. Focusing on a task requires the brain to shift out of the default mode, activate attention to external stimuli, activate working memory, as well as the ICNs required for that particular task. This switching between task and no-task task networks process, including attention shifting, is mediated by the brain's attention "reorienting system" (Corbetta et al., 2008) which involves a coordinated action of two attentional networks: (i) one ventral or frontoparietal (interruption and resetting of the ongoing mental activity by important stimuli that reorient attention) and (ii) the other dorsal or cingulo-opercular (specialized to focus attention on selected stimuli and link the selected stimuli with relevant cognitive processes, including activation of working memory specific to the task). The dorsal network generates and maintains the internal focus based on current selected goals and working memory. When a salient signal reorients attention to the new source of information (*external* stimulus-driven reorienting), output from the ventral network interrupts (as a "circuit breaker") the ongoing *internally* directed process and selections mediated by the dorsal network, which in turn shifts attention toward the novel object of interest (Corbetta, et al., 2008, p. 3). When attention and cognition are focused on the task at hand, the ventral network is partially suppressed by the dorsal network to prevent distraction by unimportant stimuli. The different patterns of recruitment are believed to be influenced by the midbrain LC-NA system. Incidentally, research has demonstrated a partial colocalization of activations, mainly in the right temporo-parietal junction (TPJ), also involved with active theory of mind and reorienting processes. This TPJ activity might be important to switch between internal, bodily, or self-perspective and external, environmental, or other's viewpoint" the latter a key ingredient of reasoning about other people's mental states or theory of mind of others (Corbetta et al., 2008, p. 13).

The most relevant to consider here is the default network, referring to the brain's tendency to revert to this pattern whenever it is not engaged in task-oriented mental activity. This network might be the neurobiological substrate for the sense of self (e.g., reference to own traits and emotions), reflections about others (e.g., theory of mind of others, empathy, moral reasoning, social evaluations), and projections of the self into the future. As Andrews-Hanna (2012) stated: "humans have the unique ability to disengage from the external world and turn our thoughts inward. . . . Through mental simulation of our past, future, and the minds of others, we travel far beyond the observable" (p. 13). Several highly connected hubs involved in other ICNs are also a part of the default network, which may allow them to coordinate other brain functions apart from the default state.

Development of the mind and punctuated homeostasis. Developmental homeostasis is a process by which animals develop more or less normally despite some defective genes and less than perfect environments. Applied to the mind, the brain's main output, developmental homeostasis drives mental development toward a quantitative range of normalcy. The latter may be defined as one's ability to resolve most conflicts internally ("good integration"), to follow a life plan ("self-realization"), and to engage in a functional exchange with the society ("functional adaptation"). These are the three main teleological targets, albeit flexible and context dependent, in otherwise probabilistic development.

Within complex self-organizing systems like personality, the tendency toward homeostasis (system inertia) competes with the tendency to change with changing conditions (adaptation and development). Such competition delivers the optimal solution for the system, which either facilitates or resists change. Personality development is punctuated by abrupt reorganizing transitions followed by prolonged periods of stability (Svrakic et al., 1996). The stability is maintained homeostatically via intrasystem adjustments, thus avoiding costly reconstruction of personality as a whole. An example would be employing defense mechanisms to redefine reality and reconcile internal conflicts. Once the changing conditions exceed the mind's capacity to resist change by homeostasis, an inevitable occurrence in mental development, the configuration becomes suboptimal. The drop in fitness triggers a self-organizing transition to a new optimum via multidirectional co-regulatory optimization processes affecting all components. In the process, new capacities/functions typically emerge to increase the adaptive fitness of the evolved system (e.g., the self-organized emergence of the sense of self in early childhood). The executive mechanisms of this punctuated dynamics are homeostasis (system rigidity) and self-organization (system development), and the pattern is called "punctuated homeostasis" or "punctuated equilibrium" in evolutionary biology (an abrupt and substantial system evolution/change towards a higher fitness level, thereafter again maintained as semi-stable by homeostasis). The early mind is characterized by frequent punctuated transitions, fueled by rapidly changing internal (e.g., growing neural and mental capacities) and external conditions (increasingly complex interactions with the environment).

There are at least three major transitions between birth and about five years of age, from the narrow world of temperament to abstract self-awareness and mentalization, continuing with slower pace towards self-organization of identity, character, and moral values. As noted, the mind becomes increasingly more rigid (homeostatic) with age but never completely loses the ability to reorganize and develop if challenged (psychoplasticity), as a function of the brain's lifelong neuroplasticity.

To illustrate the flow of punctuated dynamics, temperament is self-configured within the early mind, at the time optimal for narrow, low-complexity interactions between the infant and the caregivers, adding aspects of body exploration, emotion display, and separation anxiety, among other functions of the mind. With (epi)genetically driven transition to more complex cognition, actuated by and actuating more complex social interactions, temperament becomes suboptimal in its present state insofar as it is unable to integrate the increasingly complex reflections of the self and others. At this point, the sense of self is relatively abruptly self-organized, at first passively noticed (around two to three years of age), then accessible directly via active introspection around five years of age (Mahler et al., 1975). From a metaphysical standpoint, the development of the integrated independent sense of self at this age marks the psychological birth of a human being (Mahler et al., 1975).

As discussed in Chapter 2, personality disorder follows the same self-organizing dynamics as normal personality but with "faulty" or unfinished particles of partial object relations and the related unstable polarized affects. These severe defects are integrated into the mind and its subsystems, rendering them fragmented and their respective phenomenology and functions unrealistic and adaptively dysfunctional. Like its healthy counterpart, personality disorder is also a semi-stable equilibrium resistant to change until changing internal or external conditions render it suboptimal. Just as often as patients with personality disorder can decompensate into a reactive psychosis under severe stress, they can surprise us after prolong periods of stagnation in therapy with a sudden but sustained shift to a more integrated level of functioning.

Personality and its subsystems: sequential but nonhierarchical organization of the mind. Personality and its subsystems (temperament, self, identity, character, moral values) are theoretical constructs inferred from relatively persistent mental and behavior patterns as they are active in specific adaptive functions. The patterns include, but are not limited to, the specific ways in which a person manages anxiety, anger, and stress; achieves pleasure and satisfaction; engages in interpersonal relationships; approaches work and personal goals; plans for the future; and adheres to implicit and explicit moral standards, to name just a few of the aspects in which we are interested.

Given the hypothetical nature of personality and its subsystems, we rely on metapsychology[10] to integrate clinical observations. In our view, the system of the mind (personality) is organized into subsystems, notably temperament, the self, identity, character, and moral values. The subsystems are *semi-stable configurations of mental faculties* (cognition, emotion, motivation), self-organized within the mind over the sequential course of interactive brain and mental development to meet the increasing adaptive demands, each with a specific phenomenology and adaptive functions. We conceptualize the subsystems as co-existing, flexible, interacting, and co-regulated functional coalitions assembled for specific adaptive tasks rather than hierarchical, although a case can be made that the sense of self manages the union. The term "semi-stable" refers to the *dynamic* and *reversible* nature of the subsystems, and personality as a whole, which is one of central points in our model of personality disorder.

The punctuated development of the mind likely follows the growing capacity for information integration in a positive feedback loop. For instance, as the brain uncovers the increasingly complex world in Piagetian stages, the more complex the mind and its operations become, feeding back to the brain to further elaborate its networks. Such bidirectional interaction makes it possible for the brain and mind not only to be changed by the environment, whether internal (neurological and psychological) or external (social and physical), but also to change both environments (autoplastic and alloplastic adaptation, respectively).

By analogy to the brain's modularity, or perhaps even as a function of it, the subsystems of the mind can be thought of as relatively independent but interacting modules that cross-talk to increase the adaptive effectiveness of personality as a whole. A map of overlapping subsystems of the mind is illustrated in Figure 1.1.

Our understanding of the mind's subsystems does not go so far as to argue for the modularity of the mind, as introduced by Fodor (1983). Robbins (2017) recently reviewed the ongoing debate on mind modularity, whether limited (low-level systems underlying perception and language, among others) or pervasive (including the high-level systems of reasoning, planning, decision-making, and the like). We prefer to think of the mind as modular, not in the strictest sense but in a more modest sense of dissociability (as functionally specialized and phenomenologically discernible subsystems) and central inaccessibility (restriction on the flow of information out of a subsystem). Carruthers (2006) defined mind modules as

10. Theorizing, speculation.

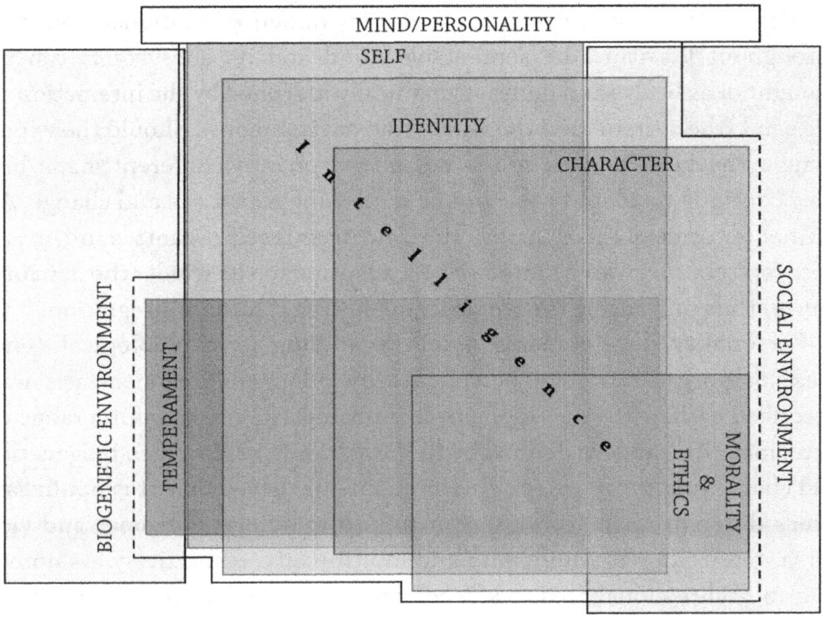

Figure 1.1 Overlapping subsystems of personality (canonical emergence of specific adaptive functions of the mind). Self-organized from mental faculties (thought, emotion, motivation) as the mind's response to adaptive demands.

"isolable function-specific processing systems, all or almost all of which are domain specific (in the content sense), whose operations aren't subject to the will, which are associated with specific neural structures (albeit sometimes spatially dispersed ones), and whose internal operations may be inaccessible to the remainder of cognition" (p. 12). Accordingly, we understand subsystems of temperament, self, character, morality, or identity all as domain-specific, interacting, co-regulated, and overlapping yet specialized adaptive functions. Each subsystem is sequentially self-organized to canonically appear within the mind during development, created by homeostatic optimization to meet the demand for increasing adaptive capabilities over time. Such sequential development is reminiscent of a canon, a contrapuntal musical composition in which each successively entering voice carries the initial theme in a slightly different pitch, here that leading theme is mental adaptation.

Put another way, despite the overlap, each subsystem, from impulsive temperament to abstracted morality, contributes a unique and dissociable adaptive function to the overall fitness of the mind, none of which are hierarchically superior to any other but which are sometimes accorded more weight than others (e.g., the subsystem of self). The emergence of the sense of self adds crucial adaptive and integrative functions to the mind but does not override the pre-existing subsystem of temperament, only contextualizes it, which continues to influence emotional priorities throughout lifespan. The semi-stable mind and its subsystems can be thought of as lively sand dunes, dynamically morphed by the interaction of the sand (the system) and the winds (the environment). Should the winds change, the dunes may move around and morph into a different shape, but they continue to adapt to the winds, combining resistance and change. As the net outcome of this dynamic, the sand mass is self-organized into existence (system survival) by interactively adapting to the winds (the dynamic dunes) thus preventing the winds from blowing it into disintegration.

Personality development: a self-organizing psychobiological complex. Self-organization of personality by punctuated homeostasis was described earlier. The development is probabilistic, allowing for a range of outcomes. The range is defined by the constraints of the given biogenetics and characteristics of a given environment. The development is nonlinear, hence different initial conditions may lead to similar outcomes and vice versa, referred to as equifinality and multifinality, respectively. As noted, in a multidirectional feedback–feedforward interaction among the three variables, genes × brain/mind × environment, each new point in development is influenced by the degree of success at the previous point, and indirectly by the degree of success at all previous points.

Based on observation of infants, postnatal mental development begins with broad dispositions to affects that define early interactive responses of the newborn. The dispositions are molded into temperament traits, the earliest traits of motivated behaviors, through associative learning. Temperament in part[11] determines the valence of internalized object relations, which we hypothesize to be the elementary particles which weave the substrate and the function of the mind, as discussed later in this chapter. The degree of integration of internalized object relations (from partial to whole) fundamentally impacts the coherence of the ensuing subsystems of self, identity, character, and morality. Under normal circumstances, internal and external conditions are "good enough" supplying a critical mass of predominantly positive affect-memory engrams[12] (representations, in psychoanalytical parlance) to neutralize the negative representations which are inevitable in normal development. With respect to subjective representations, even in the absence of any real biogenetic or environmental problems, the affective valence of experience may differ between infant and caregivers. For example, the mere act

11. The other part is quality of care.

12. An engram is defined as a group of neurons involved in the consolidation of newly formed memories by permanent changes in terms of increased of synaptic strength and dendritic spine.

of getting an infant dressed may be discrepantly experienced by the infant and the mother. Such discrepancies between the natural (infant's "view") and good care (mom's view) explain why even the most loving mother is at times perceived as frustrating by her ward. In fact, moderate age-appropriate frustration is essential for normal development of self-sufficiency, as captured by the Kohut's well known concept of transmuting internalization.

Based on a sophisticated mathematical framework, Nenad Svrakic and colleagues (Svrakic et al., 1996; Cloninger et al., 1997) formulated a quantitative model of normal and deviant personality development as a self-organizing, complex dynamic system. The model accounts for functional interactions among multiple types of influence, spanning genetic factors, family environment, sociocultural norms, and experiences unique to each individual. The model takes into account all aspects of information processing from associative conditioning of habits to enculturation about values within a unique psychological context. In this model, personality is defined as a dynamic, multidimensional system comprised of more elementary operating modular components (subsystems) which are organized in an *interdependent* way in order to carry out a particular function (personality traits). These in turn converge to govern adaptive behaviors. The satisfaction of multiple constraints results in a nonlinear dynamics, which is characteristic of all systems involving growth and development in biology, neuroscience, psychology, and sociology and occurs through a process called "complex adaptive systems."

INTERNALIZED OBJECT RELATIONS: THE ELEMENTARY PARTICLES OF THE MIND[13]

Melanie Klein (1952) formulated object relations theory as a theoretical framework to systematize her clinical observations of infants and young children. With some modifications (Ronald Fairbairn, Donald Winnicott, Edith Jacobson), the theory has become the leading model of development and functioning of the human mind. Recent advances in cognitive and molecular neuroscience, as we will show, have provided evidence for the theory, a testimony to Klein's genius. We review here some of the basic concepts of object relations theory and neuroscience that appears to support them.

13. We refer to them as elementary particles of the mind because each contains a percept, the related self-reflection, and the related affect and thus is not divisible to lower order units of mental experience, only to physiologically recorded somatosensory information (sensations/percepts, affects).

Klein's concept of phantasy[14] refers to a nonconscious,[15] preconceptual image potential of psychic life, a psychological facet[16] of biological instincts that links affects to objects and creates the world of imagination (Mitchell, 1986). Klein' viewed phantasy as essential to the development of a capacity for thinking, as the origin of thought lies in the process of testing phantasy against reality. Phantasies appear in symbolic form in dreams and play (Klein used play to make inferences of mental development). In contrast to Freud, Klein puts phantasies beneath the level of nonconscious wishes/impulses and assigns them a lasting effect on the mind: "Infantile feelings and phantasies leave, as it were, their imprints on the mind, imprints that do not fade away but get stored up, remain active, and exert a continuous and powerful influence on the emotional and intellectual life of the individual" (Klein, 1975; p. 290). In their early existence, infants differentiate little, if at all, between phantasy-based experiences and reality (a child who sucks its thumb is enacting the phantasy of feeding). Phantasy enables the mind to establish object relations, i.e., mental constructs of self and others. The concept of "internal object" refers to the mental and emotional image of an external object (person) that has been taken inside[17] the mind. The tenor of the object image is defined by the child's projected affect evoked by the interaction, negative or positive, onto the object. The projected affect is, by the mechanism of projective identification, reflected back into the mind as "self-representation." The trio together (self-image, object image, and the connecting affect) comprise an "object relation," or an intrapsychic representation of interactions between the infant and the caregivers. These rudimentary self-reflections and object perceptions combine phantasy and/or real events hence are always biased ("personal"): the categorization of the representations as positive-loving or negative-persecutory is defined by the affective reactivity of early temperament and the quality of care. Such inherently biased object relations, which are the main informant of the individual's mental functioning, may explain why each of us has a personal prism to process reality, our own "personalized reality" and a set of unique expectations defined by our personality.

14. Original spelling retained to differentiate "phantasy" (arises from genetic instincts and affects and represents the means by which infants make sense of the external world and relate to it through projection and introjection) from "fantasy" (fantasy is self-aware or phenomenally conscious daydreaming that involves wishful unreality and may include elements of the deeper nonconscious phantasies).

15. The term "nonconscious" refers to contents of the mind not reaching awareness, whereas "unconscious" refers to the loss of consciousness, a medical condition.

16. Mitchell (1986) explains phantasy using the metaphor "nonconscious commentary" on instinctual life that links feelings to objects and creates a new amalgam: the world of imagination. Through its ability to phantasize the baby tests out, primitively 'thinks' about, its (the baby's) experiences of inside and outside.

17. "Represented" (cognitive neuroscience), "engramized" (molecular neuroscience), "introjected" (psychoanalysis).

Contradictory, bad versus good self- and object mental representations are at first internalized as separate because the affects that define the valence of the experience, positive or negative, are first processed by anatomically separated subcortical structures. This normal fragmented phase in development is also known as partial object relations. Their continued separation through six months of life likely reflects a not yet fully mature prefrontal and anterior cingulate circuits which are cortical convergence zones that, when mature, integrate multimodal information, including polarized percepts and affects, and process them into the functional abstractions of the mind (concepts). In the context of the increasing prefrontal ability for abstraction, the polarized units can be integrated into a more realistic and affectively balanced experiences about own self and other people (around the first 6 months of life), now experienced as having both gratifying and frustrating features – a total affective cognitive frame (Roth and Dicke, 2006, cited by Kernberg, 2015). The timeline is corroborated by psychoanalytic observations of infants (M Klein). It is not well understood whether the integration of polarized object-relations is structural (engramized) or functional (an emerging phenomenon occurring at the level of nonconscious working memory). We believe in the latter option, whereby mature prefrontal networks which mediate working memory, here nonconscious working memory, enable operational merging of polarized units of experience into a balanced whole.

M Klein (1952) referred to partial object relations as "paranoid– schizoid" position, characterized by persecutory fears of annihilation. The mechanisms of splitting, projective identification, idealization, and omnipotence, among others, defend against persecutory anxieties of this position. As already noted, reflecting the infant's growing neurocognitive capacities increasingly capable of grasping complexity, at about six months of age, partial object relations (love-or-persecution) begin to functionally merge into unified, although still nonconscious, whole object relations (love-and-persecution[18]). The respective dyadic affects are also balanced in the process. The merger occurs and continues to mature under "good enough" conditions, which stimulate organization of brain networks (neural growth) and amass positive introjections about self and others to ensure crystallization of the mind and allow for mental growth. Both the brain and the mind are now able to process the big picture, that the self and the object are neither absolutely perfect nor absolutely persecutory but a mixture of the two, weighted toward love and gratification. The achievement is called whole object relations, or "depressive position" in Klein's terms. Both refer to the capacity of the

18. Here of course "persecution" metaphorizes the infant's perspective on everything that is not absolutely gratifying in care.

child to recognize his or her angry feelings about the frustrating but loved object (ambivalence) in a way that more accurately reflects the reality of the relationship. In such conditions, the frustrating interactions are in the minority and thus unable to threaten the positive majority, resulting in a "good internal object," a steady but nonconscious inner confidence integrated into all subsystems of the mind. Internalized objects relate to each other within the self. Phenomenologically, they are the content of one's phantasy, but this phantasy has real effects as it nonconsciously and powerfully influences one's relations toward self and others (see http://www.melanie-klein-trust.org.uk/). A complex interaction continues throughout life between the world of internalized objects and those in the real world (which are obviously also in the mind) via repeated cycles of projection and introjection (Klein, 1952).

Depressive position continues to mature throughout the lifespan. It stands as the basis of self- and object constancy (concepts of M Mahler) and mature love (the feelings of guilt and distress are an inherent part of love and deepen the love profoundly). Successfully working through sadness, guilt, and distress of the depressive position, facilitated by caring and comforting from others, is also a prerequisite for the establishment of an inside and an outside world and social life, including the capacity to recognize one's own feelings and motivations as well as those of others, notably the capacity for mentalization and the theory of mind of others. Both the dynamic nature of normalcy and the instability of the phenomenology of personality disorder derive from the dynamic and reversible nature of object relations (Klein, 1952) and the semi-stable configuration of the mind's subsystems.

Attachment patterns are not to be confused with cognitive schemata (from cognitive behavioral theory) and scripts (from humanistic theories). As defined by Bowlby and Ainsworth, attachment patterns are the child's nonconscious preconceptual internal working models of itself, an early cognitive-affective framework for understanding the world, self, and others. The patterns can be thought of as a preconceptual manifestation of the quality of internalized object relations, observed "at work" in early interactions. Incidentally, a similar, although a wider concept to schemata and scripts is that of "frame of reference" (the Schiffs, 1975), referring to one's individual filter on reality, a framework which is used to define the self, other people, and the world. At a higher level of mind organization, a cognitive schema ("I am unworthy," "I am unlovable," among others) and a life script ("try harder," "be strong," among others) refers to stable and advanced mini-systems of emotions, thinking and behavior molded through the interaction with caregivers. Both schemata and life scripts require a higher degree of mental and behavior organization than attachment and object relations (scripts develop between two and five years of age and forward, per Berne, 1972). In contrast to attachment (which is nonconscious), schemata and scripts are experienced at the level of passive, phenomenal consciousness (a "knowing how it feels") but not at the level of full self-awareness actively accessible by introspection. Both can be thought of as rudiments of adult adaptive styles.

Nonconscious working memory: where neuroscience and psychoanalysis meet.

Psychoanalysts agree that all psychological experience, a fleeting fantasy as well as the most stable attitude, is organized by object relations (Auchincloss and Samberg, 2012). These early phantasms—consisting of a self-image, an image of the other, and the affect that connects them—weave the substrate of the mind, while at the same time being the function of the mind (its affects, thoughts, motivation) much like light, which comes in discrete elementary particles, called photons in quantum physics, which exhibit wave–particle duality and combine structure and function. As the basic units of the mind, internalized object relations operate within nonconscious or very thinly conscious working memory, within the general network of cognition (both conscious and nonconscious working memory arise from within this network) (LeDoux and Brown, 2017). From here, object relations could provide personalized input that combines with other kinds of neural inputs in the assembly of the brain networks which give rise to mental faculties (cognition, motivation, and emotions), perhaps explaining the spectrum of coexisting nonconscious, thinly conscious, and fully conscious thoughts, motivations, and emotions operating in the human mind. These faculties are then self-organized into the mind's subsystems by punctuated homeostasis, as discussed. Hence we refer to internalized object relations as "elementary particles" of the mind. Recent advances in neuroscience provide support for the metaphor. Here we combine advances in cognitive and molecular neuroscience (LeDoux and Brown, 2017; Kitamura et al., 2017) and psychoanalysis (Klein's [1952] object relations theory) to postulate the processes that weave the substrate/function of the mind.

Sensory percepts (any sense) activated in the context of early interactions with objects, memories of these objects, the related self-reflections[19] activated in the interaction, and the affects associated with these interactions

19. Self-reflections are projected and reintrojected aspects of self onto objects (mother) by the mechanism of projective identification, thus inherently involving representation of objects (selfobjects). The self eventually grows out of this union as it becomes able to carry psychological functioning on its own.

are engramized via rapid synaptic plasticity during first-order information processing in, respectively: (i) primary and secondary somatosensory cortical areas (sensory percepts), (ii) left medial temporal lobe including the hippocampus (declarative memory unrelated to self, autobiographical self-reflections, and memories of related objects), and (iii) subcortical structures involved in processing and memories of affects (amygdala and the limbic system). Shortly after formation, these memories are "copied" in neocortical networks for permanent storage. Kitamura et al. (2017) showed that neocortical memory engram cells are generated over a couple of weeks after the initial fear learning, and this process of cortical "copying" is supervised (informed) by inputs from both the hippocampus and amygdala (serving as "templates" which contain initial information). The exact mechanism of the copying process is unknown.[20] At first silent, the prefrontal engrams became structurally, physiologically, and functionally mature over the subsequent few weeks. Around this time the original hippocampal engram cells become silent (perhaps later to serve as a pointer for recall of their remote copies), but those in the amygdala that store memories of autobiographical affects remain active. Hence, needing two to three weeks of continuing input from the hippocampus and amygdala to form and mature, the neocortical engramized copies of declarative and autobiographical memories become the *active long-term memories*, most likely still nonconscious, which thereon inform further mind development.

The process of long-term memory consolidation by supervised copying in the neocortex in all likelihood involves all types of memories: declarative or consciously accessible (semantic and episodic, not self-related) as well as autobiographical memories (self-related semantic and episodic, which can be nonconscious, like in object relations, or consciously accessible). All are likely associated with their respective affect states owing to the amygdala role in supervised copying. Per LeDoux and Brown (2017), for the conscious sense of self to emerge, autobiographical memory engrams (self-related sensory events, object memories, self-reflections), "flavored" by their respective amygdalar affects are first higher order represented (HOR) in *nonconscious working memory* as nonconscious self-HOR (i.e., HOR related to self). Next, the latter is yet higher order re-represented (HOR of HOR, self-HOROR) for the conscious experience of the self. The nonconscious self-HOR highly

20. The recently described role of the *Arc* gene (a virus-like acting gene, important for synaptic plasticity, cognition, and long term memory) in transmitting genetic information *via* self-assembled capsids of m-RNA that can leave the cell and deliver the m-RNA to the cytoplasm of target neurons where it can undergo activity-dependent translation and protein synthesis might play a role (Ashley et al., 2018; Pastuzyn et al., 2018). Also, immediate early genes which are activated transiently and rapidly in response to a wide variety of cellular stimuli may have a role as well.

corresponds to the psychoanalytic concept of object relations, consisting of a sensory percept, associated affect (pulled from the amygdala "warehouse"), and the self-reflection activated in the interaction. In sum, object relations are implicit early personalized "recordings" of reality, developed through early interactions, that determine how one thinks and feels about the self and others at the very basic level of the mind. Figuratively, they can be compared to nonconscious procedural memory (i.e., knowing how to do things or motor skills, like walking, talking, riding a bike), here meaning "how the mind does things," like thinking, feeling, or imagining. The novel concept of nonconscious working memory is also postulated to be a function of the general network of cognition, notably the PFCx.

Under normal circumstances (i.e., in the absence of innate or environmental risk factors), the nonconscious self-HOR consists of balanced (whole) internalized object relations which are thought to begin to merge around the first six months of life as the PFCx gradually matures and becomes increasingly able to form abstractions. Such nonconscious representations provide a thinly sense of "I" based on bodily sensations, also known as self-object boundary, a mental state that does not invoke self-consciousness. Thus, this sense of "I" is *not* experienced as self-awareness or autonoetic consciousness,[21] although it is necessary for the latter. In support of our conceptualization of internalized object relations as "elementary particles" of the mind, we cite LeDoux and Brown (2017) who note that "the presence of the self in the nonconscious representation allows for an autonoetic conscious state of the self to result from the re-representation" (p. E2020) within the *conscious* working memory. Neuroscience predicts the existence of nonconscious working memory (thus far not empirically verified) based on the available knowledge of the brain's cognitive processing, akin to the periodic table of Mendeleev which had blank pixels awaiting for the predicted chemical element to be discovered. For the conscious self to emerge via self-reflection, the nonconscious nucleus of the self (the thin sense of "I") must be successively rerepresented by the general network of cognition into a passively noticed self (the sense of "me," around two years of age) and a full self-aware consciousness of the motivated self (the sense

21. Noetic consciousness involves explicit (conscious, declarative) memory which includes semantic (facts—"what") and episodic memory of events ("where and when") that *does not* include oneself (here episodic memory is simply a complex form of semantic memory rather than a memory about the self; LeDoux and Brown, 2017) Autobiographical memory involves the self, whether episodic ("where and when") or semantic (facts and concepts—"what"). Autonoetic consciousness (awareness that the facts about what, where, and when happened to us; Klein, 2013) arises from autobiographical memory but also includes non-self related memories. To avoid misunderstanding, episodic and semantic memory related to self is referred to as autobiographical (which can be nonconscious as in object relations but also consciously accessible), while declarative memory denotes episodic and semantic memories unrelated to the self (explicit, consciously accessible by working memory).

of "me" and "my intentions" around five years of age). The exact mechanism behind these sequential higher order re-representations is not known. Likely, they occur as emerging properties by the work of the general network of cognition, PFCx to be precise. As a less likely scenario, they could be hard-wired but in a rapidly reversible, activity dependent, and dynamic way, which may be physiologically possible (e.g., Ashley et al., 2018; Pastuzyn et al., 2018). Whatever the case, at a higher level of information coalescing and processing in the PFCx (including nonconscious and conscious working memory), new conscious mental phenomena emerge (self-awareness, emotions), now consciously accessible.

The development of ICNs involved in mental faculties is informed, and thus their organization influenced by internalized object relations, a highly personalized elementary particle of the mind. Such personalized input significantly influences thoughts, emotions, and motivations, and these in turn influence memory, as their respective networks overlap and co-regulate and can be viewed as dynamic interacting systems. The personalized mental faculties are self-organized into the subsystems of the mind, *ipso facto* unique for each individual, such as the sense self, moral values, and character, among others. The brain, in other words, creates one's "personal" reality in one's mind.

The mechanism of splitting as the first organizer of the mind. Klein (1952) observed that early in development (until about six months of age) the infant's understanding of self and objects is split into two opposing experiences: *good* (i.e., gratifying, loved, loving) and *bad* (i.e., frustrating, hated, persecutory). The separation at this early age is useful because it is the first, albeit crude, organizer of the early mind insofar that it keeps the positive (gratifying) and negative (frustrating) representations split off but sorted out. The split prevents the rudimentary mind from disintegrating because it protects the gratifying introjections from the persecutory ones, thus allowing the mind to crystallize around positive experiences. As discussed, molecular and cognitive neuroscience validate, we believe, observations of mental development in children made by psychoanalysts, notably by Melanie Klein. LeDoux and Brown (2017) support the existence of nonconscious working memory in the PFCx, which could be the link between first-, second-, and third-order percepts-affects and self-awareness. This nonconscious or very thinly conscious nucleus of the mind, itself a HOR of lower order percepts and affects, is sequentially rerepresented by the general network of cognition for conscious emotions and self-consciousness to emerge. Pathological persistence into adulthood of the splitting mechanism and the related fragmentation, originally helping the mind to stay organized and crystallize, is the core pathology observed in personality disorder. Under pathological circumstances and predominant persecutory fears, merging of contradictory units of experience (bad vs. good) would gravely endanger the positive core necessary for the continuing development of the mind, creating as it were a psychological implosion. Hence, the contradictory particles continue to be kept apart by the splitting mechanism (psychoanalytic interpretation) or by the hypoactive PFCx (neuroscience interpretation), or perhaps the former is simply a function of the latter at this early stage. Whatever the case, in this "mind (matter) over matter (mind)" question, psychoanalysis and neuroscience validate each other by arriving at the same point in the development of the brain/mind. In our view, splitting can be a purely mental maneuver protecting against destructive negative experiences. We all on occasion use primitive defenses despite a presumably normal prefrontal networks.

REVISITING PSYCHIC STRUCTURES: TEMPERAMENT, CHARACTER, INTELLIGENCE, IDENTITY, SELF, AND MORAL VALUES

Modern psychology has moved away from fixed and static structures toward dynamic and reversible mental functions as they emerge, self-organize, and change within the mind while adapting to changing internal and external conditions.

How are mental functioning and its substrate related? There are no bona fide structures in the mind. We conceptualize the mind as an emergent property of the brain built of elementary units with inseparable structural and functional aspects; that is, they are both the substrate and the function of the mind. To elaborate this concept we borrow from Almaas (2001) and cite other work as indicated. As discussed, the human mind appears to originate in hippocampal and amygdalar engrams which record sensory percepts and affects created by earliest interactive experiences. As shown by Kitamura et al. (2017), the hippocampal engrams are copied into the neocortex and the process is supervised by the inputs from the original hippocampal and amygdalar engrams. The neocortical copies of autobiographical memories and the amygdalar recordings of associated affects are higher order represented in nonconscious working memory (nonconscious self-HOR), which, as discussed, highly correspond to internalized object relations, the basic units of all experience. For this reason, we conceptualize object relations as the elementary particles of the both the substrate and the function of the mind, which are inseparable in our opinion. The substrate of the mind is also its function insofar that an object relation is both an elementary particle but at the same time a function of the mind, its subliminal feeling, motivation, and thought, cognitively re-represented from nonconscious memory to autonoetic consciousness. Here, we draw analogy from quantum mechanics in that energy, momentum and other quantities of a system may be restricted to discrete values (quantization) with characteristics of both particles and waves (the wave-particle duality, as is the case with light where photons are both particles and waves). Quantum events do occur in biology, from photosynthesis to the sense of smell, but whether they have anything to do with the emergence of the mind and consciousness is a hotly debated topic. The discussion is beyond our expertise and the scope of this book, hence the previous light analogy is used solely as a metaphor for the duality of structure and function, here applied to object relations.

The relationship between a substrate and a representation that gives it its particular characteristics is like the relationship between a building and its blueprint (Almaas, 2001): they are inseparable but not identical. Just as a blueprint is more stable than the building it outlines, the substrate is slightly more stable than its function. Analogously, levels of mental functioning can be thought of as functional expressions of a particular substrate of the mind, the substrate and the function inseparable from each other, both comprised of a mosaic of more and less balanced object relations. The levels are more flexible than the substrate they express due to being directly exposed to adaptive demands ("in the trenches"). Following the same process of supervised "copies" in the neocortex, new cognitive-affective units are integrated into the substrate of the mind, either reinforcing or revising the old experiences, changing the level of functioning more readily than its substrate, which is also changing but at a slower pace. The spatialization of temporal order of experience fosters the erroneous treatment of mental processes as if they occupied space in the mind as a place or structure (Schwartz, 1981).

Demystifying the concept of the ego. Freud conceived his structural model of the psyche drawing from the postulates in chemistry and physics of the time, including the trend in the biological sciences to dissect complex phenomena into individual operating units. We suspect that, whether knowingly or not, Freud drew from the biological principle of homeostasis to formulate the concept of the ego but defined it as a distinct structure of the mind, rather than the principle of self-regulation inherent to the biological systems, including the brain and the mind.

The concept of the ego is inconsistently defined in the literature, which creates a considerable confusion about its real nature, structure, and function. We submit that the psychoanalytic concept of the ego is equivalent to the principle of homeostasis. The latter is not limited to physiology but can be applied to any complex phenomenon in nature that demonstrates a stable equilibrium in the given context, including, as we believe, the mind and its individual subsystems. Homeostasis (meaning "staying the same") refers to the universal property of a complex system whereby a variable is actively regulated to remain nearly constant, thus keeping the whole system in balance. This is achieved by multiple dynamic adjustments and regulation mechanisms within the current equilibrium. Applied to the mind, homeostasis maintains the stability of the current configuration of the subsystems of the mind, and thus the mind as a whole, until the conditions (internal and/or external) sufficiently change to make the equilibrium suboptimal, requiring change through self-organizing multidirectional optimization affecting all components and giving rise to new adaptive functions. This is why the mind (personality) and its individual subsystems are semi-stable and self-organizing by punctuated homeostasis.

Ego is defined in contemporary psychoanalysis as ... "the executive agency of the mind"[22] (Auchincloss and Samberg, 2012). It serves the function of homeostasis or self-regulation, mediating between conflicting motivations and forging compromises between them. It also serves the function of adaptation, mediating between the demands of the inner world and external reality. Finally, the ego serves the function of synthesizing all mental processes and experiences into a smoothly operating whole" (p. 69). This psychoanalytic description of "what the ego is and what the ego does" supports the correspondence between the concept of the ego and the principle of homeostasis: the ego *is* that homeostatic principle. It can be thought of as a metaphor for homeostasis. The functions of the ego (e.g., evaluation, judgment, reasoning, language, perception, symbolization, reality testing, representation, affect and anxiety tolerance, defense mechanisms, impulse control; Auchincloss and Samberg, 2012) are nothing more than functions performed by the mind through its mental faculties (cognition, emotions, motivation), especially the cognitive top-down control of affects and motivations. No specific central "structure" owns these "ego" functions, because they are performed by the mind as a whole. Defense mechanisms illustrate mental homeostasis: they can beautify reality (mature), repress reality (neurotic), or distort reality (immature) and thus stabilize the whole distressed system (the mind), avoiding costly rearrangements or unhealthy regressions to lower levels of functioning.

22. A total of about 200 authors, classical psychoanalysts, ego- and self-psychologists, object relation theorists, among many others, participated in the book, reaching consensus definitions while taking into account a collection of perspectives.

TEMPERAMENT: THE BIOGENETIC BACKBONE OF PERSONALITY

"Temperament" refers to the psychomotor characteristics and affective reactivity of the organism ("the biogenetic core of personality"). This subsystem is unique, as it is a subcortical-cortical backbone of personality, a percept-concept hybrid with strong roots in the subcortical affects but with independent aspects of conscious motivation, albeit phenomenally only, to provide emotional significance to experience and behavior. To minimize any potential misunderstandings, we outline the concepts of affects, emotions or feelings, and moods next.

Affect, mood, feelings, and emotions: different concepts used interchangeably. Affect is defined as a short-lived, usually intense, complex psycho-physiologic state consisting of subjective conscious experience (emotion, feeling), associated ideas and fantasies, and biologic and behavioral response patterns. Sensory perception of threat triggers the affect of fear, a *nonconscious brain state* within subcortical defensive survival circuits (fight, flight, freeze), only an aspect of which is the conscious emotion of fear; other aspects are defensive behavior and physiological responses. The concept of emotion is interchangeable with feeling, both referring to a conscious experience of an affect state. The emotion of fear, for example, is a subjective conscious experience of the affect state triggered by the perception of threat, a higher order cognitive representation of nonconscious sensory information processed by subcortical circuits involved in controlling fear responses within the defensive survival circuit (LeDoux and Brown, 2017). Mood is defined as a pervasive and sustained emotion, spreading over the entire self-state, including cognition, motivation, and behavior, over a relatively long period of time. In the literature, emotion is used either interchangeably with affect or with behavioral or communicative aspects of affects (Auchincloss and Samberg, 2012).

Early temperament: when human newborn begins to communicate. Early temperament is the primary avenue to communicate physiological needs and initiate interaction with the caregiver (mother), through the attachment-separation panic system, the fight-flight system, the play-joy-bonding system, the erotic system, and the feeding system, among others (Panksepp, 1998). Each of these affect reactivity systems is activated by a specific organismic need of the newborn as an automatic, preconceptual response rooted in subcortical circuits. The early affects define the subjective experience (valence) of the interaction (desirable-gratifying vs. undesirable-frustrating), communicate the state of the infant to the caregivers (e.g., behavioral manifestations of distress, interest, joy-content), and mediate pre-conceptual, affect-based cognitive framing of reality ("good" vs. "bad"). These experiences are of central importance in the early organization of the brain and development of the mind.

In the sequential course of mind development, temperament traits are the first motivated behaviors to emerge. They are observed as individual differences among infants[23] and are assessable by self-report around the age of five years (Luby et al., 1999). Heritable biogenetic dispositions to the neurophysiology of the nervous system, including general affect reactivity, are molded into stable behavior tendencies by procedural learning (repetitions) and associative conditioning during the first few years of childhood. In the process, pre-conceptual behavior reactions are strengthened into stable traits or weakened into extinction by their consequences, that is, support (reward, approval) or suppression (punishment, non-reward), respectively. Subsequent cognitive and character development contextualize the raw temperament of childhood into adult temperament traits, which continue to influence the stylistic aspect of behavior and one's phenomenally conscious preferences (automatic motivational biases—the liking and wanting and not liking and not wanting) of behavior.

The psychobiological model of temperament. We describe the concept of temperament within the psychobiological model of personality (the second major component is character) developed by Cloninger (1987), with one of us (DMS) joining several years later as a coauthor of character traits (Cloniger et al., 1993). The four temperament traits are conceptualized drawing from a number of complementary approaches, notably evolutionary, ethological, genetic, neurophysiological, pharmacological, and cognitive-behavioral. The traits are harm avoidance (HA), novelty seeking (NS), reward dependence (RD), and persistence (PE). The four traits activate behavior responses to prescriptive stimuli, such as danger (avoidance), novelty (exploration), social approval (maintenance), and frustrative non-reward (persistence), respectively. They do so rather automatically, reaching the level of phenomenal consciousness ("knowing how it feels") but rarely the level of rational decision-making as part of self-aware executive functioning. Neither high nor low ends of a temperament trait are inherently pathological, as each has adaptive advantages and disadvantages in specific circumstances. Human temperament is moderately heritable (~60%), relatively stable throughout life (although NS tends to decrease with age due to better impulse control) and cross-culturally (Miettunen et al., 2006). Complex psychobiology of each of the traits is discussed in Chapter 5, with the mechanism-based

23. An infant is a human offspring between one month and one year of age.

pharmacotherapy of personality disorder. A detailed description of the traits is provided in Cloninger and Svrakic (2017).

Harm avoidance (HA). HA is the first trait of motivated behavior to evolve in animals and is crucial for their survival. The brain's "defense motivation system" includes potentiated startle response, active defense (fight or flight), passive defense (behavioral freezing), and endocrine and cardiovascular autonomic responses (Lang et al., 1998). In humans, HA refers to *behavior inhibition* (avoidance) in response to conditioned signals of danger, punishment, and frustrative non-reward. Individuals with high HA are distressed by uncertainty, socially inhibited, fatigable, and pessimistic; avoid problems and potential danger; and excessively worry in anticipation of problems. Individuals with low HA are confident, carefree, socially outgoing, energetic, and optimistic even in uncertain situations. Adaptive advantages of high HA are cautiousness and careful planning when hazard is likely. Maladaptation appears when hazard is unlikely but danger is still anticipated, which leads to anticipatory anxiety. Adaptive advantages of low HA are confidence in the face of uncertainty and energetic optimism to resolve problems with little or no distress. Maladaptation of low HA is disregard for real danger and unrealistic optimism leading to risky behaviors, the consequences of which are potentially serious. We consider generalized anxiety disorder to be the clinical correspondent of excessively high HA, with early onset, chronic course, and most of the cognitive and emotional biases associated with high HA cited here.

Novelty seeking (NS). NS refers to a heritable bias in the *initiation of behavior*, notably appetitive approach in response to novelty and signals of reward, active avoidance of conditioned signals of punishment, and active escape from unconditioned punishment. Individuals high in NS tend to be exploratory in response to novelty, impulsive, prone to angry outbursts, easily bored, extravagant in approach to cues of reward, superficial, disorderly, and distractible in efforts. Those low in NS are described as slow tempered, uninquiring, stoical, reflective, frugal, reserved, tolerant of monotony, and orderly. Adaptive advantages of high NS are enthusiastic exploration of new situations, potentially leading to discovery and progress. Maladaptation is reflected in frequent feelings of boredom whenever there is nothing new in sight, damaging impulsivity, and frequent outbursts of anger. Persons with low NS have the adaptive advantage of being stoical, reflective, reserved, systematic, and tolerant of monotony. Maladaptation is reflected in their lack of enthusiasm, interest, and tendency to routinize activities.

Reward dependence (RD). RD refers to a heritable bias in the *maintenance of behavior* in response to cues of social reward, and is more accurately labeled as "social RD."[24] Individuals high in RD are sentimental, socially sensitive, warmly attached, and motivated by approval of others. Individuals low in RD are practical, emotionally detached, socially disinterested, independent, and indifferent about being alone. Sensitivity to social cues is the main adaptive advantage of high RD, as it facilitates affectionate social relations and genuine care for others. The disadvantage of high RD is owing to suggestibility and loss of objectivity frequently encountered with people who are excessively socially dependent. Individuals low in RD are practical, tough-minded, cold, socially insensitive, irresolute, and indifferent if alone. The advantages of low RD are personal independence and objectivity not corrupted by efforts to please others. Its maladaptive disadvantage is found in social withdrawal, detachment, and coldness in social attitudes.

Persistence (PE). PE refers to a heritable bias in the *continuation* of behavior despite failure, frustration, fatigue, and unpredictable, random reinforcement. It is observed early in life, as infants and young children vary in the length of time on a task and ability to stay with the task through frustrations (Thomas and Chess, 1984). Individuals with high PE tend to be excessively devoted to work, industrious, determined, ambitious, and perfectionistic. Those with low PE give up easily when faced with frustration, rarely strive for higher accomplishments, and show low perseverance in response to intermittent reward. High PE is adaptive when rewards are intermittent but contingencies remain stable ("intermittent reinforcement"). It is maladaptive when behavior continues even when the chances for success are objectively lost. Low PE is an adequately adaptive solution when reward contingencies change rapidly but becomes maladaptive whenever rewards and achievements are infrequent but are expected to eventually occur in the long run. If heritably excessive each of these temperament traits can turn into a trait vulnerability to personality disorder.

CHARACTER: A MIXTURE OF SELF-INTEREST AND ALTRUISM

In psychology, the term "character" (Greek *kharakter,* a "stamping tool") refers to constellations of observable behaviors, such as habitual attitudes and relationships with others, by which an individual is recognizable. Character is a relatively recent subsystem of human personality. Genetic studies are showing that human character traits are modulated

24. Conditioned reward based learning is associated with a number of other syndromes, including addiction to substances and food, pathological gambling.

by regulatory micro-RNAs not present in the genomes of Neanderthals and chimpanzees (CR Cloninger, personal communication). We conceptualize character as a subsystem of the mind, a semi-stable configuration of mental faculties (cognition, emotion, motivation) self-organized to mediate the evolutionary function of adaptation to the external environment, particularly group living. To this end, character maximizes the fit between one's emotional priorities associated with temperament and societal pressures, which advances the adaptive fitness of the mind as a whole. Kernberg (2016) speaks of character as an objective correspondent of identity or, figuratively, "who is me outside" (character) versus "who is me inside" (identity), with some overlap between the two. As character facilitates satisfaction of one's own needs just as readily as it facilitates group living, it operates to increase one's fit with the society with a healthy tone of self-interest—"functional adaptation" as we refer to it. If temperament is formed through involuntary conditioning, character is formed in some part involuntarily, based on internal models of behavior developed with caregivers[25] and partly by a choice of adaptive strategies within the given context of the individual. The choice is made at some point in adolescence, based on one's assessment, deliberate or intuitive, of the most effective ways to satisfy personal needs, achieve social recognition, and/or ensure resources in the given context. If temperament involves intense affect states of basic emotions (fear, anger, and attachment), character involves serene affect states of secondary social emotions, like empathy, compassion, and helpful behaviors, among others. We discuss the psychobiological model of character developed by Cloninger et al. (1993).

The psychobiological model of character. The model identifies three character dimensions: self-directedness (SD), cooperativeness (CO), and self-transcendence (ST), each with five lower order facets.

Self-directedness (SD) and its five facets describe responsible (disciplined), purposeful, self-accepting, self-sufficient (resourceful), spontaneous, and effective individuals, that is, those sufficiently integrated to be able to adapt behavior in accordance with individually chosen goals. These five facets of SD capture the degree of personality integration, not social adaptation, thus the dimension of SD is closer to the concept of personality health than to the concept of character and social adaptation (the trait of CO captures the latter). Individuals low in SD are described as blaming, aimless, vain, passive, and conflicted. The features are never adaptively advantageous. They combine into an operationalized portrait of a poorly integrated,

25. Internal models of behavior in attachment theory correspond to internalized object relations in psychoanalytic theory.

fragmented personality rather than its maladaptive character, although the latter is usually consequential.

Cooperativeness (CO) is a bona fide character dimension, with facets of social tolerance, empathy, helpfulness, compassion, and being principled, a mixture of prosocial and moral traits. These features are advantageous in teamwork and social groups but neutral for individuals who must live in a solitary manner. People who are low in CO are described as self-absorbed, intolerant, selfish, unhelpful, revengeful, and opportunistic, features of extreme individualism thus rarely advantageous so long as an individual lives in a group. High CO is consistently associated with high RD,[26] the latter predisposing the individual to seek gratification from others through cooperation, tolerance, and helpfulness. Cloninger et al. (1993) include in the concept of character features such as empathy, compassion, and helping behaviors, all of which are considered to be the biological roots of morality which (morality) operates as a subsystem of the mind in its own right. Although this could be questionable as a concept, it does capture the overlap between character and integrated moral values working in concert to maximize one's social adaptation.

Self-transcendence (ST) is a higher order character dimension with facets of self-forgetfulness,[27] transpersonal identification with other human beings, spirituality, contemplation, and idealism. The facets are adaptively advantageous when people are confronted with grave situations like suffering, illness, or death. They may appear disadvantageous in most modern societies where idealism and modesty can interfere with the acquisition of wealth and power. People low in ST tend to be self-preoccupied, self-centered, skeptical, objective, and pragmatic. Such individuals fit well in most Western societies because of their rational objectivity and material success. However, they may have difficulty accepting suffering, failures, personal and material loses, and death, which leads to lack of serenity and suboptimal adjustment to problems, particularly with advancing age. The concept of ST is not as clearly related to character in the strict sense of everyday social adaptation but perhaps more to everyday meditative mindfulness as the means to include intuition and creativity into activities and/or handle profound sadness and loss. As such it may be more frequent in highly integrated, self-actualized, financially worry-free individuals than in the general population (figuratively a "psychological luxury").

26. Consistently the highest correlating partner of CO is social RD.

27. Becoming "lost in a moment"—losing track of time and being absorbed by what is going on exactly in that moment of time (e.g., in creative work, a moving thought, an act of compassion).

Clarifying correlation patterns between temperament and character. Developmentally, antecedent temperament traits are a limiting factor in character outcomes (Svrakic et al., 1996). Certain combinations of temperament traits, for example, low HA (low fearfulness), low NS (low impulsivity), high RD (social attachment), and high PE (industriousness), allow full psychological development of integrated personality (high SD), enabling the individual to select and pursue his or her goals consistently while remaining functionally adapted to the society (high CO). Reversely, high HA and high NS (fearfulness and impulsivity), low PE (indolence), and low RD (social detachment) are correlated with low SD, i.e. with personality disorder or fragmented personality. Such excessive temperament coupled with self-pathology (low SD) secondarily hinder social adaptation (low CO), also a regular finding in personality disorder (this can explain the same direction of correlation patterns of CO and SD with temperament traits, albeit much less significant for CO). To summarize: (i) affect states associated with heritable temperament traits influence the valence of internalized object relations and thus indirectly the substrate of the whole personality; (ii) character traits in part develop as cognitive contextualization of temperament traits, additionally explaining their positive correlations; (iii) certain temperament configurations, notably low HA and moderate NS (optimism, energy, curiosity) and high RD and PE (social interest and hard work), facilitate mature personality outcomes (hence the association with high SD), which then facilitate functional social adaptation (hence the association with high CO); (iv) certain temperament configurations, notably high HA and NS (fearfulness and impulsivity) and low RD and PE (detachment and indolence), interfere with personality integration (hence the association with low SD and personality disorder) with a ripple negative effect on social adaptation (hence the association with low CO capturing interpersonal difficulties of individuals with personality disorder).

A comment on the psychobiological concept of character. Character is widely regarded as one of the subsystems of personality, its social interface providing an evolutionarily important function of social adaptation, this it does in concert with moral values. Character can be thought of as the external narrative of the self or, as Kernberg (2016) defines it, the objective correspondent of identity, which is the internal narrative of the self. As described, the psychobiological concept of character joins together the cause and the consequence, the degree of personality integration or health (the SD dimension) and the degree of its social adaptation (the CO dimension), here both conceptualized as character traits. Understandably, the product of the two dimensions, personality health × social adaptation, has been found to be a reliable predictor of normalcy of personality versus personality disorder. In prior research, we have shown that low SD is consistently positively correlated (~r = 0.60) with low CO in personality disorder, and the product of the two (SD × CO) represents the core impairment (intrapersonal + social) shared by all variants (Svrakic et al., 1993). A similar approach has been used by the *Diagnostic and Statistical Manual of Mental Disorders* (fifth edition; American Psychiatric Association, 2013) alternative model, with disorders of self and disturbed social relations being decisive for the diagnosis, as personal and interpersonal indices of personality pathology. In the model we present in this book, however, low SD would roughly correspond to the vertical (in depth) diagnosis, and low CO to the horizontal, adaptive style diagnosis, as discussed in Chapter 3. The inclusion of a measure of personality integration (SD) as one of the character traits has not produced invalid results in research because of the high positive correlation of mature (immature) personality and adaptive (maladaptive) character. This is largely a conceptual issue only.

INTELLIGENCE: HIGH COGNITIVE ABILITY MAKES EVERYTHING EASIER

Intelligence (from Latin *intelligere*, "to comprehend or perceive") is defined as the general mental ability to understand one's surroundings and solve novel problems, figuratively to "make sense of things," "figure out what to do," or "catch on" (Gottfredson, 1997). In addition to this general cognitive ability, there appears to be a number of specific types of intelligence which involve music, language, and spatial relationships, among others. Social intelligence is closely related to the concept of theory of mind (the ability to appreciate that others have beliefs, desires, intentions, and perspectives that guide their behavior and that are different from one's own) and also the ability to draw inferences about the mental states of others based on verbal and non-verbal cues, both crucial adaptive features for social living and interpersonal relationships. Here we focus on intelligence as a general cognitive ability which reflects contributions from various brain regions and networks and is "something of an emerging property" (Zorumski and Rubin, 2011). One's intelligence quotient (IQ)[28] derives from one's biogenetic endowment, the degree of early cognitive stimulation, and the degree of lifelong maintenance through intellectual activities. Brain processes

28. IQ—measured using problem-solving, reasoning ability on standardized tests as compared to the statistical norm or average for a certain age.

underlying intelligence involve both basic neurophysiology (e.g., glucose uptake by the neurons, reaction time in elementary cognitive tasks, among others) and higher order cognitive abilities mediated by the general network of cognition. Intelligence is an independent ability of the brain that both emerges from interacting large scale ICNs and also has a lifelong influence on the organization, function, and preservation of these brain networks and the mind. High intelligence, coupled with a reasonably integrated personality, makes everything in life easier: self-assessment, regulation of emotion, life planning and goal choosing, interpersonal relations, and effectiveness of psychotherapy, to cite just a few among many benefits. It is not only a question of quantity of intelligence but also of quality, that is, how intelligence is utilized in everyday affairs. An individual with personality disorder may have a high IQ, but his or her personality may be affect-dominated, seeking interpersonal conflicts rather than conflict-solutions, defining social reality by "feeling" it instead of reasoning all of which may reduce intellectual efficacy. Neuroscience has shown that emotion and motivation usually work in conjunction with cognition and memory but can also function independently to the extent that they can override reasoning. Cognition, by contrast, cannot function without the input of emotions and motivation, as discussed by Zorumski and Rubin (2011). Under severely pathological circumstances, intelligence may amplify trauma by the development of complex, distorted interpretations of a threatening environment (Kernberg, 2016). Cognitive systems of rationalization of pathological character traits may also reinforce the faulty adaptive strategies encountered in severe personality disorder (Kernberg, 2016).

Certain temperament types may promote or impede the development of intelligence. A child with difficulties in delaying gratification or relief of tension (the "impatient" child) can have problems in figuring out alternative options and vice versa. A child with low anxiety may be intellectually more effective and vice versa. Families who stimulate early problem-solving through play and everyday activities, attend to motivations, stimulate language development, and encourage imagination fundamentally influence the level of IQ. In a positive feedback loop, the child's developing IQ facilitates cognitive interactions with the environment described, leading to even more encouragement and more attentive care. The lifelong maintenance of intelligence is also facilitated by a positive feedback loop, whereby intellectual ability motivates intellectual curiosity which in turn increases intellectual ability. Mature character helps as well, as it maximizes external conditions for learning, emotion regulation, and problem-solving.

The dynamic relationship between intelligence, character, and temperament is captured in the concept of "emotional intelligence," originally referring to the emotional-cognitive balance that drives leadership performance (Goleman, 1995) and since revised to the point that the name has outlived the thing it denotes. Salovey et al. (2004) subsequently defined emotional intelligence as the ability to reason about emotions, and of emotions, in order to enhance thinking. The concept implies a well-organized brain capable of incorporating emotion to the benefit of cognitive proficiency and effective adaptation. In contrast, history is full of "genius psychopaths" who achieved high academic ranks but struggled in everyday life as dysfunctional partners, autocratic leaders, and so on. Some authors have questioned the uniqueness of emotional intelligence, arguing that it is not more than the *g* factor of mental ability coupled with mature personality.

THE CONCEPT OF SELF: WHEN "I" MEETS "ME"

The concept of the self has been of major interest to philosophy, sociology, and psychology throughout history and, more recently, to neuroscience. Frustratingly, we were unable to find a definition of this concept that is not lost in metaphors or plagued by ideology. As insightful as metaphors may be, they typically fall short of defining a concept with precision. For example, William James (1992: writings 1878–1899) stated that the self is what happens when "I" (the mind) reflects back upon "me" (the empirical self). This metaphor captures the essence of the self as a reflective psychic structure, but it is not factually informative. Here, we outline our understanding of the self, both of its organization and its functions, beginning safely, with some hard to dispute facts. We then review the neuroscience that could explain how the brain networks may be connected with the very personal sense of self.

The development of self: a psychodynamic timeline based on observation of children. The sense of self is believed to be activated by neuropsychological processes in early interactions, whereby the projected affect activated by the interaction with an object is, by the mechanism of projective identification, reflected back into the mind as "self-representation" (Klein, 1952). Such rudiments of self, within nonconscious working memory of internalized object relations, provide the infant with the subjective and implicit sense of "I" as the subject mentally *contrasted* to the other (~6 months of age), mainly based on bodily sensations. Around the second year of age, the nonconscious "I" is self-organized into early self-awareness by its representation (HOR) within conscious working memory (the sense of "me" and "mine") as the mental subject *co-existing* with others. The early "me" is only accessible to passive noticing (aka "phenomenal consciousness about experience;" i.e., "what is it like" to have an experience [the taste of strawberries, the feeling of safety with the mother around, etc.]). The full sense of self as intentional and purposeful ("me and my intentions") develops at about three to five years of age. It is actively accessible by introspection (aka "self-awareness" or "autonoetic consciousness"). Self-awareness is facilitated by the child's ability to appreciate others as being intentional and purposeful themselves and having feelings and motives of their own; the acquisition of the theory of mind of others and capacity for mentalization occur at approximately the same age (McAdams, 2017). Also developing at this time is the capacity for autobiographical memory, enabling the sense of identity, which allows the experience of continuity in time and space ("me, my past-present-and-future"). The subsystem of identity culminates in adolescence and is also accessible by active introspection.

The neuroscience of the self: how sensory percepts become "me." To address this topic we borrow again from LeDoux and Brown (2017) and Kitamura et al. (2017). As noted, the first-order sensory percepts, mostly activated through early interactions with objects, together with related self-reflections and the associated affects (first recorded in the medial temporal lobe memory system and amygdala, respectively) are rather quickly also engramized in the PFCx. Kitamura et al (2017) showed that these prefrontal engrams take over as the *active* long-term episodic memory. As discussed, in addition to declarative memories, these neocortical copies also include autobiographical (personal) memory (facts and episodes related to the self and associated with respective affect states provided by the amygdala). The copies inform nonconscious working memory involving the self (here as nonconscious self-HOR), or, in psychoanalytic terms - internalized object relations.

The nonconscious self-HORs distinguish self ("I") from other ("not I") based on body sensations and rudimentary self-reflections within *nonconscious* working memory around six months of age. It is a mental state "but in an extremely thin sense" (LeDoux and Brown, 2017, p. E2020) insofar as it does not invoke the conscious self or self-awareness. For the phenomenal self-awareness ("me") to emerge, a higher order re-representation of the nonconscious self-HOR (HOR of self-HOR, or self-HOROR), is necessary to be pulled into *conscious* working memory, this together with consciously accessible autobiographical memories, a scientific support for the metaphor that the sense of self indeed occurs when “I” meets “me.” In other words, the conscious sense of self depends on implicit autobiographical memory (nonconscious self-HOR harboring internalized object relations) and explicit, consciously accessible autobiographical memory, semantic (“what”) and episodic (“where, when”), which is nonconscious until retrieved into conscious working memory, where the conscious sense of self appears. The phenomenal consciousness of the self (self-HOROR) is initially accessible by passively noticing (resulting in the sense of “me” in young children) and subsequently also by active introspection (a yet higher order representation of self-HOROR, or HOR of self-HOROR, resulting in the sense of “me and my intentions”) as discussed. Of note, active introspection (the ability to examine the content of one’s mental state) involves cognitive functions of attention, metacognition, and working memory (LeDoux and Brown, 2017).

Self-representations have been described as integrated hubs for information processing, a kind of “associative glue” (see later discussion) especially “important in emotional states that crucially depend on representation of the self as part of the higher order state that constitutes the felt experience” (LeDoux and Brown, 2017, p. E2021). Without conscious self, there would be no autonoetic emotions. The brain’s growing capacity for autobiographical memory culminates in the sense of identity, the autobiographical narrative that establishes historical and prospective continuity of the self. This indicates that identity may be a function of the self rather than an independent subsystem within the mind (for a review of neurological syndromes relevant to the higher order theory of consciousness, see LeDoux and Brown, 2017, “Supporting Information,” Box 2). With the emergence of the sense of self, the mind assimilates a new module into its system, the relationships of the existing components are reconfigured and optimized, and overall mental function advances, marking a significant developmental (adaptive) step.

Adaptive functions of the self: the associative glue of the mind. Similar to other subsystems, we conceptualize the self as a semi-stable configuration of mental faculties (cognition, emotion, motivation) self-organized into a subsystem of the mind with specific adaptive functions. The subsystem of self can be thought of as an associative glue of the mind. Based on evidence from neuroscience (reviewed in Sui and Humphreys, 2015), relating the stimulus to the self (self-reference) within the task a person is performing (i) helps to bind memories to their source, (ii) increases perceptual integration, (iii) makes it difficult to re-bind a new association to a stimulus formerly linked to the self, (iv) modulates the coupling between attention and decision-making, and (v) increases interactions between brain regions. Self-reference provides a form of associative glue for perception, memory, and decision-making and, through this, acts as a central mechanism in information processing (Sui and Humphreys, 2015, p. 719). For a detailed discussion of the self as an integrative hub for information processing, see Sui and Humphreys (2015). Arising from these integrative functions is the capacity of the self to connect actual autonoetic consciousness with the subjective background information about the body (the sense of ownership of the body, authorship and control of actions, internal affects states; aka "the embodied self;" Kernberg, 2015), together creating a unified physical and mental sense of self. The integrative functions of the self open up internal space to incorporate conceptual and symbolic representations of expanding experience, internal and external. One such example are sociocultural and moral norms, added to the internal roots of character and biological morality, together forming an integrated system of character and moral values. Other integrative functions include self-assessment (a person's estimates of self toward his or her internalized standards and also the experience of being estimated by others; both constitute self-esteem), regulation of affects and mood, object love and bonding, motivations (goals), initiative (activities) including social activities, and striving, among many others, as discussed later. This illustrates the multiple and specific adaptive functions that the subsystem of self provides to the mind.[29]

Self and object constancy: the all-important milestones. The developmental milestones of self- and object-constancy (around two to three years of age) accompany the phenomenal sense of "me." Self-constancy enables the child to have confidence that the self will survive separation from the object or any temporary resurgence of the bad self. Object constancy enables the child to preserve a stable, predominantly "good" internal representation

29. The self has critical integrative functions to the extent that the awareness of emotions depends on the sense of self: in other words, without the self no emotions are possible (LeDoux and Brown, 2017). Incidentally, emotions become conscious through the same sequence of cognitive rerepresentations as the sense of self-aware self. Subcortical circuits for first-order processing of affects do not give rise to conscious emotions but instead provide lower order, nonconscious inputs that coalesce with other kinds of neural signals in the cognitive assembly of conscious emotional experiences through a series of higher order representations and rerepresentations by the general network of cognition (LeDoux and Brown, 2017).

of the mother despite his or her own contradictory affects toward whatever frustrating or gratifying behaviors she displays (Auchincloss and Samberg, 2012). Such positive representation provides nonconscious emotional support and comfort even when the mother is not around, who now represents the "good internal object." With object constancy achieved, separation can take place without much anxiety and thus the mechanism of splitting can be replaced by repression. Margaret Mahler talks about emotional object constancy, as the successful outcome of the rapprochement phase of the separation-individuation process, occurring in tandem with whole object relations, capacity for affect regulation, and rudiments of mentalization. Object constancy is further structured through other relationships; that is, it remains open-ended to an extent, as its attainment is a lifelong process.

The working self: "me" in the here and now. The sense of self is made up of multiple self-experiences (different from one's formal social roles), each experience resulting from generalizations about the self in different personal domains (sexual contacts, romantic and casual social interactions, friendships, among many others) and all coalescing into a unified and active "working self." The concept of the working self refers to a set of present self-images (or mental models of oneself) and personal goals organized into goal hierarchies (Williams et al., 2008), against a backdrop of all the corresponding autobiographical experiences of the past. Such experiences of the past thus contribute to conscious states of personal goals and self-images of the present (aka the working self). The working self and autobiographical memory are involved in reciprocal control: the working self, a powerful subsystem of the mind pivotal in information processing, controls access, recall, and encoding of specific autobiographical memories, while autobiographical memory constrains the goals and self-images of the working self, its activities and choices (Conway, 2005). The working self is reorganized in terms of active personal goals and/or self-images more or less frequently over one's lifespan. Such dynamic homeostatic adaptive revisions of the mind are to an important extent channeled by previous self-images, that is previous working selves. The working selves at different times, harboring different editions of the self with different motivational priorities, are integrated into one autobiographical narrative of the self by the function of identity, frequently involving some falsification to achieve coherence.

The virtual self: when parent's' anticipation outlines the mental self. As Kohut (1977) noted, although the infant cannot have any reflexive awareness of him/herself, caretakers react to his or her emotions *ab initio* as if he or she were a whole person, thus anticipating the later self-awareness of the child. Such "virtual self," the imagination of the caretaker, can be described as "corresponding in reverse to that geometric point in infinity where two parallel lines intersect" (Kohut, 1977, p. 96). The semantic experience of the early self (self-awareness) emerges in the course of cognitive-linguistic development (around the second year of age), which enables the child to comprehend social interactions (rituals) and language, both of which are expressed through symbols and signs that convey some affective or cognitive aspect of the experience (Allan, 1997; Mead, 1934). Accordingly, the autobiographical memories coupled with social norms are organized into a mental sense of self, i.e., what one does, what one is supposed to do, rather than a visceral one (reviewed in Oyserman et al., 2012).

The inner and the outer circle of the self: the invisible rings of the mind. We refer to self-representations within the nonconscious working memory as the *inner circle* of the self. This implicit core of the self does not change with moment-to-moment circumstances, although decisively influences the way ("how") the working self adjusts to changing conditions. In contrast, the self-aware working self forms the *outer circle* of the self, and can change goals and self-images many times over the course of a person's lifetime. One can only speculate whether Kohut (1977) had in mind the two circles of the self when talking about the self as both as an experience-distant and experience-near concept. One cannot actively access the inner circle by introspection but can analyze its continuing effects on mental functioning and behavior. As discussed, the nonconscious "inner circle" of self serves as a necessary core of the "outer circle" of conscious self to develop but retains its own sovereignty in the process. It provides a thinly conscious sense of continuity of "I," the same basic feel of personhood despite multiple self experiences or personal goals over time and across situations. The conscious longitudinal, cross-sectional, and future continuity of the sense of self is achieved by the subsystem of identity, although the strength of the self-feeling may vary in intensity in specific settings, activities, and presence of others, at least in adolescents (Savin-Williams and Demo, 1983). A failed integration of the inner circle of the self (as seen with fragmented personality) is the core psychopathology of personality disorder. In contrast, fragmentation or even liquefaction of the outer circle can occur without affecting the stable inner core (e.g., healthy postmodern fragmented self and fluid self of liquid modernity), as discussed later.

Selfobjects: when "thou" defines "me." Kohut's (1971) concept of "selfobject" denotes a dynamics wherein an external object's psychological function (rather than the object itself) is internalized and experienced as part of one's own self, where it elicits, maintains, or positively influences the sense of self. Selfobjects can be people, systems of knowledge or beliefs (political, scientific, or religious), group affiliation, daily routines (our habits and established rituals), or stimulation-seeking activities (gambling, art, addictions). To paraphrase Jacques Lacan, people begin their lives in a state of fragmentation and throughout their lives seek an external source of organization. In other words, humans organize large segments of their internal world via outside sources of calm, structure, meaning, or stimulation, which are then internalized as selfobjects.

In early development, the child's sense of self is defined and maintained by internalized, depersonified psychological functions of caretakers (admiration, reliability, connectedness, and closeness), who are thus selfobjects. The early all important "tripolar" self-image—"I am worthy," "I strive," and "I belong"—develops through interactions with empathetic, good-enough parents. Internalized parental praise gives rise to a stable sense of self-esteem (healthy narcissism), confidence, ambitions, and purpose (aka "mirroring transference with selfobject"). Internalizing idealized selfobject (a calm, strong, wise, and reliable parent) involves adopting those ideals as one's own goals (aka "idealizing transference with selfobject"). Internalized "twin-like" or "alter-ego" relationship with parents results in the capacity for authentic close relationships as well as the experience of being understood and accepted by others (aka "twinship transference with selfobject"). In the process, functions of external selfobjects are no longer needed once the child begins to possess these qualities in order to exist and function. The capacity for independent self-regulation is achieved by separation from external selfobjects, mediated by the process of "transmuting internalization." The concept refers to repeated mild frustrations of the child's narcissistic demands, be that a full denial or a compromise, sometimes planned sometimes spontaneous, but always nontraumatic (i.e., not exceeding the child's capacity at the given developmental stage to cope). Optimal frustration is the basis of a sense of boundaries later in life. Through transmuting internalization, selfobjects and their functions are gradually replaced by a cohesive self and its functions: self-regulation of self-esteem, pursuit and choice of goals, and mature relationships with others, with no need that others fulfill selfobject functions. The latter is pathognomonic of personality disorder, as these individuals, due to persisting internal fragmentation, continue to depend on others as selfobjects and seek conflicts with them to demand whatever behaviors happen to nourish this need.

IDENTITY: THE AUTOBIOGRAPHICAL NARRATIVE OF THE SELF

In psychology, the concept of "identity" (Latin: *identitas* for "sameness") refers to a sustained sense of oneself as a coherent, predictable, and authentic individual. Identity is a semi-stable configuration of mental faculties (cognition, emotion, motivation), self-organized to provide a sense of continuity of the self, which in turn advances the adaptive fitness of the mind as a whole. Figuratively, identity adds the assuring coherence of "who" to the sense of "me." It is mediated by introspectively accessible autobiographical memory. The latter enables the mind to mental time travel not only to the past but also to the future where a reliable planning of the self occurs ("prospection"). The autobiographical narrative aligns a variety of historical self-images and personal goals, from vocation, nationality, relational choices, gender roles, and religion, among many others, into a coherent story of the self frequently involving some falsification to achieve coherence, as noted. The person recognizes him/herself by these high-fidelity continuities ("identity pipelines") and is recognized by others for them ("reputation"). As the sense of self also includes *object* representations, one's identity encompasses one's integrated view of other people, as these (the consistent representations of others) reinforce the coherent narrative of the self. Temperament, character, and moral values also contribute to the sense of identity, with specific "how" and "why" facets to the sense of "who of me," a complex phenomenal experience arising from the functionally overlapping subsystems of the mind, as discussed earlier.

Widely believed to be the achievement of adolescence, the subsystem of identity logs the explicit memories (semantic and episodic) related to self since childhood (three to four years of age), around time which coincides with the development of the capacity for autobiographical memory. Most humans do not remember personal events before three or four years of age, except for flashbulb memories. The simple narrative of childhood evolves into more complex yet still fluctuating and disorganized personal goals and self-images of the teenage years. The developmental process eventually leads to identity consolidation in adolescence, as a hybridized intuitive-rational commitment to a particular working self and a particular moral value system. Functional decomposition of identity reveals two broad but overlapping identity domains, classified as *relational identity* (the extent to which one derives one's identity from personal relationships, e.g., parenting, friendships, family, romantic-sexual) and *societal identity* (the extent to which one derives one's identity from profession, work, race, ethnicity, among others). Gender identity (identification with a gender) and sexual orientation identity (identification of sexual preference) are more biologically driven and appear early in life, the former about the age of four and the latter in puberty. Neither fully fits the psychological concept of identity, although both contribute to identity coherence. Sexual-romantic identity, as listed under the umbrella of relational identity, refers to one's autobiographical narrative summarizing experience with romantic partners, both sexual and emotional.

The sense of historical coherence (identity) unites the variants of the working self over the course of a lifetime. Mature adults are able to selectively reconstruct, and in many instances falsify, their past to the point where it seems that they have planned the past and the present and can consistently plan the future, all of which provide them with a reassuring life story containing a high degree of unity, meaning, and purpose. Moreover, once a person develops an identity concept about what they are like, they will strive to verify the accompanying self-views through seeking self-verifying feedback, as William (Bill) Swann, Jr described in the 1983 article " Self-Verification: Bringing Social Reality into Harmony with the Self." By "owning" our history, past, present, and future, we maneuver ourselves into the inner position of proprietors, of creators (McAdams, 2017). By "aligning" the sense of self into a coherent chronicle, identity mediates the mind's *adaptation to the internal environment* ("inward-oriented self"). In contrast, character can be thought of as "outward-oriented self."

The sense of self is necessary for its autobiographical narrative (identity) to be told. The two are so intimately co-related that it is hard to tell whether identity is just another function of the self or, as we believe, an independent subsystem within the mind that performs a specific function, namely to connect the past, the present, and the envisioned future, an important adaptive capacity of the mind as a whole. Of note, identity modifies self and self modifies identity through reciprocal co-interaction; that is, neither is a passive reflection of the other. Identity is being continually reworked throughout the life cycle, as it not only adapts to the dynamic changes in the working self but also influences the working self in the process.

The neuroscience of identity: the "who" of "me." Autobiographical memory consists of recollected historical events in life, combining episodic (events) and semantic (facts, concepts) memory, both types explicit and consciously accessible. It is categorized into three broad areas: *lifetime periods* (school theme, work theme, marriage theme, etc., with personal attitudes and goals of the time), *general events* (specific events or a sequence of related events in one's life), *and event-specific knowledge* (visual images and sensory-perceptual features derived from individual events that distinguish real occurrences from recollections of things that never happened; Conway and Pleydell-Pearce, 2000).

Functional neuroimaging associates autobiographical memory with a core network of left-lateralized regions, including the prefrontal, parietal, temporal, and retrosplenial–posterior cingulate cortices, temporo-parietal junction, and the cerebellum, with amygdala and sensory cortices also participating (Svoboda et al., 2006; reviewed in Holland and Kensinger, 2010). The widespread activation patterns indicate that a number of co-participating regions and functions (attention, memory, emotions, perception, among others) uniquely contribute to the rich texture of autobiographical experiences. The described network of autobiographical memory overlaps significantly, albeit with some distinct features, with the general network of cognition (Conway et al., 2001). The workings of the general network of cognition underlie a number of related cognitive functions, co-emerging as rudimentary at about the same age (four to five years), with some degree of neurophysiological and phenomenological overlap among them: (i) autobiographical memory, closely related to the sense of self and identity; (ii) the intrinsic attention system involving spontaneous mentation (mind-wandering) or deliberate introspective mentation (self-generated cognition); (iii) self-projection (ability to envision the future and alternative situations, also called prospection); and (iv) mentalization and theory of mind of others.

Integrated (consolidated), diffuse (incoherent), and confused (conflicting) identity. Consolidated identity refers to a coherent alignment of all historical versions of the working self over the years, projected into the future as one's life plan. In such a well-integrated, committed internal world, occasional rogue motivations are handled with ease. Diffuse and confused identity are not synonymous. The former keeps different identity options open, as seen in personality disorder, with alternating contradictory personal goals and self-images. Confused identity refers to conflicting self-images which may lead to mental collisions leading to difficulty to recognize any personal goals or self-images, often seen in psychosis. Identity diffusion is discussed in more detail in the next chapter, "What Is Personality Disorder?"

THE SUBSYSTEM OF MORAL VALUES: THE MIND'S INNER CENSOR OF RIGHT AND WRONG

The subsystem of integrated moral values (colloquially referred to as "conscience") is defined as a semi-stable configuration of mental faculties (cognition, motivation, emotion) that defines one's personal code of values, which guides behaviors and advances social adaptation.[30] This complex subsystem is biologically rooted in the sense of empathy and reciprocal altruism, which humans share with other animals. It also includes normative standards defined by the social environment: internalized parental prohibitions and expectations (three to four years of age) followed by internalized family values (six to eight years of age) and, finally, local social norms, whether implied (culture) or explicit (law), learned and internalized during the adolescent years. Early in development, moral values provide ideals to strive for, rules to adhere to, and the inner system of distress (guilt, shame) in case they are violated. As Edith Jacobson (1964) observed, morality is depersonified, abstracted, and individualized during adolescence and finally integrated into a value system no longer linked concretely to demands or prohibitions from any particular source but oneself. Such integrated moral values allow for an impartial evaluation of oneself and others, resulting in insights, learning, and deliberate correction, rather than guilt or shame. The mind's subsystem of moral values is dynamic, insofar as it continues to develop through one's lifespan.

As noted, moral values work in concert with character (both reflect internal and external expectations) and both, if mature, promote social adaptation. Only moral values, which also evaluate the character, generate self-correction if the expectations, whether personal or societal, are not met. In what follows, we briefly describe the biological roots of morality (reciprocity, fairness, empathy, and helping behaviors), acquired normative morality, and universal, depersonified moral standards, which are all deficient in personality disorder.

The neuroscience of morality: where cognitive and emotional judgements meet. The brain network underlying moral decisions overlaps with the networks involved in the theory of mind and empathy, and all share components with the general network of cognition, each discernible by a few specific structural and functional features. The regular overlap between morality and empathy could be explained by co-activation of brain networks involved in the two phenomena, for example, seeing things from another person's' points of view (theory of mind) and experiencing others' feelings (empathy). There is suggestive evidence that moral reasoning might be

30. The term and concept "moral" refers to a set of internalized, often personal principles about right and wrong which govern behavior that cultivates and regulates complex interactions in social groups. The term and concept of "ethics" refers to (i) principles of right conduct in social, professional, and business interactions and (ii) the science of morality.

dissociable into cognitive and affective subsystems; for example, different networks may be involved in judging a robbery versus judging a rape. However, as no experience is purely cognitive or purely emotional, we understand moral reasoning as a cognitive-emotional hybrid with variable ratios of each component, especially in complex contexts. As reviewed in Pascual et al. (2013), the ventromedial PFCx is implicated in empathy, moral judgement, mediation of emotions during moral processing, adherence to values, and integration of others' intentions into moral reasoning; the dorsolateral PFCx is involved in the conscious judgment of responsibility for crimes and its punishment from a third-party perspective; these competing processes may both be mediated by the anterior cingulate cortex - ACCx (Pascual et al., 2013). Parietal and temporal structures are believed to play important roles in the attribution of others' beliefs and intentions, while anterior insular cortex and rostral ACCx, with multimodal inputs from emotional systems, are thought to mediate our visceral, "gut"-level reactions about "right versus wrong" in the social context (Zorumski and Rubin, 2011).

Biological roots of morality: inclusive fitness, empathy, reciprocity. The phenomenon of human morality has its roots in distant evolutionary instincts, which have continued through natural selection because they facilitate group living, a superior adaptive solution for all successful animal species. Helping behaviors within the group (e.g., reciprocity of altruistic actions, cooperation, sense of fairness, and penalties for violators) increase chances of survival and reproduction of individual members. The biological pillars of morality are *reciprocity* (fairness, justice) and *empathy* (concern, compassion). In addition, inclusive fitness is another basic mechanism through which pro-social behaviors have emerged and continue to thrive in evolution. Sacrifice for kin (inclusive fitness) and for people similar to us (broad inclusive fitness) are altruistic[31] in a selfish kind of way, as such behaviors increase the chances that one's own genes will prosper. Collective self-esteem or "feeling good" because of group membership is sometimes added to the psychological mechanisms facilitating group living.

Empathy: psychological *and* neural identification with others. Here, we borrow from Preston and de Waal (2002) who formulated the perception-action model of empathy. Empathy is defined as vicarious experiencing of the feelings, thoughts, or attitudes of an object, creating a state in the subject (observer) that is more applicable to the object's state than to the subject's own prior state or situation. As the proximate cause

31. Selfless concern for the well-being of others.

of empathy, attended perception of an object's state activates the subject's corresponding representations of the state, social situation, and object, and activation of these representations automatically primes or generates the associated autonomic and somatic responses, unless inhibited (Preston and de Waal, 2002, p. 4). As the ultimate cause of empathy, responsible for the evolution of the particular DNA code present in every individual member, the perception-action mechanism supports (activates) a spectrum of phenomena and helping behaviors (e.g., alarm, social facilitation, vicariousness of emotions) that are crucial for the reproductive success of animals living in groups. Empathy is a superordinate category that includes several related phenomena with the same underlying perception-action mechanism, such as emotional contagion, sympathy, helping behavior, and cognitive empathy. Empathy always involves some level of personal distress (feeling the "pain" of other) and some benefit for the subject experiencing empathy (feeling "good" in empathizing). The empathic perception of the situation of another person directly depends on his or her interdependence or interrelationship with the subject.

The shared representation of the object's state is in part made possible by the system of mirror neurons (a neuron that fires both when an animal acts and when the animal observes the same action performed by another), primarily located in the cortex (premotor and supplementary motor area, primary somatosensory cortex, and inferior parietal areas). However, brain areas and processes involved in the activation of other components of empathy also play a role in the overall neuroanatomy of empathy: factual and episodic memories (temporal lobes, neocortex), autonomic sensation (amygdala), fast subcortical processes (sensory cortex-thalamus-amygdala response) involved in contagious forms of empathy, slow cortical processes (thalamus-cortex-amygdala response) involved in cognitive forms of empathy, cingulate, orbitofrontal and ventromedial PFCx (perception and regulation of emotion, social cognition, moral reasoning), and even the cerebellum (prediction and planning of attentional shifts; Preston and de Waal, 2002). All of these areas are activated when one is observing, experiencing, or imagining an emotional state. The automatic perception-action process is subject to control and modulation, and is affected by experience and context because of the role of mental representations, which helps explain why there are different levels of empathy across individuals, ages, and species (Preston and de Waal, 2004, p. 4). With advanced development of the PFCx in humans, empathy has become a top-down modulator of a broad range of interactive and social behaviors. Incidentally, perception-action brain mechanisms are involved in other aspects of social facilitation, including our ability to learn a spoken language and understand the intentions and activities of others (theory of mind), and it even influences the development of the sense of self (modeled after those we empathize with).

Inclusive fitness: love thy relative. The evolutionary success of DNA ultimately depends on its ability to leave the greatest possible number of its copies within a population. This can be accomplished not only by direct reproduction, the well-known direct or Darwinian fitness, but also by supporting genetically close relatives (kin selection, aka "indirect or inclusive fitness"). Since other members of the group may share a proportion of one's genes, an individual can increase his or her evolutionary success by promoting such individuals as "offspring equivalents," through support, rescue, and rearing regardless of who begets them. A sibling's child, who will carry one-quarter of the individual's genes, is 1/2 offspring equivalent. Similarly, a cousin's child, who carries 1/16 of the individual's genes, is 1/8 offspring equivalent. Genes promoting behaviors of sacrifice for close genetic relatives have a higher chance of prospering. There are still other ways to promote the evolutionary success of DNA, not just through direct Darwinian and indirect inclusive fitness. Hamilton (1964) mathematically showed how indirect reproduction, i.e., supporting an identical or similar phenotypic trait in others, not blood-related members of a given population, also contributes to the propagation of similar genes. This broader definition of inclusive fitness ("love thy look-alike") helps explain why we like people similar to us. Hamilton (1964) argued that natural selection favors mutually beneficial behaviors (increasing the fitness of all involved, like reciprocity) or selfish behaviors (increasing the fitness of the actor, decreasing the fitness of the recipient). Inclusive fitness (narrowly or broadly defined), however, helps explain altruism (decreasing one's own fitness for the benefit of other) and spite (decreasing own fitness as well as the fitness of the unrelated and dissimilar recipient, as this indirectly promotes the fitness of the non-involved kin or a protégé). Helping similar genotypes and phenotypes and harming the dissimilar ones increases the fraction of the discriminating party's genes in future generations.

The emotion of love serves as the engine of sacrifice for genetic kin. Feeling love ensures that parents care for the offspring, or that an uncle protects his nephew, at the same time making these caring people feel good about themselves. Evolutionary psychology posits that most of our emotions exist because at one time they either directly or indirectly aided the survival of genes that code for them, especially fear, anger, and love. With the humanization of biological behaviors, the feeling of love has gained functional autonomy, in Maslow's sense, and has become an end in its own right rather than simply being related to the propagation of genes.

Reciprocal altruism: love thy neighbor. In reciprocal altruism, an individual acts in a way in that temporarily reduces his or her own fitness and increases the fitness of another individual. The adjective "reciprocal" refers to the expectation that the other individual will act in a similar way at a later time and a reversal of fortunes. In contrast to inclusive fitness, reciprocal altruism applies to all members of the group, not just those genetically related or those with similar phenotypic traits. It is based on long-term cost-benefit analysis, not fueled by empathy or sympathy. The majority of group-living animal species has developed at least some type of reciprocal altruism (e.g., bats, hyenas, numerous bird species, among many others). Most group animals also have developed a strong sense of fairness, justice, and equality, as primordial "morals" rooted in reciprocal altruism and cooperative efforts. A series of experiments by Frans de Waal[32] demonstrates the sense of fairness in a pair of capuchin monkeys who are not getting the same reward for the same performance. In another experiment with elephants, de Waal demonstrated a tendency to "cheat" if the opportunity arises while retaining the impression of cooperation. Inclusive fitness (helping kin), reciprocal altruism (helping with an expectation of reciprocity), and empathy (helping based on emotional co-identification) are largely independent functions, and each facilitates group living in its own specific way.

Are humans inherently good? As noted, human morality is partly rooted in biology and nature and is finalized through social communication. Preverbal human infants even at three months show more interest in "good" characters and appear to have a very elemental innate sense of fairness and justice, as shown by Karen Wynn's (2009, 2013) work. Preverbal infants consistently show attraction to a prosocial character (a positive approach response) and aversion toward an antisocial character (an avoidance response), although some of this early altruism may reflect adaptive advantage to the infant who interacts with good individuals (reviewed in Wynn, 2009). Children as young as 14 to 18 months of age have been found to help others attain their goals, irrespective of any reward from adults and without concern for reciprocation and reputation, both of which serve to maintain altruism in older children and adults (Warneken and Tomasello, 2009). Human infants also have an innate tendency to dislike those who are different and to be selfish even at their own expense (choosing less for themselves just so others get even less), exposing the very early "us" versus "them" comparisons. Fortunately, as children grow older, these negative

32. https://www.youtube.com/watch?v=GcJxRqTs5nk.

feelings wane and are replaced by generosity even at one's own expense, most likely through acculturation (Wynn, 2013). Hence, judging solely based on early empathy and reciprocity, human infants are inherently good. How then to explain the high prevalence of selfish, manipulative, exploitative, and inconsiderate people around us? What goes wrong from childhood to adulthood in many lives? Personality disorder may account for up to 10% to 15 % of these individuals. It appears that once social competition for resources and/or status enter the mind, character choices steer some people into immorality, the latter along a wide spectrum of major and minor manifestations. Character disorder (onset in adolescence or young adulthood) is a useful clinical and forensic concept to classify immoral behaviors as a chosen and self-approved social strategy.

Acquired moral norms: the civilization's self-defense. Historically, external rules of behavior became necessary as the size of human communities increased. In large groups, with complex and diverse social roles, reciprocity and fairness are not immediately verifiable, which opens the door for manipulation and cheating. Reciprocal altruism and empathy do not always suppress biological drives for dominance and aggression if one can cheat unpunished. The communities eventually resorted to explicit written codes (laws), implicit norms set by local culture, and, where applicable, religious prescriptive norms to protect the basic principles of group living—reciprocity and fairness. These external norms are subsequently internalized during psychosocial development and become a part of the integrated moral values system. Legal norms *proscribe* what is prohibited and a system of concrete punishment for the violators. Culture and religion *prescribe* both desirable and undesirable behaviors, while the reward for the adherent and the punishment for the offenders are more subjective than concrete, in that they lead an individual to feel guilt and/or shame. Much later, in the most recent history of civilization, society introduced medical treatment of deviant (amoral, destructive) behaviors deemed to result from a mental disorder rather than from a calculated choice. In sum, internalized societal and legal standards become a part of the overall moral makeup of a mature individual, working in concert but not interchangeable with biological morality and character traits. Acquired morality as civilization's self-defense may develop into its extreme of a totally socialized self (i.e., internalization of societal needs as if they were one's own), perhaps marking the end of the need for traditional prohibitive laws and prescriptive expectations, as discussed later in the chapter.

Universal morality: if it's wrong for others, it's wrong for us. In most people, the biological roots of empathy and reciprocity, combined with development of moral reasoning and acculturation, give rise to *universal morality*, also called *moral objectivism*. Meta-ethics posits that some systems of ethics apply universally because some moral values exist independently of the feeling-states of individuals within particular times and contexts. Simply put, certain behaviors are wrong regardless of the circumstances. According to Noam Chomsky (2000), universal morality is based on the principle that "if an action is right (wrong) for others, it's right (wrong) for us." This principle, if truly internalized, guides the behavior of all or most reasonable individuals regardless of their culture, race, gender, sexual orientation, nationality, or any other personal characteristic. In contrast to moral relativism (holding that moral judgments differ across cultures), and moral nihilism (nothing is intrinsically moral or amoral[33]), Chomsky considers moral universalism as an inherent capacity of human neuropsychology similar to the capacity for language acquisition. As Chomsky stated, "we're constantly making moral judgments in new situations, and over a substantial range we do it in a convergent fashion—we don't differ randomly and wildly from one another . . . young children do it, very quickly, and they also converge. . . . This is either a miracle, or rooted in our nature. . . . It's rooted in our nature just like the language is or otherwise we'd never use it in any systematic way, except just repeating what happened before." The Universal Declaration of Human Rights (United Nations [UN], 1948), and the Geneva Conventions in defining fair treatment of prisoners of war predicated this on the theory of moral universalism which, we may add, are both massively violated all the time. The stunning impotence of the UN to make a difference in the pervasive and profound ethical crisis in the modern society could be a warning that a fundamental shift to a dangerous new normal is occurring, wherein the unethical becomes the ethical by the decree of the world's military powers.

FUNCTIONAL ADAPTATION: COMMON ADAPTIVE STYLES IN A BIDIRECTIONAL WIN-WIN DEAL

The concept of *functional adaptation* involves a two-way interaction in which both sides negotiate a balanced optimum between inner needs and outside normative pressures: the individual adheres to the norms yet is authentic and accomplished ("mens sana in societatis sano"). Functional

33. Amoral means having no sense or knowledge of right or wrong (a rare occurrence); immoral refers to ignoring or deliberately violating norms one is aware of.

adaptation can be confused with overadaptation, that is, unhealthy adherence to social demands without keeping a critical mind about it. There are numerous situations in which good adaptation to a bad environment means unhealthy adaptation, for example, adapting to a bad marriage. The point we are trying to make here is that extreme conformity and extreme oppositionality are simply different faces of immaturity.

Multiple factors determine one's adaptive behavior styles in social interactions. The roots of any given style can be traced back to the formative period as the child's preconceptual, conditioned behavior which enabled him or her to express inner emotional needs and still meet the expectations set by the primary family. These early internal models of behavior, referred to as "schemata" or "life scripts" in cognitive and humanistic theories, are further modulated by temperament, advancing cognitive functions, character, moral values, and culture, eventually forming one's typical adaptive style. Temperament adds a stylistic component to behavior, making it impulsive or deliberate, shy or outgoing, sentimental or independent. Cognitive processes contextualize immediate needs or impulses within the framework of social norms, a process facilitated by the emerging subsystem of character. Character is in part influenced by the quality of internalized object relations and in part by the individual's assessment, intuitive or calculated, of the most effective ways to get ahead but also get along with other people. Moral values combine innate dispositions to empathy and fairness with external standards; they guide social behaviors but also self-assess the person thereby enabling self-correction. Environmental factors also contribute, such as family (e.g., an antisocial son models his behavior after his antisocial father) or culture (e.g., narcissism is frequent in the Western cultures, rare in African and Asian cultures). Personality assessment, importantly, involves identification of predominant adaptive styles, which are then cross-matched with the actual level of mental functioning of the person to determine normalcy and pathology of the presenting behavior style, as discussed in Chapter 3.

NORMAL, MATURE, CREATIVE PERSONALITY

We outline our understanding of these partially overlapping concepts not only to lay the groundwork for the discussion of disordered personality but also to avoid potential misunderstandings in readers of different theoretical backgrounds.

Are humans really normal? The concept of *normal* personality is mainly used in reference to social norms, that is, implicit and explicit expectations about attitudes and behaviors within the given culture or society. Normal personality, or at least the interpersonal aspect of it, is the one conforming to social norms, thus refers to the *social normalcy* of the individual. The other, more private aspect of *psychological normalcy* is not covered by this concept. Social normalcy neither necessarily denotes nor excludes psychological health. In other words, every psychologically normal person is likely to show social normalcy, but every socially normal person is not necessarily psychologically normal.

Another aspect of normal personality is the assumption of its normal (Gaussian) distribution in the population. The question is whether this assumption applies to the human mind. Statistical methods often assume that quantitative human traits are *normally distributed*, which is why the term "normal" personality is used in the first place. Although widely considered a rigorously proven theorem, the assumption has not really been confirmed when it comes to psychological traits. The assumption of normal distribution indeed holds for many features in biological organisms. Nature was very generous in a few cases, very stingy in a few cases, and rather even-handed in the vast majority of cases. As a general rule, the more random factors that are involved in producing a certain feature, as is the case with personality, the more likely it is for this feature to be normally distributed. Moreover, all other patterns of distributions tend to converge toward normalcy as the number of observations approaches infinity. Human psychological features do not deviate much from these general rules, with some exceptions. The more biologically driven the feature is, the more likely its normal distribution. Genes that drive temperament development appear at random in a population, and their propagation is regulated by natural and social selection. Since temperament traits are formed before they are fully exposed to the normative pressures by the society (around five to six years of age), they are likely normally distributed in populations of children.

During subsequent personality development, society exerts normative pressure to suppress the extremes on both ends of a temperament trait. Children with extreme NS are "corrected," that is, diagnosed and treated as ADHD or conduct disorder, those with excessive HA as anxious or depressed, and those detached with excessively low RD as schizoid or autistic. The only exception to such normative suppression are children with high (but not excessive) RD, who are "allowed" to develop without corrective medical or social intervention. The ethical implications of the loss of authenticity of children having been corrected by such psychological engineering is a major concern but beyond the scope of this book. These normative pressures do not directly affect the general normal distribution of temperament traits, but they do affect the narrow ends of the bell shape by clipping off the extremes. In the long run, however, some skewness toward genes coding for high RD may be expected. Notwithstanding, our temperaments are normal at present.

Some character traits are not normally distributed. In prior research (Cloninger et al., 1993) we found out that all character scores tend to be skewed toward high values. The CO scores, capturing helpfulness, empathy, and acceptance of diversity, indicate that the vast majority of people are very cooperative, the minority are just cooperative, and those not cooperative at all are hard to find. The social desirability artifact was addressed in the cited study but was hard to eliminate. In addition to social desirability, the skewed distribution toward high CO can be in part explained by negative social selection against *low RD*: reward-dependent children are easy to condition to conform to social norms and thus likely to become cooperative citizens, while low RD children may be treated for autism or schizoid manifestations. The SD scores were also skewed toward positive values (resourceful, purposeful, responsible), although less significantly, perhaps reflecting a combination of personal desirability (positive bias toward oneself), social desirability (it is desirable to be perceived as self-sufficient), and the fact that low scores on this trait reflect severe personality pathology, found in not more than about 10–15% of the population. The ST traits was the least skewed of the three, perhaps due to low personal and social desirability of the descriptor items.

Mature personality: from solidity to fluidity. The concept of mature personality extends the social concepts of normalcy by introducing internal criteria of psychological well-being. Mature personality is thus synonymous with a high level of mental health. Criteria for maturity are informal and vary in the literature but converge toward an ability to deal with conflicts internally, maintain consistency of self-image and stable self-esteem, experience coherent identity, and exhibit principled moral standards, and character that is not merely fitting the social norms but extending into activities for the common good (aka "extended self"). Mature or "high integrity" individuals are comfortable with themselves, follow authentic personal goals guided by a strong sense of internal direction that appreciates but does not depend on approval by others. Such personal health is also reflected outside, as mature individuals do not envy others, fully enjoy bilateral cooperation, are tolerant of diversity, and are inspirational to many. They are warmly appreciated by their families, a few but intimate friends, as well as by the extended social environment at work and in the local community. These concept of maturity may sound idyllic in comparison to the narrative of mental health in the postmodern and liquid modernity eras, as psychological concepts are rapidly changing. The current liquid modernity emphasizes transiency rather than stability and loose connectedness via cyber-networks versus solid connectedness in the real world. As Bauman (2000) and Palese (2013) noted, liquid modern humans appear to be excluding themselves from traditional networks of support, while also freeing themselves from the restrictions or requirements those networks impose. Nomadism becomes a general trait as a person flows through his or her own life like a tourist, changing places, jobs, spouses, values, and sometimes more—such as political or sexual orientation. Does stable integration obscure the unique perspectives of the fragmented or fluid self? Are not the standards for mature personality today more related to one's capacity for flexibility, tolerance, and containing and less to the stability (or perhaps inflexibility) of the one's chosen adaptive style? Notwithstanding, the new liquid maturity still means stable core integration of the substrate of the self, while its liquidity in the outer circle enables the person to handle transient trends in the outside environment and transient disturbances of internal homeostasis. Such liquid maturity is capable of creating ever new ways of adaptation, albeit a liquid adaptation. In short, maturity is a dynamic process, not a mastered and fixed developmental stage. The operative definition of new maturity would be the capacity for fluid change rather than solid stability.

The inner sense of meaning: available to everyone, discovered by few. Maslow postulated that the opportunity for self-actualization emerges after basic physiological and safety needs are met. This hierarchy is to an extent true, but is not decisive. It is the internal attitude of the individual that determines whether he or she self-actualizes, as illustrated by countless examples of underprivileged but highly self-actualized individuals, like Mahatma Gandhi. Existentialism posits that defining the fundamental meaning of one's existence begins with the human individual naturally striving to understand one's own self and the world beyond simple physical needs and pleasures. The primary virtue of existentialism is authenticity. Each individual, not society or religion, is solely responsible for giving meaning to his or her life and living it passionately and sincerely, that is, authentically as famously noted by Kierkegaard. The specific meaning one gives to his or her life may vary from person to person, but it always depends on a strong sense of internal direction which provides clarity of emotion and motivation, as well as freedom of thought, that is, an integrated, courageous mind. It is the sense of meaning itself that drives the person, and meaning can find its substrate anywhere where humans exist; in other words, finding one's meaning is not necessarily tied to privilege, as summarized by the adage "happiness is hard to find inside one's self, and impossible anywhere else". In the contemporary world, a mature person may experience confusion arising from the discrepancy between his or her authentic needs and socially dictated "needs" and "desires." Such feeling of social intrusion is likely just a temporary phase in the transition towards a completely socialized personality, as discussed. Notwithstanding, an increasing number of people, the young included, are finding meaning outside the "linked in" world, at remote places away from social networks. Simply put, the ongoing grassroots redefinition of privilege highlights the importance of having time for oneself, not goods (the "less is more" maxim).

Creativity: a gift of nature or self-actualization at work? Self-actualization in the Maslow's meaning may be confused with extraordinary giftedness. The former implies the highest level of mental health, acceptance of and deep relationship with others, the latter (giftedness) not necessarily requiring a relationship with others or even mental health. Indeed, many creative geniuses throughout history were either immature or mentally tormented (e.g., the creative geniuses of Nikola Tesla, a lifelong loner; Salvador Dali; Marcel Proust; among others). Edvard Munch, who painted "The Scream," one of the most recognized masterpieces in the history of art, wrote in his diary: "My fear of life is necessary to me, as is my illness. They are indistinguishable from me, and their destruction would destroy my art."

Self-actualized people reach their full potentials but may not be creative according to the standard of producing socially valuable products, science, or masterpieces of art. Both creativity as a source of beauty and awe and creativity in turning everyday activities into events of love and meaning reflect one's psychological maturity and self-actualization and do not necessarily require natural giftedness. Such *creativity as attitude* is intrinsically valuable so that nothing of demonstrable social value need be produced, although the two are not entirely excluded from one another (reviewed in Barron and Harrington, 1981). *Creativity as achievement* (i.e., producing socially valuable products or masterpieces of art) requires artistic or scientific talents not necessarily reflecting one's psychological health but largely dependent on one's neurogenetics, that is, a gift of nature. The current trend of *pseudo-creativity* refers to private internet postings of pieces of "art" (tweets, photographs, texts, etc.) or merely personal opinions related to social themes, feeding off trends and attracting followers. A survey from a few decades ago indicated that more than 80% of Americans believe that they have something important to say and should write a book. Everyone is given a chance to be an author today, as countless blogs allow people to express themselves. On the negative side, such open access is blurring the criteria for bona fide contributions to art, science, and culture.

Is it possible to be healthy and unhealthy at the same time? We can only offer a speculative answer to this question, using anecdotes about creative individuals and those with personality disorder as examples. An extraordinary inborn aptitude, physical or mental, endows the individual with a talent-specific intense perceptiveness, a powerful organizing force from the early phases of mind development (e.g., Mozart). The resulting strong sense of internal direction leads to a personalized designation of meaning that is not fundamentally dependent on external circumstances. This means that, for gifted individuals, interactions with others are less relevant for personality development, as the power of internal direction drives the development toward the specific outcome, reducing the importance of outside support and feedbacks. The talent also provides a mental sanctuary for the person to find comfort during turbulent times, personal struggle, or struggles with other people. In the developmental process dominated by an inborn talent, other aspects of personality may remain underdeveloped, such as character traits, sociability, self-regulation of mood, mature sexuality, or affect regulation. These neglected aspects become in fact psychological deficiencies existing side by side with the dominant creative self. The way Albert Einstein, an incredible mind perhaps with a deficient capacity for empathy, treated his first wife Mileva Maric (she was born a cripple due to a disease that displaces the hip bone, giving her a limp) would probably qualify as abusive by today's standards. Some creative artists have used mental struggle as inspiration—Salvador Dali and Edward Munch, for example. Of note, adaptive regression in the service of the ego, as Freud eloquently coined the phrase, can be a highly desirable component in creative processes, especially in fine arts. In contrast to artists, creative scientists depend less on their inner world for inspiration, as their creativity inherently involves externally defined criteria and goals. The most notable exception is Nikola Tesla, who allegedly came up with creative ideas in his dreams. Both creativities, scientific and artistic, rely more on intuition than on sensory perception, however.

The towering dominance of inborn talents in creative geniuses is similar and yet fundamentally different from personality disorder, wherein a pathological but dictatorial self-concept takes over the organization of the mind, leaving behind fragmented residuals along with the underdeveloped authentic needs of the individual. The artistic self of a creative genius is also dictatorial but far from being an alien, insofar as it is rather a natural organizing talent. As we have seen in our practice, an individual with fragmented personality who is also talented has a better course and quality of life.

We discuss here the controversy about Vincent Van Gogh's life and mental health, both widely used to portray a "mad genius." In our opinion, his life and work not only epitomize the idea of authenticity but also illustrate that a creative genius does not always mean successful adaptation by popular standards. The unwavering sense of internal direction defining his unique understandings of life, art, truth, and people around him gave passionate meaning to Vincent's world long before he became an artist. He was at first an art salesman (too honest for his own good), then a priest passionately giving to those in need, selfless and sacrificing to the point that the parishioners thought of him as the "second coming of Christ" (Stone, 1934). During the last few years of life, he was ridiculed by the citizens of Arles—"mad redhead" they called him—while continuing to create some of the most powerful paintings in the history of art. The power of his mind was able to penetrate beyond the physical limits of ordinary senses and instill life into inanimate reality, its movement and texture, so powerfully represented in his paintings of starry skies at night. Vincent's ultimate, uncompromising authenticity made him look bizarre to ordinary people, who bluntly rejected him. Crowds in general, and especially crowds in those rigid conservative times, are defensively ruthless to those they cannot understand. Vincent was painfully aware of but not discouraged by the mockery. He continued to crave love and the closeness of a soulmate until the moment he gave up and committed suicide. Today, there is no consensus on Vincent's health issues; opinions range from temporal lobe epilepsy and various medical conditions to bipolar disorder and borderline personality. Our guess is therefore as good as anyone else's. It is, however, monumentally mistaken to put the word "borderline" next to Vincent's name. We have yet to meet a borderline with such innate and consistent fiery passion for love, art, and life, irrespective of the fact that it eventually lead to Vincent's psychological cremation by the intolerant society of the time: hence the motive to argue against the absurdity of diagnosing Vincent as having a personality disorder. An unambiguous sense of internal direction is unknown territory for fragmented individuals. Such sensitive and internally directed individuals as Vincent are, first, rare in the history of mankind and, second, uncompromisingly honest and thus seen as difficult by others. We choose to believe that Vincent was a genius who followed the internal direction of his enhanced sensitivity with unparalleled passion and authenticity. His greatest talent was to passionately exist identified with his deep understanding of life. "My life and love are one" he wrote to his brother. The art of painting was merely the medium to express this understanding, which was also recognizable in everything else he was, in every atom of his being, from work and relationships to feelings. Irving Stone so appropriately titled the biographical novel about Van Gogh's life and work *Lust for Life*. Van Gogh did not have a personality disorder: he had an authentic personality, at its highest substantiation of existence.

A fine line between genius and psychosis? It certainly appears so. Creative people and patients with Schizophrenia have a reduced D2 receptor binding potential in the thalamus compared with less creative people and healthy controls (de Manzano et al., 2010; Talvik et al., 2003). The decreased D2 receptor densities in the thalamus, the brain's "traffic control" center, lower thalamic sensory gating, thus increasing information flow to the rest of the brain. Perhaps this thalamic permissiveness can explain the ability for novel and *ipso facto* somewhat unusual associations related to creativity (MacKinnon, 1962) and bizarre associations related to psychosis (in the latter, the overflow of sensory information might overcome the brain's ability to process it effectively). As discussed, complex mental functions are born through the dynamic and coordinated interaction of large-scale functional networks: the default network (wakeful but resting state) and task-positive networks; the two systems are anti-correlated, but not completely, during active and resting brain states. The default mode network, active during daydreaming, ruminating, or mind wandering, is particularly important for creative ideas (the aha! moment in the shower). Strong functional connectivity within networks coupled with flexibility in switching between the default and task networks (the earlier mentioned brain's "circuit breaker") appear to be instrumental for turning daydreaming and mind wandering into creativity, while the opposite (weak functional connectivity and difficulty switching between non-task and task networks) seems to be the case with psychosis. As Gregoire and Kaufman (2016) summarized: "The creative brain is particularly good at flexibly activating and deactivating these brain networks, which in most people are at odds with each other. In doing so, they are able to juggle seemingly contradictory modes of thought—cognitive and emotional, deliberate and spontaneous. This allows them to draw on a wide range of strengths and thinking styles in their work." In contrast, individuals with Schizophrenia show increased connectivity within the default network and difficulty switching between the default network and task-positive networks, which is referred to as dys-connectivity (Zhou et al., 2007) and may be suggestive of a functional disintegration in the intrinsic brain functional activity, perhaps accounting for some of the cognitive and psychotic symptoms in Schizophrenia. Figuratively, individuals with psychosis are "mentally stuck" in the default mode, whereas creative individuals use this mode to feed novel associations to the task networks and turn random mind wandering into creative outcomes.

Is creativity keeping mental illness alive in the population? It certainly appears so. Creativity is conferred, at least in part, by common genetic variants and comes with an increased risk of psychiatric disorders conferred by these same genetic variants (Power et al., 2015). One of the most puzzling features of the group of Schizophrenias is the stable global incidence (~1% worldwide) despite negative selection pressure, the latter due to reduced fertility of the patients. One explanation for the epidemiological resilience of Schizophrenia is that creative relatives of affected patients, who (the relatives) carry the polygenic liability but do not have the illness, could compensate reproductively for the low fertility of the patients, thereby maintaining genetic polymorphisms conferring Schizophrenia in the population. In a study of 300 000 subjects with Schizophrenia and their nonaffected siblings, the siblings, but not the patients, were overrepresented in creative professions (Kyaga et al., 2011).[34] The patients had no increased rate of overall creative professions compared with controls, but an increased rate in the subgroup of artistic occupations. Interestingly, a surprisingly high prevalence of Schizophrenia is found among children of Nobel Prize winners (A Einstein and J Watson, among others).

SOCIAL TRANSITIONS AND THE CHANGING CONCEPTS OF MENTAL HEALTH

Throughout history, technology has promoted both social progress and psychological evolution. Among countless examples, control of fire and cooked food, as predigestion, provided extra time to our ancestors to do more with their brains, such as develop spoken language and tools (a gorilla spends 50% of the day eating and digesting raw food, 30% resting, 6.5% changing location, and only 3.6% in social activities). Similar technological leaps in the evolution of humans occurred during the agricultural and industrial revolutions and are occurring during the current digital revolution and information age. In this section we address the impact that the modern, postmodern, and the current liquid modernity periods have had on human personality and psychopathology and the scientific conceptualization of both.

From modernism to postmodernism: from "how to fit" to "what to choose." The increasing prevalence of personality disorder, now estimated to be about 10% to 15% in the community and about 50% in psychiatric patients, co-occurs with the social transition from conservativism (classical and modern) to social liberalism (postmodernism). A plausible hypothesis that draws upon our model of personality disorder may, at least in part, explain its recent increase in prevalence, from a virtually unknown problem in the conservative period.

Based on classical writings (S Freud, C Jung, E Jones), neurotic phenomena were the dominant "psychopathology of everyday life"[35] in the

34. Familial cosegregation of creativity and bipolar disorder was also found but not for unipolar depression.

35. Here we are paraphrasing Freud's famous book *The Psychopathology of Everyday Life* that popularized the concept and the intrapsychic dynamics of neuroses in a theory-light manner.

conservative period, both classical and modern, while individuals presenting with fragmented personality were rarely mentioned. The dynamics of neurosis is thought to be activated whenever nonconscious impulses threaten to break through into consciousness, which would force the individual to face his or her unacceptable "dark side." The main adaptive task for people in the conservative eras was to find indirect ways ("how") to fit their forbidden impulses and preferences into one of the few top-down enforced lifestyles ("task of correct appearance"). Facing pressure for cookie cutter-type uniformity, many of the outliers ended up overadapted (aka "conformism"), engaging in nonauthentic feelings and behaviors solely aimed to fit or, more precisely, not to differ. Faced with shame, guilt, and inferiority, they nonconsciously repressed their drives and struggled with anxiety and neuroses. The minority of others creatively sublimated their secret, unacceptable sexual preferences (e.g., Leonardo da Vinci, Oscar Wilde) or disguised atheism through religiously non-commiting philosophical acceptance of a "higher power" as the organizing principle of the universe, managing this way to "fit but not commit." Not surprisingly, people of this period are called "the silent generation." Figuratively, conservativism was the age of repression, guilt and neuroses.

The baby boomers of the 1960s embraced diversity, promoted social tolerance,[36] and dethroned and demystified sexuality, which had been one of the stumbling blocks of adaptation in the conservative eras. The main adaptive question became *what* to choose among multiple alternatives ("task of correct choice"). The "uneasiness in civilization,"[37] once arising from the conflict between individual needs and societal norms, was transformed into the uncertainty of identity in the postmodern culture, wherein an individual seeks to match his or her real strengths with available opportunities. Such self-examination in the context of weak norms and nondirective society may have catalyzed dilemmas about meaning, purpose, direction, and identity, all fostering the psychopathology of personality disorder. The emphasis here is on the qualifier "fostering" (or contributing) as we do not claim a causal relationship. Figuratively, postmodernism was the age of personality disorder: it liberated people from guilt and neuroses, but the lack of external structure increased the risk of disorganization in fragmented individuals. The latter can achieve organization internally (through the dictatorial deviance) and/or externally (through highly structured, directive, and uncompromising environments, e.g., strict social norms, religious and other

36. "Make love, not war" was the slogan of the hippie generation.
37. The English translation of Freud's work is *Civilization and Its Discontents*.

cults, and ideological extremism). Such environments palliate the psychopathology of personality disorder by superimposing external structure on the fragmented substrate. The group's ideology is internalized as one's own motivation around which personality fragments are organized providing an imported but compensatory self image. In some cases, individuals indoctrinated into deviance committed heinous crimes (e.g., the Manson family cult). Organized but person-sensitive groups, such as art communities or humanitarian activist movements may help integrate fragmentation by allowing the affected members to self-determine own strengths within the overall spectrum of the group's activities. Such sensitivity to individualized needs is simply not plausible in large organized societies. The liberal postmodern culture provided little normative guidance to help organize those with fragmented personality, which may in part explain the epidemics of personality disorder over the past 50 years. On the positive side, the nondirective postmodern society encouraged creativity in well- integrated individuals, perhaps explaining the explosion of innovative breakthroughs in the latter half of the 20th century. The 1960s have been described by historians as a single decade encompassing the most significant changes in history, capitalizing on the postwar baby-boomer's creativity with a fondness for change: they started the space age (man in space, manned lunar orbit), the digital era, and computer technology (single chip microprocessor); gave a social voice to youth; invented the laser, fiber optics in communication, heart transplant and internal pacemaker technologies, supersonic airliners, the picture phone, video games, the LED light—among many other examples.

In her book *The Neurotic Personality of Our Time*, Karen Horney (1937) signaled the transition from the age of neuroses to the age of personality disorder. The "neurotic personality" in the title itself implies the transition. The same text written today, perhaps only retitled into *The Disordered Personality of Our Time*, would provide a good illustration of the types of behaviors we associate with personality disorder. Among Serbian authors, equally brilliant insights into neurotic personality were reported in the 1962 book *Šta su neroze?* (What Are Neuroses?) by Mirko Švrakić, father of one of the authors (DMS) of this book. Table 1.1 summarizes social transitions from conservativism to social liberalism and their impact on adaptive strategies, personality, and psychopathology.

As transformations of human society and the science of psychology continue through our current period of liquid modernity, the main adaptive task nowadays is to be included, rather than to belong or to make a truly authentic lifestyle choice. One's mindset, self-image, and identity are changing in a fluid manner, activated and retracted in part by trends

Table 1.1 SOCIAL TRANSITIONS AND PSYCHOPATHOLOGY: SUMMARY

Period Variable	Classical and Modern Western Conservativism (Ended Mid-20th Century) Strict and Rigid Norms	Postmodernism (Social Liberalism) (Mid-20th Century–2000's) Loose and Flexible Norms
Adaptive direction and lifestyle selection	**Top-down** preapproved templates ("cookie-cutter" society) **"adaptive collectivism"**	**Bottom-up** build-it-yourself **"adaptive individualism"**
Adaptive task	**HOW to fit** (task of correct appearance)	**WHAT to choose** (task of correct choice)
Adaptive strategy (individuals)	**Conformism and overadaptation** (the mandate to fit) **Repression and neurosis** (most non-fitters)	**Exploration and experimentation** (for integrated) **Pathologization into extremes** (for fragmented): ***internal* extremism** (PD) ***external* extremism** (cults, activist groups, etc.)
Effect on psychopathology	**Fostering the dynamics of neuroses** Guilt and anxiety (for those not fitting) Protective against PD (high external structure)	**Fostering the dynamics of personality disorder** risk of fragmentation (weak external structure) Protective against neuroses (social tolerance)
Effect on personality	**Low individual liability for adaptation** (external structure as "shortcut" to adaptation) **Suppression of creativity** (major inventions—few and far between)	**High individual liability for adaptation** (weak external structure: self-examination) **Freeing of creativity** (high rate of inventions) **Consumer mentality** (for vulnerable and poor) (cheap immediate pleasures and kitsch culture)
Effect on society	**Suppression of diversity**	**Tolerance of diversity**
Colloquially	**Age of neuroses**	**Age of personality disorder**

Legend: PD = personality disorder

spun off by virtual social networks. Such fluidity of the self is discussed later.

Postmodern decentralization of personality: the healthy fragmented self. The postmodern fragmented self and, for that matter, the fluid self of the liquid modernity period, are not necessarily pathological phenomena. Rather, each may represent functional adaptations to the fragmented and fluid real world, respectively. Cyberspace social networks are a social model built upon cyber-social relationships. Glancing over internet-posted fragments of information about a person and equally quickly casting approval or disapproval, appear to have taken the place of traditional social relations. The connections among the linked-in are weak and impersonal, kept alive by trending topics. The impression is that people have begun to expect more from technology than from one another (Turkle, 2010), at least in some parts of the world (particularly in the West). Within a span of only 20 years (1985–2005), the average number of close confidants decreased by about one whole person, from 2.94 to 2.08, while the number of people saying that they have no one to share their personal stories with almost tripled within that same time period (McPherson et al., 2006). At the same time, the average number of followers on Twitter in 2016 has shown an increase of 340% since 2012. Functional adaptation during postmodernism required the individual to tolerate diversity and uncertainty, as well as the multiplicity of one's self-image to keep up with the fragmentation of the previous "analog" society. For these adaptive tasks, a solid, consistent, and monothematic narrative can become an obstacle. The postmodern fragmentation of the self can be thus viewed as an adaptive psychoplastic response to the postmodern society and culture, most notably to the increased role of abstract symbols in the development of the sense of self. Postmodernists (e.g., Gergen, Jameson, Baudrillard, Denzin) agree that the centralized self of the conservative eras has been compartmentalized into the fragmented self of the postmodern era as the new normal. The postmodern fragmented, "decentered" self has no essence, is emotionally flat, lacks depth, and is saturated with incoherent and unrelated abstract self-images activated by the media (Tseelon, 1992). Gergen (1991) writes that signs and symbols which are created by culture and education furnish people with "a multiplicity of incoherent and unrelated languages of the self" (p. 6). This self is transient and fractured, with no future and perhaps no past. We submit that in most instances such adaptive postmodern fragmentation takes place in the outer circle of the self, sitting upon a stable integrated core and thus, as it were, a healthy fragmentation.

This healthy fragmented self is expressed in many independent, frequently contradictory experiences of self, undeservedly dubbed "multiphrenia" (Gergen, 1991). Such healthy multiplicity of selves might open the door for creative personal characteristics to become materialized. As mentioned, the postmodern period is regarded by many as the most creative period in human history, with numerous and giant leaps in science, social rights, information technology, and health care, among many others. In respect to social issues, postmodernism also marks the "privatization of ambivalence" (Bauman, 2000), that is, the acceptance of boundary crossing, which the modern period fought hard against through its intolerance of diversity. Boundaries are still being constructed to exclude strangers, not at the state level but by vaguely defined "aesthetic communities" (groups of people who chose to identify as "members" of a culture without a strong denominator ["neo-tribes" who discriminate against strangers as "different" and "non-fitting"]).

Is there a health risk associated with the postmodern fragmentation of self? To the best of our knowledge, the postmodern fragmented self does not per se increase one's risk of mental disorders, and it actually may have helped one's adaptation to the fragmented society. The concept of personality as a stable structure historically has mandated psychotherapy to integrate any existing fragmentation, regardless of the context. Our model of a semi-stable mind as well as our concept of functional adaptation, both personalized, context and time sensitive, enable us to discuss "pathological" not as a failure of integration per se but as a failure to accept and functionally express one's fragmentation or, more recently, one's fluidity. Tolerance, multiplicity, containing, and expression have become key concepts in modern psychology. The paradigm of liberated normalcy is illustrated by the adage that it is "insane not to go mad in a mad world" so expressively foreshadowed in the second half of the past century by *Catch 22*, a satirical novel by Arthur Heller (1961) adapted into a popular cult movie of the 1970's. Tolerating one's own and containing others' different and contradictory personality fragments is easier in cyberspace than in the real world, as the former handles the fragments with ease, not necessarily needing to confront their historical discrepancy. The match between the postmodern fragmented self and cyberspace society appeared perfect. However, the things are changing fast.

Liquid society and the fluid self: the mandate of being included. The current culture has been called "liquid modernity" (Bauman, 2000) not as a successor of postmodernism but rather as a continuation of the modernization of human existence, wherein a person changes his or her mindset (values, political orientation) and social position (jobs, spouses, homes, countries) in a fluid manner. The liquid mindset is that of shifting rather than that of staying, of desire rather than need, of provisional instead of permanent commitment, of transience rather than stability (Palese, 2013). The adjective "liquid" is used to draw contrast with "solid" in modernism and "fragmented" in postmodernism. The fluid state of the outer self allows for its transient identifications with a trending choice and subsequent retractions into itself. Two lines tie the individual to the society: first, contemporary consumerism perpetuates progress and modernization by producing new desires; second, by doing the first, the individual becomes incorporated into the products he or she consumes; the person is both a consumer and consumed (Palese, 2013). Such a dynamic is reminiscent of a swarm: it provides a perfect balance between liberty and dependence, fear and security, living and belonging (Palese, 2013). Liquid modernity, as a continuation of modernization of human life, overcomes some of the major existential dilemmas of postmodernism: the uncertainty of choice has been resolved by the transiency of choices.

Sociobiology may provide clues for the social and psychological evolution of humans. Eusociality is the most advanced forms of group living and helps explain the ecological dominance of insects and perhaps can shed some light onto the future of human evolution. Modern sociobiology, founded by EO Wilson, challenges the generalizability of inclusive fitness to all organized groups and takes a different stand on altruism and sacrifice. Nowak et al. (2010) describe a scenario wherein the primordial founder of a colony who happened to be near a food source develops a genetic mutation to feed its offspring, a common nurturing phenomenon called "progressive provisioning." Another mutation could result in offspring that stayed near the nest, rather than leaving, and did things instinctively recognized as "need to be done" (like protecting a fertilized egg, regardless of the ownership). These behaviors happened to be good for the whole group. Sociobiology offers a new theory of eusociality that reduces the significance of genetic relatedness in cooperation and social behaviors but views the colony (society) as a larger entity for evolution and favors its success above all else. Individual member is viewed as a single cell in the composition of the group. Whether or not the theory stands the test of time, it certainly fits the current trends in human social evolution, now in the phase of liquid modernity, where weakly connected individuals have a role to play, or rather an opinion to cast in cyberspace, without much personhood (globalization of choices, depersonification of individuals).

The traditional concepts of stable self, identity, individual, and individuality are not only rapidly losing meaning in the liquid society but also turning into obstacles to the relentless change. As noted by Palese (2013), instead of being a fact, the self and identity have become a task, a self-building project to find one's role, both as a good consumer and as a competitive product in the global market. In such self-building, the liquid individual excludes him/herself from traditional networks, resulting in fragmentation of real-world society. Instead, cyber networks (social media) provide "identity updates" required in order to be included, as the "need for inclusion is nothing more than legacy of the abandonment of the authentic sense of belonging" (Palese, 2013, p. 2). Such identity updates are mediated by those trending on virtual social networks and can be thought of as cyber selfobjects that activate the sense of self of those to whom they are linked-in. As in real swarms, people flock on social networks, scatter and gather again, from one aim or movement to another, rarely including the same group of people (Palese, 2013), literary turning individuals into momentary units of a trend. The unified choice averages out to reflect every member but no member in particular. Individuality and uniqueness have become disruptively rogue, threatening the flow of the trend. These global cyber networks have weak intragroup bonds as people are transiently organized around a theme, akin to synchronous and instantaneous changes in the direction of a swarm. The idea of society is kept alive by trends, although it is not the people but the *choice* that aggregates. Incidentally, social networks are becoming increasingly interconnected and able to share social trends, and thus likely to eventually coalesce into a global swarm of human choices, a collective mind of humans.

In what would represent a radical change, human swarms could oust explicit social communities, their leaders, and status hierarchy. These have been the traditional forms of human group living as well as the major source of human intolerance. Real swarms do not even have status hierarchy: working self-propelled, the units of a swarm alternate between leaders and followers, based on nothing more than the direction of the flight, usually only for the duration of the flight (Bauman, 2000). Such self-sufficient, hierarchy-less organization renders as nonessential commands from above as the swarm does not need them to form or to survive (Bauman, 2000), perhaps the best possible form of democracy there is. Alternatively, a swarm-like organization of humanity may lead to presently unknown forms of mental dysfunction or sources of struggle.

The past might not have been as different as one today might think it was, and liquid modernity might not be as modern as it appears to be at first sight. In 1892 Leo Tolstoy (2010) wrote in his diary: "How deceptive and impossible adapting to life is. There is nothing stable in it. It is the same as if one wanted to adapt to running water. Everything—personality, family, society—is changing, dissolving, transforming, and morphing like clouds." This 150-year-old insight is a reminder that the human mind and the societies it creates move along a spiral with a widening radius, a sort of psychological twister carrying the expanding knowledge upwards, revisiting old problems with more advanced understandings. Today a new form of cloud (the iCloud[38]) floats around us, the virtual world for storing data, including personal information

38. "iCloud" is a household name for a cloud storage and cloud computing service in the virtual world (which we, for some reason, always imagine to be above) with about 782 million users as of 2016.

about identity and activities ("cyber collection of identities"), providing computing services and e-mail communication. It is also a metaphor for virtual social networks, where liquid people find and get updates for their identity, thus connecting these two distant periods (classical and liquid) by the shared existential theme of identity.

The linked-in and the linked-out. The poor of the world are not capable consumers and most lack access to cyber-identity updates. They are in predominance: about half of the world's population does not have internet access and lives on less than $2.50 a day. The poor are defined *primarily* as bad consumers (other features are irrelevant) and are thus not linked-in, as they cannot fund the inclusion (Palese, 2013). Separated from cyber selfobjects, they are left with very few options by which to build identity: defiant and deliberate isolation from the linked-in (resulting in self-perpetuating ghettos), "blue-collar" crime (an affordable road to identity, both personal and group), cheap culture (vicariously living through the lives of celebrities and fictional stories), and, eerily reminiscent of Aldous Huxley's *Brave New World*, cheap physical pleasures (fast-food related obesity is believed to account for about 40% of overall obesity in the United States). The poor of the East and South may have an advantage for now, because their still pristine communities keep them closer to the original "analog" sources of the sense of self and identity.

NOSTALGIA FOR THE OLD: TRADITION IS CONTINUALLY RECREATED

Many discussions of the evolving human self are imbued with nostalgia for the traditional selfhood constructed through direct social relations. Modern culture and its symbols and signs are abstract, divorced from group interaction, but, as Allan (1997) points out, what they mean to humans depends on how they are used in interaction. Both the postmodern fragmented self and the fluid self of liquid modernity are natural adaptive outcomes of the psyche-environment interaction, rooted in the same interactive self-reflection as the traditional self but in a new cultural setting of depersonified social rituals, the increasingly abstract "language" of the culture, and the dislodging of social interactions into the virtual world. Both the postmodern fragmented self and the fluid self of liquid modernity are built on top of an integrated inner core of whole object relations, which provides a thinly conscious but unmistakable trans-situational continuity (the sense if "I") not disturbed by sociocultural transitions. Such a healthy inner core is able to withstand adaptive transformations of the conscious outer working self, whether fragmentation or liquefaction. In contrast, personality disorder reflects a fragmentation of the inner core of the self, at the level of the elementary particles (the polarized sense of "me" and the fragile sense of "I") affecting the mind as a whole and its subsystems.

The baby boomers of the analog era, the force behind the explosion of innovations in the 1960s, may feel uneasy in the super-transient liquid modernity, perhaps explaining their nostalgia. Many report a sense of fragmentation of time and activities as well as superficiality in social contacts, and describe as especially annoying the pressure to be linked-in in order to keep one's identity up-to-date. Multitasking (performing tasks in parallel) and task-switching (tasks performed in the same time frame but not at the same time), both almost a mandate of today's society, may generate a sense of incompetency and incompleteness in the baby boomers. Incidentally, tenacious focusing on the job at hand still appears to be optimal for quality and efficient outcomes, even in the digital era. The baby boomers appear to be mentally functioning at an analog level, needing a stable ("solid") psychological safe haven within the self by which to process and integrate fragmented daily experiences. The Y generation (millenniums or echo boomers, born between 1980 and the mid-1990's) and the Z generation (born between the mid-1990s and 2012) appear to be perfectly comfortable with the fluidity of the digital age, both socially and psychologically. The romance may not last for long, as bioenhancement is likely to become a reality in the near future, requiring new adaptive skills. Bioenhancement is hardly new. The telescope and the microscope have expanded the reach of our senses in the not so distant past. The new technologies, such as the brain-chip interface, improve our memory and cognition, this time extending the reach of our minds. Like never before, bioenhancement might be dehumanizing, as it blurs the boundary between persons and things (Bess, 2015). In the process, Bess argues, bioenhancement is altering the notion of personhood, ultimately turning humans into commodities. However, bioenhancement is also an inherently human endeavor; it continues the long historical process of controlling ourselves and our world, expresses our natural desires for new capabilities and richer experiences, and pursues our potential to be more than we are now, which is what gives life meaning, at least according to Messerly (2017). This is the near future that the Y and Z generations, and any other subsequent generation coming, will face and we believe successfully adapt to. Until it's time to move again.

CHAPTER 2

What Is Personality Disorder?

DISEASE, ILLNESS, SICKNESS, OR DISORDER: NONE OR ALL OF THE ABOVE?

Everyone has an idea, albeit largely intuitive, of what illness or disease is. However, an attempt to apply these concepts to personality disorder turns into a complicated task. Four terms in the English language refer to impaired health: illness, sickness, disease, and disorder. The concept of illness contrasts with wellness by referring to a subjective experience of ill health. By definition (e.g., *Diagnostic and Statistical Manual of Mental Disorders* [DSM], International Classification of Diseases [ICD]), personality disorder causes clinically significant personal distress and/or social difficulties. Thus the concept of illness could apply. The concept of sickness refers to the accepted status that a syndrome has for an individual (in terms of ability to live a productive life) and for a society (in terms of regulations for assistance and care). Many individuals with personality disorder erratically perform at work, engage in crime and addictions, seek interpersonal conflicts, inadequately raise their children, and usually expect more from others than they themselves are ready to contribute. Therefore, the concept of sickness could apply as well. The concept of disease refers to a condition that, first, deviates from a biomedical norm and, second, is amenable to biomedical intervention (Scully, 2004). Neuropathology of personality disorder has been recognized, most notably as a suboptimal cortical regulation of moods and behaviors (reviewed in Lieb et al., 2004; Siever and Weinstein 2009; New et al., 2008; Kernberg, 2015), while mechanism-based pharmacotherapy can be tailored to harness homeostasis and modulate subcortical temperament traits (discussed in Chapter 5). Hence, the concept of disease could also apply. Semantically[1], there is no essential difference between the terms "disease" (deviation from normal) and "disorder" (deviation from order). The term "disorder" is more value-neutral and less stigmatizing than the other terms, a clear advantage in sensitive circumstances. The term has been actively promoted in the past couple of decades to mitigate the stigma historically attached to mental dysfunction, whether in the form of self-shame or in the wider social context. For example, the DSM classifies Schizophrenia (traditionally considered an illness) into "Schizophrenia Spectrum and Other Psychotic *Disorders*." All of these concepts and terms—illness, sickness, disorder, and disease—apply to personality disorder, although none captures the compensatory, healing essence of the syndrome. If for no other reason but destigmatization, the term "disorder" seems most adequate. For the same reason, we advocate that the term "personality" be dropped from "personality disorder" and the term "adaptation disorder" be used instead (elaborated later).

WHEN IS PERSONALITY "DISORDERED"?

We first review the official standing of the American and international psychiatric associations (the American Psychiatric Association [APA] and the World Health Organization [WHO], respectively) and then discuss alternative nosological and classificatory options.

Official standing of the American and international psychiatric associations. According to the fifth edition of the DSM (DSM-5; APA, 2013), personality disorder is diagnosed when the following criteria are met:

> *Criterion A*: "Long-term patterns of internal experience and behavior that markedly deviate from the individual's culture." The patterns are manifested in two (or more) of the following areas:

1. Cognition (manner of perceiving and interpreting self, others, events);
2. Affectivity (range, intensity, instability, appropriateness of emotional responses);

1. Here the term is relating to meaning in language or logic.

3. Interpersonal relationships (problems in social functioning);
4. Impulse control (disturbance in control—impulsivity, inconsiderateness, transgressions).

Criterion B: Maladaptive behavior is pervasive, expressed in a broad spectrum of functioning, not just in an isolated segment or relationship (e.g., not just at work, but within family, with friends, etc.).

Criterion C: The pattern of internal experiences and behaviors causes subjective difficulties or leads to greater disturbances in social, professional/work, or other important aspects of functioning.

Criterion D: The pattern of internal experiences and behaviors is stable, of relatively long duration, perceived during adolescence or early adulthood. The pattern persists throughout life, with a tendency of improving in middle and later years, especially in persons with borderline and antisocial manifestations.

Most classifications distinguish 10 clinical categories of personality disorder: schizoid, schizotypal, paranoid, borderline, narcissistic, histrionic, antisocial, obsessive-compulsive, dependent, and avoidant. The following four points are noteworthy here.

1. We do not conceptualize "borderline" as an independent subtype but rather as a level of mental functioning shared by all clinical variants of personality disorder.[2] In fact, individual variants of personality disorder can be thought of as different clinical expressions (different "faces") of the underlying borderline personality, referred to in this book as fragmented personality. We prefer the latter term because it highlights intrapsychic fragmentation as the essence of personality disorder. The term "borderline" has been overused and misused to the point of confusion. It refers to a type of personality organization (Kernberg, 1975), to a group of "difficult" patients on the border between neurosis and psychosis (clinicians), or to a separate category of personality disorder (DSM, ICD), the last two concepts plagued by stigma and therapeutic nihilism.
2. We do not view the DSM avoidant personality disorder as an independent variant. Hypersensitivity to negative evaluation or rejection, feelings of inadequacy, fear of intimacy, and ambivalence about

2. We prefer the term "variant" over "subtype" to avoid the impression of distinct categories.

social contacts are transdiagnostic and may nonspecifically appear in all variants of personality disorder.

3. We combine the DSM passive aggressive and dependent subtypes into the negativistic-dependent variant of personality disorder, based on our clinical observations that submissiveness and passive aggression regularly co-occur in this particular variant. The identity of the patient is fused with his or her selfobject (corresponding to the archaic "merger" transference[3]), and the patient reacts with negativism, bitter complaints, and/or sulking if his or her expectations for protection are not fully met which may expose his or her own profound fragility and helplessness, a narcissistic injury. This variant of personality disorder shows a significant overlap with "character neurosis"[4] because the compensatory solution to inner fragmentation (i.e., almost total dependence on a selfobject) also creates a conflict (troubling experience of one's own fragility and helplessness) resulting in passive aggression (as an attempt to control the selfobject).
4. DSM-5 classifies schizotypal personality disorder, despite strong evidence for its place among the Schizophrenia spectrum disorders, where it is classified in the ICD.

A noteworthy difference between the DSM and the WHO's ICD system is that the DSM classifies narcissistic personality disorder, whereas the ICD appears to be ambivalent toward it and classifies it secluded from other subtypes, together with dubious entities such as "haltlose," "immature," and "psychoneurotic" personality disorder. It is believed that the WHO does not consider narcissistic personality disorder prevalent enough worldwide, excepting the rich Western countries, to merit an equal classificatory status with other subtypes.

The basics: epidemiology, comorbidity, professional challenges. Personality disorder is common by the standards of the WHO, with a prevalence of about 15% in the general population and about 50% in psychiatric patients (Svrakic et al., 1993, 2002). It is also a chronic disorder, which is widely considered difficult to treat. The early symptoms of fragmentation are recognizable in childhood as precursors to personality disorder (reviewed in Bozukluklarının et al., 2015), become fully evident in late adolescence, and then persist for decades, causing profound personal

3. A subtype of mirroring transference, a very early need to feel safe and secure in the reliability of other, which protects against overstimulation.

4. Defined as personality disturbance in which personality traits are the functional equivalent of neurotic symptoms (i.e., create an intrapsychic conflict).

struggles, pervasive interpersonal problems, and occasionally crime and addictions. Personality disorder acts both as a predisposing influence and a comorbid condition in a range of psychiatric syndromes, for example, substance use, affective disorders, brief psychotic disorders, impulse control disorders, and eating disorders, among others. Such high prevalence, chronic interpersonal conflicts, erratic work performance, long but uncertain treatment, and significant comorbidity have turned this syndrome into a significant health and social issue. Most clinicians express academic interest in its psychopathology, but only a minority proceed to obtain expert training in psycho- and pharmacotherapy. Patients are typically treated by general psychiatrists, with symptom-centered medications and little if any psychotherapy, leading to understandably disappointing outcomes. The latter are perpetuating the myth that personality disorder cannot really be treated. It is not a cliché to say that therapeutic nihilism is incompatible with a valid working alliance and a productive patient-clinician relationship. As with other specialty patients, clinicians who are not well versed in personality disorder are best advised to limit their involvement beyond formulating a working diagnosis and to delegate further care to colleagues who specialize in the field. Such referrals are routine practice in all health care and ultimately benefit the patient.

Persons with personality disorder are commonly labeled as "aggravating," "demanding," or "conflict-prone." They challenge the limits of a clinician's knowledge, therapeutic skills, and even personal integrity. Alternatively, they may be seductive or charming, may appear helpless, and may elicit inappropriate blurring of professional boundaries, giving rise to a personal interest on the part of the clinician to condemn or rescue the patient. Supervision is recommended, not just to recognize the countertransference feelings but in order to use these feelings as a tool in psychotherapy. In return, by developing a therapeutic relationship with these patients, many clinicians mature both professionally and personally and above all learn a great deal about the human mind. In many instances, working with these patients can make the clinician feel as though he or she is in therapy as well.

FROM PSYCHODYNAMICS TO ATHEORETICAL DIAGNOSIS . . . AND BACK TO BOTH

In the 1950s, then new diagnosis of personality disorder was based on psychodynamic formulations (DSM; ICD, ninth revision). Although insightful and valid, psychodynamic criteria were difficult to operationalize for research and reliable interrater clinical diagnosis. To mediate the reliability problem, the third edition of the DSM (DSM-III; APA, 1980) introduced an operationalized, polythetical,[5] and purely descriptive, atheoretical approach. In a sweeping rejection of psychoanalysis, the DSM-III eliminated its flagship, the neuroses, and trivialized them as merely a superficial concept of "anxiety disorders." By mandating personality assessment on Axis II, the DSM-III raised the clinical awareness of personality disorder and galvanized research, albeit initially mostly concerning epidemiology and comorbidity. Ironically, the intended increase in diagnostic reliability did not materialize, due to heterogeneous and overlapping criteria. Despite countless studies based on the DSM-III criteria, the conceptual understanding of personality disorder remained at the rudimentary level of behavior descriptions.

With minimal changes, the subsequent revisions of the DSM (APA, 1987, 1994, 2000, 2013) and the 10th revision of the ICD (ICD-10; WHO, 1994) retained the same or minimally revised categorical criteria for personality disorder, and, consequently, the same problems remained: *intra*categorical heterogeneity of criteria (ranging from specific behaviors to subtle experiential phenomena), *inter*categorical overlap with low discriminant validity of the categories (shared symptoms by different subtypes, multiple diagnosis for a single patient), and arbitrary cut-off decisions about the number of criteria sufficient to receive the diagnosis. The descriptive DSM-5 and ICD-10 criteria reduce the depth of the diagnosis and leave unanswered clinically relevant questions with respect to differential diagnosis and treatment planning. For example, neither provides relevant information to differentiate the nature of the patient's chronic social anxiety, aside from minute symptomatic differences and arbitrary duration of symptoms between social phobia and avoidant personality disorder. Is it a conflict-driven expression of neurosis or a deficit-driven expression of personality disorder? The treatments, of course, greatly differ for the two. The DSM-5 (APA, 2013) criteria are reprinted from the fourth edition,[6] and both largely correspond in substance to the ICD-10. Much of the previous discussion of the DSM system applies to ICD-10 as well, with some noted exceptions. With the aforementioned problems in mind, many have questioned the construct validity of the DSM and ICD concept of personality disorder, that is, whether it is a true psychopathological

5. A total number of criteria and the minimum number required for diagnosis; these are arbitrary cut-offs with little empirical support.

6. The DSM-5 alternative model is discussed later in the chapter.

construct with meaningful associations with other constructs of relevance. In support of its substantive reality, large-scale studies provide evidence that the DSM construct of personality disorder predicts important psychosocial functioning constructs, such as subsequent Axis I disorders, suicide attempts, violent and criminal behavior, and interpersonal conflicts, among others (reviewed in Wilson et al., 2017). Recent, more sophisticated models take into account intrapsychic (self) and interpersonal (social) impairments in personality functioning as proposed in DSM-5 ("alternative model for personality disorder," Section III: "Emerging Measures and Models") and the 11th revision of the ICD (ICD-11), both discussed later.

The simplistic, symptom-centered approaches in the DSM and ICD eventually became an obstacle to development in the field, unable to keep pace with the evolving dynamic and integrative conceptualization of mental syndromes, a weakness especially relevant for personality disorder. In the past 15 years, psychodynamic assessment of personality disorder has made a comeback, supported by neuroscience (as discussed in Chapter 1) and by the strong movement for a personalized diagnosis that is embodied in psychodynamic analyses. Several psychodynamic diagnostic manuals have been developed aiming to increase the construct validity and provide clinical sophistication to the categorical diagnosis of personality disorder. The two most prominent are the *Psychodynamic Diagnostic Manual* (PDM; PDM Task Force, 2006) and the *Operationalized Psychodynamic Diagnosis* (OPD; OPD Task Force, 2008). Each is discussed in brief next.

1. The PDM was created to provide practitioners with a tool to diagnose their patients in depth using operationalized psychodynamic concepts. To this end, the PDM diagnosis is organized around three dimensions: Axis P—patterns of personality and disorder, Axis M—mental functioning, and Axis S—manifest symptoms. Here we are mostly interested in Axes P (personality) and M (mental functioning) because they dimensionally assess the degree of personality integration and profiles of mental functioning, from normalcy to psychopathology. These help clinicians understand the complexity and individuality of each patient, to wit what one *is* rather than what one *manifests*.

Axis P defines four levels of personality organization, from healthy, via neurotic, borderline, and psychotic, based on the assessment of the following seven capacities of personality: identity, object relations, affect tolerance, affect regulation, super-ego integration and ego-ideal, reality testing, ego-strength and resilience. Of note, "ego" denotes homeostatic functions of personality, "super-ego" the subsystem of internalized moral values and ideals.

Axis M in the PDM describes profiles of mental functioning that are defined using dimensions that cover different and crucial areas of personality (mind) and mental functioning, including

- Capacity for regulation, attention, and learning
- Capacity for mature relationships and intimacy
- Quality of internal experiences (level of self-confidence, self-assurance, self-respect)
- Affective experience, expression, and communication
- Defense patterns and capacities
- Capacity to form internal representations
- Capacity for differentiation and integration
- Capacity for self-reflection and self-observation
- Sense of morality: capacity to construct and use internal moral standards and ideals.

2. The OPD diagnostic system also ventures beneath the surface of descriptive diagnosis. The system is based on four psychodynamically relevant diagnostic dimensions (Axes I–IV) and one axis (Axis V, mental and psychosomatic disorders) the latter to diagnostically include the syndromal-descriptive diagnoses listed in Chapter V (F) of the ICD-10. Axes II, III, and IV (interpersonal relations, conflict, and structure[7]) yield a personalized psychodynamic diagnosis that makes it possible to define the foci to be worked on in therapy, provide therapeutic strategies tailored to the patient, and tools for measuring change; that is, the focus is both on diagnosis and on therapeutic process. We are here interested in the OPD Axis IV: Structure, as it assesses the degree of personality integration. The OPD operationalizes structure via six component categories:[8] self-perception, self-regulation, defenses, object perception, communication, and bonding. The level of personality integration is assessed based on mental capacities and vulnerabilities across these six component dimensions (aspects) each with four subdimensions. The first three dimensions relate to the patient's self, while the other three relate to the patient's object relations:

- Self-perception (subdimensions: self-reflection, self-image, identity, differentiation of affects);

7. As already mentioned, we use the concept of dynamic subsystems of the mind with inseparable substrate and function instead of structure, but here keep the latter term to preserve the originality of the manual.

8. These six "categories" of structure, as they are labeled in the manual, are in fact dimensions of structure, each varying quantitatively.

- Self-regulation (subdimensions: affect tolerance, self-respect, regulation of instinctual drives, anticipation);
- Defenses (subdimensions: type, result, stability, flexibility of defense mechanisms);
- Object perception (subdimensions: subject-object differentiation, empathy, perception of whole object, affects related to objects);
- Communication (subdimensions: contact, understanding the feelings of others, communication of own feelings, reciprocity);
- Bonding (subdimensions: internalization, separation, variability, accepting help).

The OPD differentiates four levels of integration of structure (well-integrated, moderately integrated, poorly integrated, disintegrated). A low level of integration is typical of personality disorder and implies poorly developed mental inner space and substructures, to the extent that the conflicts are worked out in the interpersonal sphere, rather than mentally (internally).

The operationalized psychodynamics in the two manuals (PDM, OPD) are helpful in clinical practice because they assess the patient's level of mental functioning on the basis of parameters that are highly relevant to psychotherapy. The manuals are not intended to replace the DSM and ICD diagnosis but to bridge the gap between descriptive precision (the DSM and ICD) and individualized clinical differentiation (the PDM and OPD). For example, the OPD is also used in the new field called "psychoanalytically informed neuroscience" (Kessler et al., 2013) created to help transfer psychodynamic constructs into neuroscience, thereby combining reduction and expansion as well as reliability and validity.

DIMENSIONS OR CATEGORIES: AN OUTDATED DEBATE

Historically, psychology has been interested in normal personality, psychiatry in personality disorder. Psychology has relied on dimensional analysis to explain personality, a method by which observation of complex phenomena is reduced to simpler and more economical units or factors ("dimensions" or "traits"). Applied to personality, factor analysis of self-reported[9] phenomenology and behaviors identifies common traits in a population that vary quantitatively among individuals ("everyone has these traits, but they vary

9. Some researchers have factor-analyzed all English words describing behavior in a dictionary as observations (units) for factor analysis ("if a word is recorded, it implicates prevalent behaviors").

in strength"). In psychiatry, the approach has been far more categorical ("affected" or "not affected"), as with all medical models of disease, which facilitates the decision to "treat" or "not treat." Advances in one discipline have not been fully realized in the other, despite both sharing a common subject in personality. This is perhaps due to the "narcissism of small differences" as the two disciplines have been mutually entrenched for years in asserting independence over their respective turfs, to the detriment of both.

Categorical models (ICD, DSM) partition personality disorder into distinct, clearly separated subtypes, an essentialist approach based on the postulate that each subtype represents but few essential features, determined *a priori* by clinical insights (top-down assumption). This pigeonhole approach is ill suited to address such a complex, dynamic, and quantitative a phenomenon as human behavior. A cynic might go so far as to label this approach black-or-white thinking, one of the essential features of the syndrome it seeks to classify. Categorical diagnosis describes severe, prototypical cases that meet all or most of the diagnostic criteria, at the expense of being able to handle atypical, mixed, or mild cases, which are much more frequent. Due to overlapping criteria, an individual patient may fit several DSM-III subtypes of personality disorder at once, making treatment planning and priorities difficult to establish in such cases.

Dimensional models define a number of continuous behavior traits, based on factor analysis of observable behaviors, and specify individual differences as quantitative variations along these traits. Quantitative traits eliminate the problem of multiple and overlapping diagnoses and are as easily applied to common atypical and mild cases as they are to the rare prototypical and severe cases. Factor analysis is a bottom-up[10] approach, searching for higher order, umbrella dimensions to summarize observable single but co-occurring or interdependent behaviors. Human personality is assessed *a posteriori* at the confluence of its component dimensions and their facets. Despite claims that the identified dimensions capture fundamental psychobiological processes of personality ("the nature carved at its joints" is the popular slogan), most dimensional models ignored the neurobiology behind the dimensions; this, in our view, is reflective of the state of neuroscience at the time more than a partisan omission on their part. Be that as it may, all dimensional models of personality remained phenotypical. Moreover, these models do not address what is it about some traits that makes them pathological? No behavior dimension is specific to personality disorder; rather, each represents a more or less extreme variant

10. It is considered a bottom-up approach—because smaller units of observation are organized into larger encompassing units (dimensions).

of normal behavior, without any natural (i.e., nonarbitrary) breaks to separate pathology from normalcy. The extreme standing is not sufficient to be neither pathological nor dysfunctional: for instance, a socially inhibited, shy person can be both well adapted and fulfilled. Similar arguments stand for emotional reactivity, dissociality, and excessive devotion to work, all of which have also been proposed to represent "pathological" traits of personality disorder (Livesley et al., 2007). This presents a strong argument against separating the study of normal personality from that of maladapted personality. In fact, the continuum between normal and maladaptive variants provides a unique opportunity to study maladaptive personality syndromes in the context of a rare but optimal experimental design in which controls and subjects both share the same underlying continuous traits.

At one point, at the tail end of the last millennium, all models of normal personality were dimensional and all models of personality disorder were categorical. The models were not interchangeable, because one (dimensional) was concerned with individual differences and the other (categorical) with individual similarities, just one of many incompatibilities. Psychiatry and psychology have now reached a state of healthy cooperation, reflecting both integrative trends in sciences in general and the growing need to overcome the stalemate in the field. By consensus, dimensions have "defeated" categories in their ability to define, describe, and measure personality disorder, although the subtypes still remain informative for psychotherapy strategy planning. Most categorical models have been dimensionalized, that is, factor analyzed into dimensional representations of the original DSM categories of personality disorder (Zimmerman et al., 2011; reviewed in Trull and Durrett, 2005). Most dimensional models have been adjusted to account for individual categories as unique configurations of the specified dimensions (Cloninger et al., 1993). Finally, shared dimensions underlying normal temperament and personality disorder have been identified, providing a platform for studying normal and pathological variants within a single model of personality (Cloninger et al., 1993).

The essence and the appearance of personality disorder: central impairment and its facets. Many authors (e.g., Wakefield, Kernberg, Svrakic, Cloninger, Divac-Jovanovic, among others) have long argued that the central problem among individuals suffering from personality disorder is not their extreme behaviors. Rather, as the argument goes, the etiological essence of personality disorder lies underneath the surface, in the vulnerable organization of personality. The latter is the core deficit pathognomonic for the diagnosis, while extreme behaviors represent the manifesting facets or variants. This shared core deficit can be thought of as the "personality factor" behind the maladaptive behavior and cannot be captured by diagnostic models based on extreme traits alone. In prior research (Svrakic et al., 1993) we reported that a shared personality impairment coupled with extreme behavior dimensions is vital to validly distinguish normal personality from personality disorder: low character dimensions were found to be indicative of any personality disorder ("diagnosis"), whereas extreme temperament dimensions were found to distinguish the subtypes ("differential diagnosis"). Similarly, Divac-Jovanovic et al. (1993) showed that a common "borderline" dimension underlies different adaptive styles of individual subtypes of personality disorder (at the time we used the term "borderline," which we now refer to as "fragmented" personality).

The "alternative model for personality disorder" in DSM-5 and the new ICD-11 proposal have adopted the core impairment and its manifesting variants approach. The DSM-5 proposal defines the core problem (Criterion A) as significant impairment in self-functioning (problems with identity and self-direction) and interpersonal functioning (lack of empathy and intimacy) which are shared by all subtypes. The two impairments are highly correspondent to the concept of low self-directedness (SD) and cooperativeness (CO) as decisive factors leading to diagnosis (Svrakic et al., 1993). Similar to our approach, the DSM-5 alternative model provides a scale, called "level of personality functioning," to assess the severity of impairment, from mild to severe, and sets moderate impaiment as the threshold for the diagnosis of personality disorder. The DSM-5 descriptors of moderate impairment correspond to the concept of fragmented personality in this book. Criterion B defines five "pathological personality traits": negative affectivity, detachment, antagonism, disinhibition, and psychoticism. Six traditional categories of personality disorder are retained (antisocial, narcissistic, borderline, obsessive-compulsive, avoidant, schizotypal) each defined as a specific configuration of these five pathological personality traits thereby resulting in a dimensional-categorical hybrid. If an observed pathological trait does not fit into the category of personality disorder diagnosed based on specific configuration of other traits, it is used as a qualifier (e.g., impulsivity in avoidant personality). This model unnecessarily complicates the diagnosis by defining variations in core impairments (problems in identity, self-direction, empathy, and intimacy) which are presumably specific for individual subtypes (while at the same time shared by all subtypes), and combines these "specific core problems" with specific configurations of traits to define individual subtypes. Notwithstanding, the DSM-5 proposal combines psychodynamic and descriptive assessment and cross-matches behavior traits with variable severity of personality pathology, a true advance in the field. On the other hand, the proposal relies on a highly questionable concept of pathological behavior traits and relies on every bit as questionable selection of individual subtypes of personality disorder.

Several valid subtypes are eliminated, notably histrionic, paranoid, schizoid, and dependent, while the schizotypal subtype, a documented Schizophrenia spectrum syndrome, is retained. Whether the proposal manages to attain traction in research and practice remains to be seen.

The new ICD-11 model of personality disorder, released in 2018 after a number of delays (WHO, 2018) contains the following important changes:

1. Traditional categorical subtypes of personality disorder are eliminated. Conceptually, personality disorder is defined as "problems in functioning of aspects of the self (e.g., identity, self-worth, accuracy of self-view, self-direction), and/or interpersonal dysfunction (e.g., ability to develop and maintain close and mutually satisfying relationships, ability to understand others' perspectives and to manage conflict in relationships) that have persisted over an extended period of time (e.g., 2 years or more)".
2. As the first order of diagnosis, "personality status" (in fact, personality health vs. pathology) is quanitatively assessed for severity varying from "not disordered" (healthy personality) to "personality difficulties," "mild disorder," "moderate disorder," and "severe personality disorder." These severity levels are distinguished based mainly on the quality of interpersonal functioning (in the final ICD-11 version, the role of self-dysfunction is given some weight, although the dysfunction is poorly defined).
3. As the second order of diagnosis, clinical subtypes of personality disorder are further qualified based on a combination of five pathological traits or patterns: negative affectivity/poor emotion regulation, social and emotional detachment/disinterest, dissociality/narcissism, disinhibition/impulsivity, and anakastia/rigid perfectionism. As already noted, these patterns are continuous with normal traits, thereby requiring an arbitrary cut off to determine the point at which normalcy ends and pathology of behavior begins. Note that both ICD 11 and DSM-5 alternative model include comparable "pathological" traits (negative affectivity, social detachment, antisociality, disinhibition-impulsivity), but, as the fifth trait, the ICD 11 describes anankastia while DSM-5 describes psychoticism (the ICD 11 classifies psychoticism as Shizotypal personality within Schizophrenia spectrum disorders). Finally, ICD 11 adds a descriptive dimension of emotional, behavioral, and interpersonal instability (ICD-11 calls it "borderline pattern") in an apparent abandonment of borderline as an independent category of personality disorder (in our opinion this dimension should have been used to determine the severity of personality pathology, as the first order of diagnosis). If the clinician for any reason cannot assess these symptom dimensions (e.g., does not have the time or resources), he or she retains the option to rate only the status of personality, from healthy to

severe personality disorder which makes such diagnosis overly general and thus not very useful for treatment planning.

Field trials of the ICD-11 model revealed that most people show "some degree" of impaired interpersonal functioning labeled "personality difficulties" (Yang et al., 2010). These are classified as "subthreshold" levels personality pathology, as "circumstances that are neither disease nor injury but still merit diagnosis or pose a problem," much like resistance to antibiotics or being a carrier of a problematic genetic trait. The ICD working group views this as an opportunity to destigmatize personality disorder with the idea that since almost everyone shows some form of interpersonal difficulties, those with a personality disorder will not stand out as much (Tyrer et al., 2011), a questionable line of reasoning. The inclusion of "some degree" (verbatim quantifier) of interpersonal difficulties into the world's leading classification system of mental illness carries the risk of abuse and worsens the already advanced psychiatrization of life in Western countries. In what represents a step forward, the ICD-11 system diagnoses personality status (normalcy vs. pathology) separately from behavior clinical symptoms. It remains to be seen whether personality pathology can be reliably diagnosed mainly based on the quality of interpersonal functioning (in ICD 11, self-dysfunction is vaguely defined and open to subjectivism). Both the DSM-5 alternative model (a categorical-dimensional hybrid) and the ICD 11 model (purely dimensional) propose a conceptually questionable core impairment of personality disorder, insofar as both mix together self dysfunction and interpersonal pathology, the cause and its consequence, much like Cloninger's psychobiological model which clearly influenced both classifications. The decision to use only the "pathological" ends of continuous traits in both models is even more questionable, for reasons already discussed.

SEMINAL CONTRIBUTIONS TO THE MODERN CONCEPT OF PERSONALITY DISORDER

Following the introduction of personality disorder into DSM and ICD classifications, literary every paradigm in psychology and psychiatry put forward an explanation of the causes and development of the disorder. We thus confine ourselves to a discussion of the seminal contributions and contributors.

Psychodynamic concepts that have stood the test of time. Here we review object relations theory, the contributions of O. Kernberg and H. Kohut, and attachment theory.

Object relations theory has clarified psychodynamic pathways that lead to severe personality pathology. The centerpiece of this theory, namely the internalized object relations which are the basic units of all experience, seems to be supported by neuroscience, as discussed. There appears to be a general consensus that biogenetic and/or environmental imperfections trigger specific psychodynamic processes which in turn steer mental development into a compensatory syndrome of personality disorder. The process is known as developmental homeostasis. Early object relations (integrated at around six months of age – combine phantasy and real interactions; Klein, 1952) are the substrate for more complex mental experiences by the mother-child interaction during the separation-individuation stage (from six months to about two years of age; Mahler et al., 1975). Mental life arises from these early interactions, which provide the foundation for regulation of emotions, thought, motivation, and behavior, including social behavior. The theory establishes a link between inadequate mother-child relationships during the rapprochement subphase and developmental personality problems. The mother-child relationship can either promote individuation or downgrade object relations to partial. The former is mediated by good-enough mothering while the latter is caused by early adversity (abuse, neglect, trauma) or a heritably heightened negative affect reactivity. In the context of less-than-perfect development, which is the most common scenario in the general population, internalized object relations vary along a continuum from polarized to realistic and range from fleeting to enduring (Auchincloss and Samberg, 2012, p. 175). This explains why practically everyone's mind harbors more and less realistic images of the themselves and others, which are *dynamic* and *reversible* in nature (Klein, 1952). Personality disorder, rooted in partial object relations, is also a dynamic and reversible syndrome, moving in and out of remaining diagnosable over time (McGlashan et al., 2005). The average short-term test–retest reliabilities are 0.54 for specific subtypes and 0.56 for any personality disorder, even with structured interviewing. Longer term test–retest reliabilities are found to be 0.51 for any personality disorder and 0.34 for specific subtypes, which, together with significant diagnostic change over as little as six months, indicate a diagnostic reversibility of the syndrome (reviewed in APA, 2012). However, personality disorder is not quite a state condition, but is captured by the concept of semi-stability as it fluctuates with changing internal or external conditions, stabilizing and destabilizing. Such results call for a dynamic nosology of personality disorder as advocated in this book.

Otto Kernberg was the first to recognize that individual clinical subtypes of personality disorder may represent different phenotypic manifestations of the same core defect of personality, which he called "borderline personality organization." Although Kernberg centered his approach around the static concept of structures, his insights, both clinical and theoretical, are highly relevant for the concept of and psychotherapy principles found in severe personality pathology. His postulate that positively charged object relations serve as the core for crystallization of the developing mind (Kernberg, 1975) is now supported by neuroscience, except perhaps that the precise process is higher order cognitive representation, rather than crystallization (which nevertheless captures the general idea). More recently, Kernberg (2015) proposed a general developmental framework that integrates psychoanalytic object relations theory with neurobiological aspects of social cognition, the theory of mind, and the complex issue of empathy, yet another testimony to his talent for eclecticism and synthesis. Kernberg's Structured Interview for Personality Organization (STIPO) (Clarkin et al., 2007a) is a remarkably useful guide in developing a precise diagnosis of personality fragmentation. The basic principles of transference-focused psychotherapy, developed by Kernberg and colleagues, are integrated in the majority of contemporary psychotherapies of patients with personality disorder (Chapter 4). We incorporate much of Kernberg's work as the foundation upon which we build our formulations.

Heinz Kohut made groundbreaking insights into the psychological architecture of personality disorder. Kohut's (1971, 1977) brilliant concept of selfobjects captures the essence of never-ending relationships with important figures who have participated in the formation of our mental life, notwithstanding long physical separation. Our mental separation from important objects can only vary in degree; complete separation is close to impossible, even in mature relationships. Individuals with personality disorder manifest an excessive and persisting dependence on selfobjects who serve to define and maintain their self-image. This explains the proclivity to stir interpersonal conflicts, which actively seek to demand that others stay in the role of selfobjects or begin to assume the role (alloplastic adaptation). Kohut recognized the coexistence of the dominant grandiose self and the split-off real self in narcissistic personalities, a duality of the self now believed to characterize other variants of personality disorder as well. Kohut is often criticized for underestimating the internal, heritable determinants of psychopathology in comparison to the role of unresponsive-unemphatic selfobjects, i.e., bad parents.

Attachment theory (John Bowlby, Mary Ainsworth) focuses on the quality of the child's attachment pattern to the early caregiver as the foundation that shapes, but does not irremediably compromise further mental development, insofar as it remains open to modulation by sufficiently strong and consistent corrective influences. Attachment is defined as a preconceptual motivation which directs the child to seek proximity with a familiar caregiver when alarmed, typically with the expectation of protection and emotional support. Individual differences in attachment are molded on the one hand by the sensitivity of the caregiver and, on the other hand, by the innate dispositions of the child.[11] All infants become attached if provided any caregiver (nature), but they vary in the quality of the attachment (nurture): those securely attached receive comfort when alarmed and thus feel confident to explore the world. Pathologically attached children, whether anxious-ambivalent, anxious-avoidant, or disorganized-disoriented, are inadequately if at all comforted when alarmed and thus lack such confidence. To maintain his or her instinctual relationship with the primary caregiver, the child abandons the opportunity to explore other people and their minds, even his or her own mind. Defective mentalization is one of the pivotal aspects of adult personality disorder: not understanding one's own feelings and motives and the feelings and motives of others is the central problem in interpersonal relationships. Subtle but chronic misinterpretations of reality, social and internal alike, are therefore common. Only a very small minority of "borderline" (fragmented) individuals show secure attachment, while all others show a diverse and unresolved attachment pathology (Agrawal et al., 2004).

The psychobiological model pioneered the basis for epistemic iterations. Cloninger (1987) pioneered a psychobiological approach to personality by associating observable behavior dimensions with discernible neurobiological circuits involved in different forms of learning and memory. Personality is conceptualized thus as consisting of two distinct but bidirectionally interacting components—temperament ("biological core") and character ("social interface")—each mediating specific adaptive functions. The two components are related at multiple levels: *origination* (character in part arises as contextualized temperament), *development* (character outcomes are limited by antecedent temperament traits), and *adaptive function* (temperament provides emotional drives to mental life while character optimizes their fit with social norms). The traits are quantitative in the sense that everyone has them; they are just more or less pronounced. The extremes, or high and low ends of temperament traits have specific adaptive advantages and disadvantages; that is, they are not inherently pathological. In contrast, low ends of character traits are maladaptive in most cases, except for self-transcendence, which is largely peripheral to everyday social adaptation. Cloninger's model defines a platform for studying normal and pathological variants within a single psychobiological concept of personality. Given the limiting effect of antecedent temperament on character outcomes (Svrakic et al., 1996), heritably excessive temperament

11. Innate dispositions have not been in the forefront of the attachment theory.

traits or, more precisely, the underlying subcortical circuitry associated with them, are referred to as trait vulnerabilities for personality disorder. The disorder is diagnosed based on dysfunctional character ("case") as the core impairment shared by all subtypes, while the differential diagnosis is made based on specific configurations of temperament traits (behavior "style"). Placing the diagnostic weight on dysfunctional character (a composite of immature personality and suboptimal social adaptation, as discussed) has helped increase diagnostic specificity insofar as it reduces the possibility that individuals with heightened temperament traits but who are self-directed and cooperative (i.e., no personality pathology) are diagnosed as having a personality disorder ("no personality pathology—no personality disorder"). Prior to this model, a socially shy individual avoiding contacts with strangers, who is otherwise productive and functionally adapted, stood the risk of being diagnosed as having a personality disorder. The two-step diagnosis has other advantages over dimensional and categorical approaches, perhaps the most important of which rests in the ability to formulate more precise treatment ramifications. For example, character is more susceptible to psychotherapy and temperament to pharmacotherapy, but both are treated simultaneously given their bidirectional influences. Temperament not only shapes the clinical picture but also acts as an early trait vulnerability to developing a personality disorder, and mechanism-based pharmacotherapy is now possible (Chapter 5).

The psychobiological model has set a new standard in the fields of personality and personality disorder. It has outmoded categorical and factor-analytical dimensional models not only because of its conceptual sophistication, two-step diagnosis, or its ability to guide treatment but also because it proposed an association between overt behavior and its underlying neurobiological processes. At the time of its original publication, Cloninger's (1987) proposal was criticized by many as reductionistic. In the meantime, however, psychobiological approach to mental syndromes has emerged as a consensus theoretical orientation provided that it is formulated as testable hypotheses. As knowledge progresses through epistemic iteration, one of the effects is to reconcile inconsistencies in the fit between behavior dimensions and their suggested neurobiology (Kendler, 2009). Thus Cloninger's postulates about neurophysiology of temperament have been either confirmed or expanded and refined in subsequent research. For example, whole brain resting-state fMRI data, analyzed by machine learning - pattern recognition techniques, can be used to develop connectome-based predictive models of a person's temperament traits of NS, HA, RD, and PE. Specifically, the four traits are reliably predicted at the individual level based on the strength of functional connectivity within frontal-subcortical circuits, concentrated on the hippocampus, basal ganglia, prefrontal cortex (PFCx), and cingulate gyrus (Jiang et al., unpublished data). Cloninger's model does not account for intrapsychic dynamisms underlying the syndrome of personality disorder, because the traits are true operationalizations. However, a high degree of personality integration (expressed as high SD) has been shown to correlate with high maturity of defense mechanisms and vice versa (Mulder et al., 1996), a finding that validates both models (psychodynamic and psychobiological). The pivotal aspect of the diagnosis (i.e., low character traits) actually captures two distinct but functionally related aspects of personality pathology, namely the intrapsychic cause (low SD, indicative of immature personality) and the attendant interpersonal consequence (low CO, indicative of interpersonal problems). This does not undermine the diagnosis of personality in health and disorder because of close covariation between personality integration (SD) and its social adaptation (CO), but is more of a conceptual issue, as discussed. We view SD as vertical in-depth diagnosis of personality pathology vs health, and CO as horizontal diagnosis of social (mal) adaptation.

Are psychodynamic and psychobiological models mutually exclusive? The answer to this question is unambiguous: they are not. The models are compatible and complementary, and in some areas overlapping. Both define the core impairment shared by all variants of personality disorder: fragmented personality in the psychodynamic model and poorly integrated self and the ensuing uncooperative character (low SD and CO) in the psychobiological model. Both models place heritably heightened negative affects at the root of personality disorder: in most psychodynamic models, these disruptive affects are fear and anger; in the psychobiological model they are excessive novelty seeking (NS; anger), excessive harm avoidance (HA; fear), and excessively low reward dependence (RD; detachment[12]). Both models recognize the importance of early environments in mental health and disorder, including the power of environmental factors to either correct or further pathologize biogenetic dispositions as well as to independently steer development toward personality disorder. However, only the psychodynamic model is developmental in terms of defining the mental details of interactive dynamics leading to personality disorder or, figuratively, the "molecular psychology" of personality development and disorder. These two popular models have influenced clinicians to combine psychodynamics and psychobiology into a unified treatment of personality disorder. Largely influenced by the psychobiological model, psychotherapists now generally value pharmacotherapy that regulates affect intensity and activation (e.g., anxiolytic, antidepressant, mood stabilizing medications, among others). Largely influenced by the resurging psychodynamic models, even

12. Detachment is a heightened but reversed (mirror image) of attachment.

die-hard biological psychiatrists now accept psychotherapy as an effective treatment for individuals with personality disorder. Throughout this book we combine these two models in an attempt to consolidate knowledge about the psychodynamics, pathodevelopment, and psychobiology of personality disorder.

ON ETIOLOGY OF PERSONALITY DISORDER: "BAD GENES" AND/OR "BAD ENVIRONMENT"

There appears to be a general agreement that the main etiological factors for personality disorder are heritably heightened affect states (excessive fear, anger, detachment) and adverse environmental factors (substandard parenting, childhood psychological trauma), acting singly or in concert. These are discussed in turn.

Heritably heightened affect states. There is accumulating evidence that the newborn's heritably heightened negative affect reactivity can frame the majority of early interactions in a negative light, frequently irrespective of the real quality of these interactions. Such innate bias toward negative self- and object experiences impacts the development of all primary affect systems, as identified by Panksepp (1998): separation-bonding (panicky, insecure attachment, detachment), fear and anger (both heightened), the erotic-lust affective system (infantile), seeking-exploration (suppressed), and the play-joy-bonding system (distrust).These early subcortical affect systems can be thought of as intrinsic brain value systems that automatically inform emotional learning, such as adaptive and instinctual responses to threat versus care (usually referred to as temperament traits), and have a critical impact on further brain and mind development. For example, excessive fear and anger are associated with displeasure, distress, and sense of urgency and danger even in the setting of good care, and may initiate early defensive fantasies, all of which combine to influence the specific way in which the brain (i.e., large-scale functional networks) and mind (beginning with internalized object relations) organize in personality disorder. Along similar lines, an emotionally detached, "slow to warm up" infant may create a reciprocal feeling of emotional alienation in the caregiver, a dynamics known as evocative gene-environment correlation, thereby increasing the likelihood of early defensive withdrawing into autistic fantasy, as a nonconscious defensive maneuver. In other words, early affects influence the architecture of the same cognitive networks by which they are eventually to be controlled. Under pathological conditions, such bidirectional influence creates a positive feedback loop between excessive subcortical reactions and subeffective cortical control, affecting both the top-down feedback regulation of affects and higher order cognitive integration of early object relations. Childhood precursors of personality disorder, present as early as six years of age, include hostile, paranoid worldview; intense, unstable, inappropriate, or flat emotion; impulsivity or rigidity; overly close or distant/avoidant relationships; extreme or absent sense of self; and peculiar thought processes and behaviors, among others (reviewed in Bozukluklarının et al., 2015).

Excessive temperament traits of HA, NS, and low RD are, in a sense, the "carriers" of the biogenetic affect-related risk for personality disorder, hence they can be thought of as trait vulnerabilities. The traits are hardwired in subcortical circuitry and conditioned into behavioral biases several months after birth; they are preconceptual, that is, operate before cognitive networks are interactively organized and are in fact essential for the higher forms of cognition to organize, as discussed. The traits are heritable (up to 60%) and have been demonstrated to reduce the probability of mature character outcomes (Svrakic et al., 1996), a yet another demonstration of the adverse impact of early effects on personality development. The most frequent trait vulnerabilities are excessive HA and NS. The former (HA), characterized by proneness to anxiety and fearfulness, increases the risk of most variants of personality disorder, particularly of paranoid, negativistic-dependent, anankastic, and narcissistic variants. The latter (NS), characterized by propensity to anger and impulsivity, is the main trait vulnerability for the antisocial and histrionic variants. We have also shown (Svrakic et al., 1993) that low RD, which captures low social interest and detachment, represents a trait vulnerability for the schizoid variant. Coexisting traits of excessive HA and NS create "approach-avoidance" conflicts, whereby a new situation is experienced both as attractive and threatening. The approach to one alternative (novelty) increases the appeal of the other (safety) and vice versa. In patients thus afflicted, owing to the chronic mental exhaustion and frustration associated with this stalemate pattern, outbursts or episodes of acting out are common. This combination is hence referred to as "explosive temperament" and carries the highest biogenetic risk of personality disorder. We have noticed a high prevalence of somatic complications with these explosive individuals, perhaps reflecting chronically high autonomic arousal under stress.

Table 2.1 illustrates configurations of temperament traits specific for individual variants of personality disorder, in which some traits act as primary trait vulnerabilities for a variant, while others act as modifying traits which contribute to and perpetuate the phenomenology of the subtype.

Neuropathology of personality disorder: hypersubcorticality and hypofrontality. Heritable DNA polymorphisms and/or early experiences influence gene activity and expression in the neurons. Through G × E interaction, environmental influences epigenetically silence or activate

Table 2.1 TEMPERAMENT PROFILES OF PERSONALITY DISORDER VARIANTS

Personality Disorder Variant	Temperament Trait Vulnerabilities and Modifying Traits			
	Harm Avoidance	Novelty Seeking	Reward Dependence	Persistence
Antisocial	**Low** (modifying trait)	**HIGH** (main trait vulnerability)	**Low** (modifying trait)	**Variable**
Histrionic	**Low** (modifying trait)	**HIGH** (main trait vulnerability)	**HIGH** (modifying trait)	**Low**
Narcissistic	**HIGH** (main trait vulnerability)	**Variable**	**HIGH** (modifying trait)	**High**
Anankastic	**HIGH** (main trait vulnerability)	**Low**	**Moderate**	**HIGH** (modifying trait)
Negativistic-dependent	**HIGH** (main trait vulnerability)	**Low**	**HIGH** (modifying trait)	**Variable**
Schizoid	**low** (modifying trait)	**Low** (modifying trait)	**Low** **(main trait vulnerability)**	**Low** (modifying trait)
Paranoid	**HIGH** (main trait vulnerability)	**Variable**	**Low** (modifying trait)	**HIGH** (modifying trait)

Upper case: HIGH end of trait
Lower case: low end of trait

inherited gene variants involved in neurodevelopment. Such "nature *and* nurture" modulated genetic and epigenetic activity is a defining factor in how the brain and mind self-organize. With personality disorder, G × E interaction operates in the context of biological and/or environmental pathogens, which singly or in concert mediate an aberrant organization of the brain and the mind. Specifically, stress affects network development and topology in two ways: mild stress drives random brain networks toward scale-free, crash-resistant connectivity, whereas severe and persistent stress may fracture scale-free connectivity (Zorumski and Rubin, 2011). Juggling genetic and environmental imperfections, developmental homeostasis may lead to specific aberrances in brain organization (hypoactive PFCx, dysfunctional frontolimbic networks) with aberrant regulation and organization of cognitive processes, poorly restrained affect reactivity, and volatile impulse/action patterns (reviewed in Siever and Weinstein, 2009; Lieb et al., 2004; New et al., 2008), all of which may become neuropathological roots of personality disorder and continue to shape its clinical presentation. As discussed, heightened subcortical affect states and hypofunctional PFCx likely perpetuate each other in a positive feedback loop, maintaining in the process not only the mental but also the neural pathology of personality disorder. Numerous other features arise from such hypofrontality coupled with hypersubcorticality—impaired executive function, lack of empathy, underdeveloped prosocial emotions and helping behavior, and low capacity for mentalization, among others. All contribute to the psychopathology and interpersonal patterns of personality disorder.

The importance of early care in mental health and disorder. There can be no doubt that the roots of personality are established during the first few years of life, within the narrow world of early interactions between the newborn and the caregivers. The early interactions are largely biological-intuitive for both sides, the infant and the caregivers, and thus do not covary much with sociocultural periods. Although the philosophy of child-rearing continues to evolve, new insights never challenge the value of attuned loving care. Interfamilial differences in delivering care reflect socioeconomic status, subculture, educational level, family functionality and intactness, and psychological health of the parents.

In addition to heritable dispositions, inadequate early care may account for the fact that there have always been and shall always be children at increased risk for developing a personality disorder. Research shows that these children have a high frequency of adverse early life events, such as physical or verbal abuse, neglect (a form of abuse), and/or psychological trauma. Severe psychological trauma in childhood (e.g., sexual or physical abuse, loss of a parent, among others) is a potent factor, capable of acting alone. It is defined as a severely distressing event or several events which may generate an overwhelming amount of stress that exceeds the child's ability to cope with or integrate the emotions involved with the experience. Such traumatization is a frequent but underestimated factor in the development of personality disorder. Neuroimaging studies show that early psychological trauma is associated with enhanced limbic activation to emotionally valenced faces in depressed and healthy children (Suzuki, et al., 2014), documenting subcortical reactivity and, indirectly, prefrontal hypoactivity, both of which are regularly found in personality disorder.

Inadequate, but not necessarily flagrantly abusive parental practices, possibly arising from the parent's mental or marital problems or education level, may appear less dramatic in comparison to abuse or trauma but are also quite significant. As Kohut and Wolf (1978) noted, "it is not so much what the parents *do* that will influence the character of the child's self, but what the parents *are*." (p.416). Just a few of these suboptimal parental practices include lack of positive reinforcement; affectionless control; inadequate reactions to the child's emotional experiences, either turbulent (overreactions) or trivializing (underreaction, devaluation, dismissiveness); disregard for the emotional states of others (a negative model to the child); rigid or overregulation of one's own emotions (affectionless, distant parents); and a tendency to invalidate painful experiences of the child by shaming or blaming the child for such experiences. Under such immature care, the child may fail to develop the capacity to recognize, define, and modulate his or her own emotions; tolerate or process emotional or interpersonal stress; and trust his or her own experiences as valid.

The monumental importance of parental psychological stability for mental health and disorder in children is supported by research. Among children living in poverty, Luby et al. (2013) have identified structural changes in the brain, specifically smaller volumes of the amygdala (a key structure in emotional health) and the hippocampus (critical to learning and memory, the superhub in brain networks) that can lead to lifelong problems such as depression, learning difficulties, and limitations in the ability to cope with stress. The Luby et al. study also showed that *the extent of structural changes* was comodified strongly by quality of parenting, that is, whether parents were nurturing or not. Children who were nurtured and loved were somehow protected against the impact of poverty on their brains. This important study has confirmed what we have suspected all along: quality of care during the first several years of life is critical to establishing the foundation for healthy personality and mental health in general. This holds true not only for nonpsychotic psychopathology but also for a powerful modifying influence on the risk for Schizophrenia spectrum disorders (Tienari et al., 2004). Reflecting a growing awareness of the importance of early care, an increasing number of families are raising children in a way that is attuned to what the child's mind needs, rather than simply rushing to prohibitions that would limit the child's initiative, imagination, or creativity and raise anxieties during the preschool years. As a colleague said, "I'd rather live with a broken vase than with my daughter's suppressed drive to explore."

Do specific traumas have specific mental consequences? The vulnerability-stress model recognizes specific diatheses that make an individual susceptible to certain psychopathologies under particular pathogens (specific trauma, stress). A meta-analysis identified a possible link between specific traumas in childhood and the risk of specific phenomenology (variants) of personality disorder (Hankin and Abela, 2005). A few of these links that do not represent linear causality but rather depict general directions of behavior modeling include the following:

- Physical abuse and neglect may be linked to the antisocial variant;
- Sexual, emotional, or physical abuse or neglect may be linked to the borderline variant;
- Neglect, without other forms of abuse, may be linked to the dependent variant;
- Sexual abuse alone may be linked with the histrionic variant;
- Emotional abuse along with another form of neglect may be linked with the narcissistic variant;
- Emotional abuse and excessive parental control may be linked with the paranoid variant.

We note again that the causal relationship between specific traumas and specific variants of personality disorder has not been examined in a systematic manner; these are clinically relevant correlations that should not be taken to carry implications of causality.

DEVELOPMENT OF PERSONALITY DISORDER: SELF-ORGANIZATION WITH UNFINISHED PARTS

The cause and subsequent development of personality disorder involves multiple interacting forces, combining biogenetic dispositions, pathogenic environment, suboptimal brain and mind organization, and self-organizing punctuated homeostasis. Pathological development follows the same self-organizing dynamics as described for normal personality but incoporates dichotomized (polarized) elementary particles of partial object relations into the mind. The emerging field of developmental neuroscience integrates cellular and molecular mechanisms of brain development with hands-on observations of personality development. Here we discuss its application to personality disorder.

Bad enough conditions exceed the mind's ability to assimilate imperfections. In most cases, less-than-perfect parenting or heritably strong affect states are incorporated into the brain and mind with no major consequences; that is, the development still falls within the quantitative range of normalcy (aka "developmental homeostasis"). The latter is achieved through self-organizing processes of homeostatic optimization and may be reflective of "scale-free" attributes of the brain and the mind (discussed in Chapter 1). The problem arises when the genetic or environmental pathogens are excessive, that is, "bad enough," or when the risk factors co-occur and potentiate each other, whether additively or synergistically. Such excessive pathological ingredients may overpower the mind's homeostatic ability to assimilate imperfections, resulting in some specific cases in personality disorder. For this to happen, negative-affect charged mental representations have to be massive enough to endanger the positive ones, and to continue to do so over a prolonged period of time. In a vicious circle that maintains inner fragmentation, excessive negative experiences perpetuate the operation of splitting, which continues to keep them separate from positive experiences, and thus prevents the neutralization of those same negative experiences that necessitated its operation in the first place. Polarized negative units of experience flood the mind with persecutory fears and revengeful aggression; lost among them are scarce positive experiences amplified by primitive idealization. Again, the split between positive and negative representations may reflect a defensive maneuver of the mind or a hypofunctional PFCx in the context of stress, or the former might simply be a function of the latter.

Bad circumstances may subside, but their impact on the brain and mind is rather enduring, albeit not fixed. To illustrate the point we borrow from Frances Champagne (Champagne, 2008; Champagne and Curley, 2009). Poor parental care (here neglect) epigenetically silences genes coding for glucocorticoid receptors (GR) in the hippocampus. The underrepresented GR receptors hinder the normal hippocampal suppression of the hypothalamus-pituitary-adrenal (HPA) "stress axis."[13] Without this regulatory hippocampal suppression of the HPA axis, cortisol (the "stress hormone") is continually produced by the adrenal glands despite its high levels in the plasma, facilitating negative affect states even in low stress conditions and creating stress-vulnerable adult phenotypes. The described susceptibility to stress rooted in poor parenting increases the risk of a spectrum of adult anxiety and

13. There are numerous functions of GR in the brain, one of which is called a *GR-dependent gene expression,* which is central to a number of functions vital for survival. GR receptor is a transcription factor and modulates activity of a large number of genes, among others those involved in mood and emotional behaviors, cognitive functions (e.g., consolidation and flashbulb memory formation), and addictive states.

mood syndromes, not just personality disorder. Attenuating or accentuating neurophysiological effects of parental care on stress vulnerability have been demonstrated in both animals (Champagne and Curley, 2009) and humans (McGowan, 2009). Of note, good care promotes GR expression in the hippocampus and resistance to stress and mood and anxiety syndromes.

Fragmented personality: the core impairment of personality disorder. The concept of fragmented personality is central to our model and thus will be repeatedly revisited. Despite our best efforts, some redundancy is unavoidable. We believe that the term "fragmented personality" is more informative than "paranoid schizoid position" (Klein, 1952) to illustrate the essence of personality disorder, although the concepts are correspondent. Both presume reversibility and shifts between more and less integrated periods of mental functioning, depending on external (e.g., loss, stress) and internal factors (e.g., successful resolutions of crises, learning). The term "fragmented" is also more informative than the term "borderline" to capture the inconsistencies and incoherences in one's experience of self and others as well as the turbulent social relations that follow.

A normal phase in early development until about six months into life, fragmented personality (partial object relations) pathologically persists in individuals with personality disorder. However, object relations are neither fixed nor absolute. A person may function at the level of partial object relations in romantic relationships but at a more mature level in other interpersonal aspects, as we have observed. Similarly, a person can move between partial and whole object relations in situations of stress or loss followed by successful resolutions. It is the *predominance*, the *relative resilience*, and the *pervasiveness* of fragmented functioning that define fragmented personality at that period of time and in that given context.

The splitting mechanism (underlying normal early fragmentation) is only a temporary, albeit important organizer of the developing inner world of the newborn, which is soon to become suboptimal to meet the demand for handling more complex adaptive tasks as the system of the mind normally develops. Complex biological systems, such as the human brain and mind, arise as the most functional configuration of available component parts or processes. In personality disorder, polarized ("unfinished") particles of experience *are* the available building components, operating within nonconscious working memory from where they are integrated into mental faculties and the subsystems of the mind. Specifically, the intrinsic connectivity networks involved in the assembly of mental faculties are informed by such dyadic fragments which render the faculties biased (e.g., "black-or-white" thinking, polarized emotions, contradicting motivations) which are eventually self-configured into the subsystems of the mind, thus rendering the whole system (personality) dysfunctional from the standpoint of adaptive efficacy. The result is an inconsistent sense of self, insufficiently contextualized temperament, and character traits subserving internal organization at the expense of social adaptation. Coterminous with the aforementioned one may find a diffuse and incoherent identity accompanied by unprincipled and corruptible moral values.

Splitting: a barrier to growth but the hero of survival. Inner fragmentation does not significantly disturb the simplicity of mental life in the first six months of infancy, at least not observably. In the context of pathological conditions, however, the continuing fragmentation renders the mind suboptimal in terms of its ability to incorporate more complex representations of the self and others. In order to function otherwise, it would require a more realistic, less polarized understanding of the world, which would normally be achieved by higher order cognitive merging of the dichotomized extremes thereby enabling the infant to recognize the "big picture," that good and bad coexist in the same object and self. If such recognition were to happen in the context of predominant negative experiences, it would overwhelm the few positive ones, jeopardizing in the process the positive core of the mind necessary for mental growth. Such risk perpetuates the operation of splitting, which is both a barrier to growth and the hero of psychological survival: it protects against the chaos of disintegration by maintaining primitive order, figuratively a "divide and survive" strategy. Such a quick fix clears the space for other immature defenses to operate, including denial, projection, projective identification, and primitive idealization, among others. These mechanisms interfere with normal development: they further cement the defensive distance between the weak core of positive experiences on the one side and overwhelming negative introjections on the other side. In our view, it is at this point in "at risk" development that omnipotent fantasies come to the rescue. The end product is what is called personality disorder. Fairy tales do not always come true: here, good does not triumph but is rather overpowered by evil and hibernating in the background. The tale of "Sleeping Beauty" rescued by the prince adequately metaphorizes the real selves of our patients, dormant for the most part, but liable to be "rescued" years later, whether in therapeutic relationship or by a mature loving partner, which would both be represented figuratively as belated selfobjects who mediate inner integration.

When rescuing fantasies organize the mind: the birth of personality disorder. Persisting fragmentation of personality can be thought of as an internal stalemate which stands in the way of the developmental progress necessary to achieve a balanced self-image. Instead, contradicting, short-lived polarized units of motivations, emotions, or thoughts cancel each other out before they get a chance to consolidate with sustained consistency. However, *a* self has to develop within the mind of a human being; this is a phylogenetic given. We hypothesize that the drop in fitness associated with the stalemate of fragmentation activates developmental homeostasis to self-organize the mind by any psychological means or available components. One must keep in mind that a child attaches not to objects or experiences that give him or her pleasure but to those that reduce pain (Cyrulnik, 2008). Mentally endangered by negative affects and persecutory experiences, the child will self-stimulate to safety through omnipotent rescuing fantasies which thereby reduce pain. More precisely, it is the nonconscious homeostatic optimization mechanisms that employ omnipotent fantasies to organize the inner fragments and stabilize the mind; hence we refer to the process as psychological survival through personality disorder. These defensive fantasies may involve his or her own grandiosity (power, wealth, beauty), a fantasized powerful protector, revenge and getting even with the world, or safety of detachment, each of these a defensive self-ideal. These are seen as childhood precursors of personality disorder, as early as six years of age (reviewed in Bozukluklarının et al., 2015). Over time, variant-specific fantasies (narcissistic, histrionic, dependent, etc.) organize inner fragments into a highly unrealistic and dictatorial but compensatory self-image, leaving the rest of the fragmented mind (the real self) split off (such duality is discussed later). The dictatorial self staves off disintegration but further pathologizes personality by shunting it into deviance. Personality disorder can thus be thought of as a homeostatic attempt by the mind to heal itself by self-organizing into an inner dictator which fuses the fragments with the power of fantasy and unrealistic exaggerations. As JC Perry and G Vaillant once discussed, just as fever and callus formation are the body's physiological reactions to insults or disease, personality disorder may well be the mind's effort to heal itself through fantasy and exaggeration ("organize by all possible means").

THE DYNAMICS OF PERSONALITY DISORDER: FRAGMENTED PERSONALITY IN SEARCH OF PSYCHOLOGICAL SURVIVAL

In contrast to Kernberg (1975), who classifies "low" and "high" level of "borderlines," we consider all bona fide cases of personality disorder as severe and fragmented. Next we analyze specific aspects of the mind's subsystems in personality disorder.

The dual self of personality disorder: when deviance protects vulnerability. Suggestive evidence for the hypothesized compensatory role of personality disorder comes from the regularly observed duality of the self within the mind of these patients. The term "duality" is intended to illustrate that the individual has a dual-self system, one pathological and dominant and the other hidden and real, both of which coexist side by side: a rudimentary real self, harboring impotent rage, resentment, insecurity, and fear, is split off from the dominant compensatory self, harboring variant-specific omnipotent fantasies and extremized images of self and others. The dictatorial pathological self organizes the inner fragments, as it were, by the brute force of omnipotent fantasy, which becomes a pathological amalgam that holds the mind together. The compensation comes with a price tag of deviance, inauthenticity, and self-serving interpersonal relations. Figuratively, personality disorder can be thought of as "better any organization than no organization," where psychopathology is the lesser of two evils (the alternative is disintegration).

Characteristic duality is observed in therapy with all variants of personality disorder: a dominant pathological self, whether grandiose, theatrical, antisocial, anankastic,[14] negativistic-dependent, schizoid, or paranoid, compensates for the underlying fragility of the real self. The two selves coexist but are barely aware of each other, divided by "vertical splitting" and mutual disavowal (Kohut, 1971). The respective phenomenologies of these selves are also dual, with the deep sense of insecurity, exceptional sensitivity to (mis)perceived rejection, envy, boredom, and impotent rage bleeding into the precarious cohesion of the dominant pathological self, which is basically an impersonation of a fantasized defensive image. Hence the peculiar coexistence of contradictory features such as grandiosity and inferiority, theatricality and shyness, dependence and aggression, among others, all of which form important diagnostic clues. Most patients are aware, albeit distantly, of their own fragility and inauthenticity, which stirs up disturbing disintegration and existential anxieties. The therapist may find that he or she communicates only with a compensatory part of the patient's mind but at the same time affectively also resonates with the part harboring diametrically opposite feelings and self-image. The self-duality is recognized by patients, albeit vaguely, but the recognition has no emotional relevance (due to the splitting mechanism) and thus no significant impact to self-initiate inner integration. Instead, these patients usually try to better disguise their inauthenticity by nongenuine adoption of socially desirable behaviors, further entering the territory of "as if" personality described by Hellen Deutsch. They may seek treatment, at least initially, not to change but to perfect their cover-up. The task of therapy involves undoing the alien self and thereby opens the space to uncover, develop, and strengthen the unknown real self

14. Formerly obsessive-compulsive personality disorder (OCPD). However, the syndrome does not include frank obsessions and only moderate behavioral rituals (compulsions). The term "anankastic" reduces possible confusion with OCD and captures the essence of the disorder (the term derives from Greek ἀναγκαστικός—anankasticos, for "compulsive" rigidity).

within the safe milieu of psychotherapy, in contrast to the patient's unsafe early environment. However, such work brings with it the threat of disintegration by overriding the separation of the two selves and is associated with the risk of internal implosion and chronic disintegration anxiety, a source of resistance to therapy.

We use the narcissistic variant of personality disorder to illustrate this dynamics. Here, the pathological grandiose sense of self-importance is built around primitive idealizing fantasies (beauty, brilliance, success). These may or may not be connected to reality by some objective, albeit frequently exaggerated individual quality. The grandiose self is manifested through entitlement, interpersonal exploitation, arrogance, idealization of the powerful, devaluation of the weak, counterattacks toward the critical, and psychological exhibitionism in pursuit of admiration ("I am admired therefore I am"). Such highly unrealistic self organizes the fragmented mind into the pathological but psychologically safer narcissistic personality disorder. The residual real self is split off, disorganized, envious, revengeful, with vaguely defined (if any) interests of its own. Obscured by compensatory grandiosity, but thinly present in self-awareness, narcissistic persons feel endangered and inferior, struggling to find external support for their unstable self-esteem and chronic dysphoria (Svrakic, 1990). The duality is presented in Table 2.2.

Table 2.2 NARCISSISTIC DUALITY: COEXISTING CONTRADICTORY FEATURES, DOMINANT AND HIDDEN

GRANDIOSE SELF DOMINANT, OVERT	real self split off, subliminal
Grandiosity	Inferiority, insecurity
- free floating (omnipotence, omniscience)	Pursuit of metamorphosis ("new beginnings")
- structured (tied to a personal feature/skill)	Fatigue by living (Sisyphus type futility/pessimism)
Exhibitionism	Hypochondriasis
(mirroring in admiration)	Black-or-white perspective
MENTAL FACULTIES	
EMOTIONS	
Secondary	Primary
Exaltation (idealization)	Envy
Disappointment (devaluation)	Boredom (chronic)
Aggression (eruptive, provoked)	Vengeful resentment (impotent, unprovoked)
Dysphoria (default mood)	Emptiness (lack of meaning)
	Lack of prosocial emotions

(continued)

Table 2.2 CONTINUED

GRANDIOSE SELF DOMINANT, OVERT	real self split off, subliminal
COGNITION	
Autocentric	Deficient
Egocentric perception of reality (defined through one's own needs) Sense of specialness Omnipotent fantasy Hypersensitive to failure (shame)	Lack of genuine interest Lack of curiosity Superficiality Stereotypic Pervasive cynicism/skepticism
MOTIVATION	
Pseudosublimation (exhibitionistic motivation for work)	Lack of Commitment (lack of endurance, lack of initiative)
INTERPERSONAL RELATIONS	
Turbulent, conflict seeking (unstable) Entitlement Arrogant, haughty demeanor Pathological intolerance to criticism	Basic disinterest, lack of empathy, fairness, and reciprocity Distrust of others Need for protection, nurturing Search for a transformational object (selfobject)
MORALITY	
Entitlement, egocentricity, exploitation Ethical herostratism* (opportunistic, corruptible) Pathological lying (leaving the impression of success and power) "As if" ethics (leaving the impression of morality) Ethical "blindness" (does not recognize effects of own immorality on others)	Global ethical poverty Ethical cynicism (does not believe others are genuinely ethical)

** In reference to Herostratus, the ancient Greek arsonist whose name has become a metonym for someone who commits a criminal act in order to become noted

In general, an individual with any variant of personality disorder is said to be compensated when his or her expectations are satisfied and thereby provide support for the compensatory self-image, whether narcissistic, histrionic, or any other. Being compensated does not mean being mature but simply that the unrealistic self-image has at the moment won the battle for internal organization, bringing more stability in everyday life and mood, within their families, with coworkers, as parents, and so on.

The role of excessive temperament: when subcortical forces drive the mind. Temperament, the first motivated behavior of a human newborn, fundamentally influences the affective valence of early interactions and continues to provide emotional significance to behavior and guide automatic reactions to stimuli throughout life. Normally, cortical feedback loops to subcortical circuits mediate top-down cognitive control of affect states and instinctive behavior reactions(aka "corticalization," "cognization," or "contextualization" of behavior). In personality disorder, with a hypofunctional cortical feedback, affects and behaviors are poorly contextualized on a daily basis, perhaps the reason Kernberg (2015) describes these patients as more "reflexive" than "reflective." Moreover, affects can break out of prefrontal control and self-perpetuate into rage or extreme fears with potentially disastrous consequences (aka "amygdala hijack"; Goleman, 1996). The most serious psychological consequence is the collapse of the splitting mechanism and annihilation of the positive fragments (figuratively, psychological death), risking disintegration into psychosis and self-harm. Excessive temperament traits profoundly limit the emotional spectrum toward oneself and others: these individuals are usually angry (at themselves and someone else), fantasize or act out revenge, feel betrayed, fear the loss of a selfobject, or are detached and disinterested. Envy and boredom are regular companions. A few powerful selfobjects are idealized but not genuinely loved.

As noted, excessive HA and NS and low RD (fearfulness, impulsivity, detachment) not only increase the risk but also modify the symptomatic presentation of personality disorder, as illustrated in Table 2.1. Low HA and low RD are trait modifiers for the antisocial variant, adding fearlessness, lack of empathy, and disregard for norms to the core impulsivity (NS is the main trait vulnerability). High persistence (PE) is a trait modifier for the anankastic and paranoid variants (excessive HA is the main trait vulnerability for both). With the anankastic subtype, high PE adds perfectionistic external order to contain internal apprehensive anticipations. With the paranoid variant, high PE adds perseverance to a distrustful lifestyle and relentless litigation in pursuit of justice. This variant is also modified by low RD, thus adding restricted emotionality to the mix. With the schizoid variant, a generally hypoactive temperament (low NS, HA, PE) contributes stoic rigidity, low anxiety, and inertia, respectively, to the syndrome already set in motion by low RD (disinterest, detachment), here the main trait vulnerability. In contrast, high RD is in general a protective factor against personality disorder. It not only fosters rewarding positive interactions but makes other traits (excessive HA or NS) easier to attenuate via associative conditioning. High RD, however, modifies the phenomenology of some variants, notably histrionic and narcissistic, both characterized by excessive dependence on social approval.

The subsystem of character: an outside spectacle subserving internal organization. Normally, character traits coupled with moral values optimize the fit between one's internal needs and normative social pressures, both thereby mediating social adaptation. Most people therefore willfully adjust their adaptive behaviors to respond as close as is healthy to the feedback from the environment.[15] With personality disorder, character traits persist in social deviance despite negative feedback, as if the behavior were subserving some vital internal need at the expense of better adaptation. For these individuals, the primary operating environment for social behavior is not external but internal, where it compensates for inner fragmentation ("inside oriented character function"). The behavior is thus primarily conditioned based on its inner effectiveness, while external adaptation becomes of secondary importance. Figuratively, "me" primarily needs to organize "I" and uses others as supporting actors in the struggle to stay compensated. For example, a paranoid personality scans the environment to detect signs of malevolence, typically misattributed; these signs are then used by the compensatory paranoid self to maintain the paranoid frame of reference. Any other, more realistic interpretation of others would challenge the definition and maintenance of the paranoid self, which is vital to stay compensated. The same self-serving dynamics but with specific themes (antisocial, narcissistic, etc.) is seen with all variants. Indeed, one of the most peculiar features of personality disorder is that these individuals have difficulty learning from interpersonal fiascos but rather keep repeating the same pathological patterns despite and in denial of the isolation and dislike they incur from others. The real gain is psychological, i.e., internal organization, rather than external adaptation and genuine sociability.

Poorly integrated moral values: corruptible and opportunistic morality. As one of the subsystems of personality, integrated moral values provide the experience of conscience, the mind's inner voice that guides morally principled behavior. The moral values work either in concert with character to mediate social adaptation, or independently from character, in which case the role is to self-evaluate ("moral censor"). There is

15. Uncritical adaption is equally pathological as maladaptation

generally a high correspondence between the level of personality integration and depersonification of moral values. With severe personality pathology, moral values remain biased and "personal," because persisting split-off idealizing and persecutory self- and object representations work against integration (Kernberg, 1975). This is observed as moral permissiveness (aka "opportunism" or "corruptibility") as well as prejudiced, nonprincipled moral values, which are characteristic of all variants. Here belongs moral relativism, as these patients feel justified to distort or break rules to facilitate inner integration. Diffuse moral defects are manifested more as egosyntonic "soft" immorality in interpersonal relations (manipulation, deceit), not so much as violations of legal norms, except occasionally in the case of the antisocial variant. In such a morally impoverished world, reality testing vis-à-vis one's interpersonal relationships is impaired, mostly due to the reduced capacity for self-evaluation and lack of remorse following immoral actions. Another feature of poorly integrated moral values is that individuals can be hypertrophied (rigid and punishing) in certain areas (e.g., relationship with friends and family) and completely permissive in other areas (Kernberg, 1975) An antisocial man functioning at the fragmented level may be horrified by the thought of disrespecting his parents, while at the same time is involved in organized prostitution chains and other major violations of the law.

Whatever happened to empathy and reciprocity in personality disorder? Most adults with personality disorder manifest defects in reciprocal altruism and empathy, two of the biogenetic pillars of morality. At least some lack of empathy can be biogenetic, e.g., callous, unemotional prepubescent boys who manifest cruelty from early childhood, a deficit thought to be associated with a mutation of the oxytocin receptor gene (Dadds et al., 2014a). However, most adults with personality disorder did not exhibit a striking lack of empathy and fairness in childhood, which is suggestive of intact biological capacities. For some reason, these capacities are not maintained moving forward, which is likely a function of pathological neuropsychological development. A fragmented child is defensively oriented, battling to stay compensated by any and all means possible, an inherently egotistic situation, while empathy, altruism, and moral values are of secondary importance. The latter are simply not omnipotent enough to organize the inner fragments which become subservient to the unlimited power of fantasized exaggerations. We speculate that the subcortical perception-action circuitry involved in empathy and the related prosocial phenomena are simply *not used enough* to stabilize synaptic contacts in the Hebbian sense (the process is regarded as the neuronal basis of unsupervised learning). Simply put, neurons that do not fire together do not wire together, and these individuals literally do not train their brains to be prosocial, despite a normal potential. The prosocial motivation eventually goes dormant but is not lost, as in autism. As an indirect proof of the concept, these individuals can develop empathy and feel good about this capacity in psychotherapy.

Soft immorality versus acts of crime: a discontinuous distribution of a continuous liability. In general, people do not perfectly adhere to their own moral rules but cheat to a lesser or greater extent, particularly when the chances of a reward are high and the risks of punishment are low. Anyone can be tempted to create advantage for him/herself by manipulating the truth or by selectively violating sociolegal or moral norms. Such impulses are residuals of our biological selfishness naturally selected for self-preservation but long suppressed by the mold of civilization. The question is not whether a person will have immoral impulses but how often, in what context, to what degree, and most importantly will they act upon them. Normally, during the moment of temptation, the inner censor of conscience activates distress and guilt, creating a moral conflict and a rational rejection of immorality (a prefrontal function). The person *chooses* not to act upon the temptation and not to cross the line, regardless of whether he or she would be caught (in most people this becomes a second nature). Where morality is weakly internally censored but mostly controlled externally by the fear of consequences, the individual may succumb to the temptation if the likelihood of being caught is low. Such transgressions may occur on a regular basis creating a pattern called "moral opportunism." The key point here is that the majority of people are capable of "soft" moral transgressions (e.g., white lies), and many of more serious immoral behavior (manipulation, exploitation), but only a few cross the line into crime and violence ("criminals"). Such discontinuous distribution of a continuous liability may reflect, one the one hand, a threshold effect (most people are subjectively disturbed by the idea of crossing the line) and/or on the other hand, the exponentially more severe punishment for serious crime and a correspondingly higher fear of consequences.

Identity diffusion: the hallmark of diagnosis. Identity assessment (discussed in Chapter 3) is increasingly used as it has become one of the pivotal tools in making a clinical diagnosis of personality disorder. Identity diffusion, the hallmark of the diagnosis, is best described as an *incoherent life narrative*, a blurry "who" of "me" which also extends into the blurry narrative of others, who are seen as personless silhouettes (deficient theory of mind) excepting the few who come to vivid prominence as selfobjects.

Identity diffusion is manifested as chronic and profound yet distant (split off) uncertainties regarding "who am I in fact" and "where am I going in life." This is accompanied by conflation of one's own thoughts with those of others, feeling false and/or empty, coexisting contradictory images of self and others, a sense of unfulfillment, intolerance of loneliness, ambiguous gender identity without gender dysphoria, oscillating identification of sexual preference (unstable sexual identity), among many other features. Some of the features (e.g., body and gender uncertainties) imply early problems with identity. Instability, another feature of diffuse identity, refers to frequent shifts in views and values (which become especially prominent whenever an individual finds him- or herself in the orbit of a strong person, "chameleon-like"), as well as to frequent consideration of contradictory alternatives in work and life, and lack of sense of continuity over time. Contradicting behaviors and relationships are difficult to logically string together. As an important diagnostic clue, the interviewer has difficulties resonating with the patient's incoherent story but rather feels confused by it. Many fragmented individuals find and cling to outside sources of structure through either role absorption or joining doctrinized social groups. Neither external structure nor personality disorder truly consolidate identity; they merely serve to mask identity diffusion, although they help to palliate to some extent the individual's struggle to stay compensated.

CLINICAL PRESENTATION OF FRAGMENTED PERSONALITY: THE CORE PROBLEM AND ITS PRECARIOUS SOLUTIONS

Personality disorder is experienced intrapersonally, expressed interpersonally, and diagnosed in both contexts. Here we discuss (i) the phenomenology, symptoms, clinical signs, and interpersonal relationships and (ii) seven discernible variants of personality disorder, each typifying a specific compensatory solution to inner fragmentation.

Phenomenology, symptoms, clinical signs. Experiential and presentational dynamics specific to personality disorder arise from the fragmented substrate of the mind reverberating through mental functioning. The characteristic aspects of emotions, cognition, motivation, and interpersonal relationships of individuals with personality disorder are discussed next.[16]

16. The term "phenomenology" refers to the structure of subjective experience, "symptom" to a subjective experience noticed by the affected individual as unusual or deviant, and "sign" to objectively observable manifestations.

Stable instability of the mind: emotions, thought, motivations, and behavior. A popular slogan among clinicians is that "the only stable thing about fragmented personality is its instability." The pervasive instability of the self is experienced as a chronic sense of mental fragility ("I feel as if I could fall apart any minute," a patient of ours once said), and as a profound preoccupation with one's own inner space (outside events not directly related to self-image may be seen as "distractions"), often to the detriment of memories of interpersonal events ("I remember how I was dressed but not how my date for the evening was dressed," another patient once said). Mood instability is manifested as unpredictable swings between opposite emotions, fueling matching shifts in cognition, motivations, and behavior. Default dysphoria, intense envy, unforgiving anger, boredom, and emptiness are ever burgeoning in the background. Within this setting of polarized personality, negative (positive) stimulation easily activates negative (positive) images and anger (elation). Depending on the valence of the activated self- and object images and affects, these individuals tend to oscillate between periods of optimistic exaltation (new idealizations of new people and of the associated self-image) and disillusionment owing to failures and frustrations along the way (devaluing themselves and others, including those previously idealized). These "down" periods can be manifested as atypical depression (discussed later) and/or may stir volatile interpersonal conflicts and/or self-injurious acting outs and suicidality. The unpredictable mood turnarounds are difficult to understand, as they seem to appear from nowhere, driven as they are by an idiosyncratic internal agenda rather than by anything appreciably based in reality. One important exception to such mood instability is the schizoid variant, in which emotional detachment serves as the compensatory solution to fragmentation. A schizoid person withdraws emotionally from the overly complex real world into the world of autistic fantasy, which enables him or her to be in full control of mental experiences ("unilateral adaptation"), while appearing outside as socially disinterested, affectively blunted, and hypoemotional.

With other variants, mood oscillations may be dramatic and may last for weeks at a time. For this reason they are easily mistakable for bipolar II disorder, where mood swings may be frequent, brief, and sometimes reactive. Although clinically similar, mood swings within bipolar II and fragmented personality differ in a fundamental way. The former refers to episodes of pathologically strong moods (hypomania, depression) which are able to overpower the otherwise normally functioning PFCx and usually interrupt rather healthy periods of mental functioning. The latter by contrast involves a hypofunctional PFCx failing to control subcortical affects (elation, dysphoria, rage), which arise as "limbic" reactions to idiosyncratic and/or misattributed perceptions of success, failure, or provocations. The distinction also includes a number of phenomenological, longitudinal, and cross-sectional differences between the two conditions (reviewed in Parker, 2014).

Triggers for human emotional reactions are thought to involve a mismatch between a perceived stimulus and one's expectations, an assessment made rapidly and not necessarily conscious or correct (Zorumski and Rubin, 2011). One should keep in mind that people process sensory information through a personal prism, which is basically a set of unique expectations reflecting one's unique personality features. In personality disorder, one's expectations are extremized in order to be able to feed the needs of an exaggerated self-image, which makes these individuals susceptible to fail own expectations. As the most intense emotions are triggered by failures, individuals with personality disorder manifest negative emotions (dysphoria and anger in particular) more frequently and more intensely than positive emotions (elation), although the latter can be rather impressive as well.

Poor self-regulation of mood and affect states. With fragmented personality, as discussed, positive and negative affect states have not been cross-neutralized, owing to a hypofunctional PFCx. In the context of such hypofrontality, polarized affect states, particularly the negative ones, are easily activated by negative stimulation and have a tendency to self-perpetuate out of control, culminating in panic, despair, anger, and aggressive outbursts. Alternatively, following a positive stimulation, positive affects also easily escalate into exaltation and euphoria ("joie de vivre"). The patient typically has difficulty containing his or her affective reactions (to calm down) without the help of others. As a manifestation of acting out, at least its communicative function, dangerous behaviors may occur without much thought or concern about the consequences. Common are threats of suicide and/or self-harming gestures, reflecting diverse motivations, for example, a profound exhaustion with psychological fragility, an infantile (demonstrative) demand for care by a selfobject, or an attempt to strengthen one's own psychological boundary, among many others. We recall one of our patients saying that cutting through the skin on her thighs or arms "brings relief" because the pain helps her "verify" the boundaries of her own body. Another patient stated that "the adrenaline rush during a high speed joy ride enables the physical danger to define the borders of my psychological being."

Acting out: a defense mechanism, resistance to change, or way of communication? The concept of acting out refers to phenomenology and/or behavior that dramatize or symbolically realize nonconscious transference fantasies or defenses against them in an interpersonal setting (Auchincloss and Samberg, 2012). Some consider acting out to be a defense mechanism in its own right (the nonconscious is expressed through behavior and hence protects itself against being uncovered by the conscious mind), while others view it as a resistance to change (resistance because acting out is "used" to impede self-reflection a necessary step before correction), and yet others as a way of communication that conveys important clues for therapy (Auchincloss and Samberg, 2012). Resistance and the communicative function of acting out are difficult to separate though. In the context of neuroses, acting out is a defense mechanism that symbolically materializes aggressive or sexual impulses in order to gain relief from tension or anxiety associated with the conflict ("acting out of a conflict").

Core dysphoria: the default mood of personality disorder. Dysphoria, deriving from Greek for "difficult to bear," refers to a variety of chronic and pervasive but ill-defined negative moods, all common with individuals with personality disorder: emotional distress, emptiness and boredom, resented neediness and dependency, sense of mental fragility and inadequacy, irritability, deeply rooted sense of abandonment, self-destructiveness—in short, a "miserable state of mind," a patient once said. Such miserly moods in turn fuel negative interpersonal attitudes, for example, sarcasm, envy, bitterness, resentment, cynicism, active and passive aggression, among many others. We refer to this experience as "core dysphoria" because it seems to be rooted in the fragmented personality core; the dysphoria is understood to result from the exhausting, never-ending and ultimately futile struggle for inner stability (Pazzagli and Monti, 2000). Neuroimaging studies provide suggestive evidence for the causal association of personality fragmentation and chronic low mood in personality disorder. Frontal lobe abnormalities, both structural and functional, have been demonstrated in medication-naive female adults with early-onset dysthymia and depressive personality disorder (Lyoo et al., 2002).[17] More than two-thirds of subjects (32/44) in the Lyoo et al. study met criteria for depressive personality disorder, a controversial entity characterized by "mood traits" of negative reactivity, low self-esteem, critical attitudes, hypersensitivity to rejection, difficulty being angry, orality, and introversion, among others. Another way to state the results of this study is that a dysfunctional frontal lobe was associated with intrapsychic and interpersonal features indicative of profound personality pathology (fragmentation) in young adult females

17. The study mixed together subjects with dysthymia and/or depressive personality disorder, a questionable decision from a methodological standpoint.

who were selected for dysphoria. The frontal dysfunction in Lyoo et al. was hypothesized by the authors to represent a developmental pathology of the brain, whereby a smaller frontal cortex volume during adolescence in turn resulted in a smaller genu part of the corpus callosum, hindering the interconnection of the frontal regions of the brain. Such hypofrontality in regulating self-image, mood, and anxiety, perhaps caused by those same moods and anxieties in the first place, is a pivotal component in both the development and perpetuation of personality disorder, as discussed.

Recurrent atypical depression and dual depression. The constructs of atypical depression and "borderline" (fragmented) personality overlap, the latter (fragmented personality) in most, but not all cases, is at the root of the former (atypical depression). A study using dimensional approach to clarify the association between personality disorder and atypical depression showed that a mixture of cognitive and mood traits which are characteristic of fragmented personality, like high neuroticism, impulsivity, anger, hostility, and low deliberation, are common to both atypical depression and cluster B and C variants of personality disorder (Chopra et al., 2005). Episodes of atypical depression are distinguished from typical major depression based on (i) preserved reactivity to pleasurable stimuli (the patient responds to "good news"), reversed vegetative symptoms of (ii) increased appetite or weight gain and (iii) hypersomnia, (iv) heavy or leaden feelings in limbs, and, as the cardinal feature, (v) profound and chronic rejection sensitivity, not limited to mood disturbance. In the context of personality disorder, atypical depression is understood to reflect a psychological "dive" below the level of core dysphoria, perhaps caused by periods of profound disappointments. Rejection or abandonment sensitivity refers to a chronic, intense, irrational expectation of rejection and rapid overreaction to it, without a reason or indication that this might in fact happen. The phenomenon is believed to be rooted in the continuing need for selfobjects, whose rejection is dreaded as it actually threatens not only the integrity but also the survival of the self (selfobjects of course define *and* maintain the sense of self). The dynamics is indicative of an early developmental deficit and is highly suggestive of personality disorder. Many view rejection sensitivity to be a transdiagnostic link between personality disorder and episodic atypical depression. As an important clue for differential diagnosis versus typical depression, persons functioning at the fragmented level have an uncanny lack of guilt, lack of concern for others, and lack of genuine sadness when, for example, facing a relationship break-up. What may appear as depression on the surface is in fact impotent rage, resentment, revengeful wishes, or feeling of defeat by external forces (Kernberg, 1975).

Numerous reports indicate that patients with personality disorder can and do have episodes of typical depression as well. Both types of episodic depression, typical and atypical, can be superposed on core dysphoria, a phenomenon dubbed "double or dual depression."

Is (borderline) personality disorder an atypical mood disorder? Given the significant overlap between atypical depression and borderline (fragmented) personality, a frequent question has been whether "borderline" is simply a facet of a chronic unipolar major depression, just adding a component of atypicality to the latter. In our opinion, this is not the case. Fragmented personality is a developmental phenomenon with chronically low mood arising as a consequence of inner fragmentation, rather than the other way around. After all, not every fragmented individual is chronically depressed, many are just unstable or impulsive, and most alternate between dysphoria, elation, and impulsivity. A casual look at the long-term traits of borderline personality in DSM-5 reveals that only a few traits relate to depression, and most to interpersonal turbulence and psychological instability: rejection or abandonment sensitivity, impulsivity, persistently unstable self-image (identity disturbance), chronic feelings of emptiness, intense interpersonal relationships which alternate between extremes of idealization and devaluation, among others. Similarly, Parker (2014) has argued, based on empirical analysis, that the primary feature of atypical depression is a personality style of rejection sensitivity and that some of its "atypical" features (i.e., hypersomnia, hyperphagia) are homeostatic self-consolatory responses to a dysregulated state of mind marked by anxiety, irritability, and depression, rather than symptoms per se. Parker concludes that personality disorder might be in a spectrum with atypical depression when shared features of interpersonal sensitivity, emotional dysregulation, and abandonment preoccupations are taken into account. We quote this eloquent argument, fully applicable to fragmented personality:

> Let us assume that there is a relatively distinctive personality style marked by disturbed interpersonal relationships, identity disturbances, behavioral dysregulation and preoccupations with being abandoned and rejected. When sufficiently severe and dysfunctional (i.e., as a consequence, the individual and/or those around that person suffer) we may accord it "personality disorder" status. As such it provides a predispositional diathesis to heightened and variable responses to stress. In certain circumstances, the individual might respond by "acting out" with vituperative anger and hostility and not be depressed at all. In other circumstances, the individual may "act in" and experience an extreme reactive depressive state, "atypical" or otherwise. In essence, the obligatory

> predispositional component in such a diathesis-stress model is the personality style that may or may not lead to a depressive state. (p. 253)

This is not to say that adult-onset mood disorders do not profoundly affect personality, in some cases even at the fundamental level of object relations, but this they do only transiently and do not outlast the episode of mood disturbance ("transient fragmentation," as discussed later).

Anxieties of the vulnerable: biological and functional, state and trait. We use the terms "trait" to refer to stable individual dispositions to behave or feel a certain way ("how the person typically is"—a longitudinal view) and "state" to refer to temporary changes in attitudes and behaviors which parallel changes in internal and external conditions ("how the person currently is"— a cross-sectional view). Anxiety, an unpleasant experience of apprehensive anticipation of danger or failure, includes a number of associated features, for example, a deep but ill-defined feeling of insecurity, difficulty concentrating, arousal, hypervigilance, and feelings of unreality, among others. Biological trait anxiety refers to anxieties associated with excessive temperament traits (specifically high HA), whereas functional trait anxiety refers to anxieties stirred by the dynamisms within the fragmented mind. A rich variety of trait anxieties, from biologically anxious temperaments[18] (trait vulnerability in negativistic-dependent, narcissistic, paranoid, and anankastic variants of personality disorder), pervasive uneasiness about physical health (hypochondriasis) and psychological safety (disintegration anxiety), intense separation anxiety (resulting from unfinished individuation and attachment pathology), metaphysical anxiety concerned with authenticity of existence (existential anxiety), unique abandonment anxiety (reflecting the vital need for selfobjects, distrust in own ability, lack of self and object constancy, among other causes), and chronified state anxieties (e.g., persistent social phobia) characterize personality disorder. These are discussed in some detail next.

Abandonment and separation anxiety: losing selfobject versus losing object. Separation anxiety refers to excessive fear about being separated from an attachment figure who provides support and comfort (fear of losing an object), while rejection or abandonment sensitivity is about the fear of losing the selfobject who defines and maintains the sense of self (and thus the fear of losing self), the deeper of the two phenomena. Both are common with all variants of fragmented personality (except schizoid), usually heavily intertwined, and both are exacerbated by episodes of

18. High HA or anxious temperament is clinically presented and diagnosed as generalized anxiety disorder (GAD).

atypical depression and/or flare-ups of dysphoria. As these individuals are "stuck" in the separation-individuation phase, having not achieved a full separation and even less so individuation, they show a peculiar intolerance of being alone. They cling to the therapist and other important objects, neither as an act of love nor as an authentic bond, but rather as an act motivated by their needs for support and/or maintenance of the sense of self by a selfobject. With respect to separation anxiety (losing an object), the phenomenon of "separation avoidance" refers to the pattern wherein these patients quickly "attach" to someone and equally quickly "detach" while they are attaching to someone else, having no unattached periods; they are figuratively social butterflies. As an example of abandonment anxiety, a patients of ours (MDJ) felt the urge to exchange SMS messages with me every weekend to "reaffirm she (the patient) existed." In the latter stages of therapy, the patient was able to "feel" herself without relying on my messages. The therapist must accept such symbiosis initially (although it can last for a while) as the way for the patient to develop trust that a safe relationship and a reliable object who is going to "be there when needed" are indeed possible.

These patients attend therapy sessions in sequences, intermittently, sometimes with long breaks in between. The maxim "less is more" applies here: although both sides have agreed on the need for long-term treatment, for these patients less therapy is better in certain phases, for example, when the therapeutic process stirs disintegration anxiety. The therapist should accept these interruptions and not interpret them as resistance (which they really are), because disintegration anxiety (the real reason for the break) can be incapacitating and carries the risk of deeper regressions. These patients nonconsciously cling to their intuitive rule of safety—"better fragmented than disintegrated"—and most eventually return to therapy. We consider it a major milestone when the patient is able to raise the level of his or her anxieties from disintegration to separation, which is suggestive of inner integration approaching ambivalence. Because of these chronic, profound, and diverse anxieties, the phenomenology of fragmented personality can impress as one of "continual crisis." Fortunately, these patients are never as bad as they look when doing poorly.[19]

Fragmentation anxiety: disintegration and existential variants. Continual danger of disintegration and struggle to compensate through an unrealistic self-image create anxieties specific for personality disorder, regardless of the variant and even in the context of low baseline

19. They are also never as healthy as the look when they are doing well (this of course does not apply to those engaged in therapy).

disposition to anxiety (low HA). These trait anxieties arise as a function of (i) fragmented personality, which fuels doubts about own psychological safety (disintegration anxiety), or (ii) of the precarious cohesion of the compensatory self, which fuels doubts about one's own authenticity and purpose (existential anxiety). Both anxieties are likely unique to humans who, in developing self-awareness, opened the door to self-doubt, thereby expanding the repertoire of fear-inducing stimuli to abstract threats, such as concerns about one's own psychological cohesion, anticipation of failure, and metaphysical questions of purpose and meaning. The bed nucleus of the stria terminalis, an extension of the amygdala (the "fear center"), is believed to be the main brain region involved in such nonexplicit, more general, sometimes unrealistic or irrational anticipations of danger for this reason called anxiety and not fear. With dependent, narcissistic, paranoid, and anankastic variants, fragmentation anxieties are superimposed on the underlying anxious temperament and high HA ("dual anxiety").

The natural course of fragmentation anxieties is fluctuating, a function of the fluctuating degree of compensation achieved by compensatory functioning. Because of such a waxing and waning course, fragmentation anxieties may be misdiagnosed as *state* anxiety, frequently misleading treatment away from the root cause of the problem. As state anxieties and trait fragmentation anxieties differ in a number of fundamental ways, so do the corresponding treatments: state anxiety equally relies on medication and psychotherapy (e.g., cognitive behavioral therapy [CBT]) while fragmentation anxiety requires long-term reconstructive psychotherapy with only sporadic and short-term use of medications during periods of exacerbations. Such "comfort pharmacotherapy" is favored because surges of fragmentation anxiety can lead to the formation of new symptoms, the deepening of existing symptoms, or to regression. A warning signal is when an individual with fragmented personality reports that he or she is "never anxious." Such claims of total absence of anxiety indicate primitive defenses, notably denial and dissociation of affects, usually coupled with certain "macho" adaptive styles, especially antisocial.

Disintegration anxiety: psychological equivalent of the fear of dying. The most disturbing type of trait anxiety includes an eerie and profound feeling of mental fragility experienced by the patient who is struggling to maintain a cohesive sense of self. The patient experiences a disturbing uneasiness about his or her psychological safety. Kohut (1977) calls this "disintegration anxiety" and describes it as ill-defined (relative to specific anxieties) yet intense and pervasive, rooted in the patient's "dawning awareness" that the cohesion of his or her self is precarious and could easily disintegrate under adverse psychological circumstances. Should the precarious compensation provided by the unrealistic self-image fail, the patient is left defenseless against psychological collapse, resulting in a serious loss of initiative and self-esteem, a sense of utter meaninglessness (Kohut, 1977, p. 103) or, figuratively, psychological death. The fragmented personality core is at a continual risk of disintegration or, as Kohut calls it, loss of structure, leading to disintegration anxiety. In a book published posthumously, Kohut (1984) considers disintegration anxiety one of the deepest anxieties a human can experience, a psychological correspondent of the fear of physical death. The central content of this anxiety is difficult to describe. As Kohut (1984) points out "the attempt to describe disintegration anxiety is the attempt to describe the indescribable. But since it is a profound human experience, it is not an exact verbal definition that is called for, but rather an attempt to evoke a taste of the experience in question" (p. 16). Describing a similar observation, Klein (1952) talks about the "fear of invasive malevolence" with the paranoid-schizoid position (i.e., fragmented personality), which (the fear) is experienced as coming from the outside but ultimately deriving from the projection of the person's disintegration fears (imminent annihilation) causing paranoia, a phenomenon typical of all variants of personality disorder.

A special form of disintegration anxiety is *hypochondriasis*. Although cognitive anxiety (aka the "mental side of anxiety") is the most common type, a significant minority (up to 25%) of individuals with personality disorder present with the "somatic side of anxiety" as well. The latter refers to bodily symptoms reflecting autonomic arousal associated with anxiety, gastrointestinal distress, palpitations, vertigo, and headaches, fatigue, among others. In DSM-5, "somatic symptom and related disorders" is an umbrella category covering somatic symptom disorder,[20] defined as preoccupation with somatic manifestations (which are usually minimal and medically unexplainable), and "illness anxiety disorder" (aka "hypochondriasis"), defined as excessive concerns that one has a serious but undiagnosed disease (usually based on misinterpretations of normal or minor bodily sensations). The former (somatic symptom disorder) can be thought of as "disease conviction anxiety" resulting in demands for treatment while the latter and deeper (hypochondriasis) as "health worry anxiety" resulting in demands for diagnostic workups and does not respond to reassuring findings. In contrast to neuroses, where somatization serves as a defense mechanism, hypochondriasis arises from the core problem of fragmentation, a form of disintegration anxiety, and a deeply rooted

20. Formerly somatization disorder.

distrust in one's own health, whether mental or physical (it has been called "body psychosis"). Hypochondriasis is thus usually suggestive of personality disorder, particularly narcissistic, histrionic, antisocial, and paranoid. Reconstructive integrative psychotherapy is the treatment of choice; relaxation techniques and CBT may be helpful. Antidepressants are not very effective, especially not the monoamine oxidase inhibitors (MAOIs). Maintenance and relapse prevention studies confirm the value of continuing medication long-term in treatment responders.

Existential anxiety: a dim but unmistakable awareness of own pretense ("as if"). This form of trait anxiety arises from the ultimate inability of individuals with personality disorder to develop an authentic sense of meaning and true calling. Like disintegration anxiety, existential anxiety is rooted in the core pathology of personality disorder, the fragmented self and diffuse identity in particular. The patient, whether compensating by fantasized exaggerations (unrealistic deviant self) or by reliance on external sources for internal structure (e.g., ideological groups, cults), lives by the dictate of false motivations, beliefs, and assumptions, which provide protective but transparently artificial existence. He or she does not really trust his or her lifestyle, which feels like a fabrication; sorely lacks authenticity and passion, and profoundly doubts his or her purpose. As pointed out by Mollon (n.d.), the patient rigidly clings to these artificial solutions as if they were his or her own, even when these solutions are felt as dictatorial and cause pain. Most patients recognize their "as if" personality which is suggestive of some, albeit subconscious, awareness of their own impersonation according to the dictate of the compensatory self. Subconscious here means subliminal in the Jungian sense to refer to mental experiences consistent with phenomenal consciousness accessible to passive noticing, rather than active introspection. Such storing of the "as if" recognition within the subliminal enables the individual to, as it were, "avoid eye contact" with the psychological alien in their inner world, but, for most, especially amongst the highly intelligent, the precariousness and make-believe quality of their lives is transparent and deeply disturbing.

Anger and aggression: the default affect-behavior complex of personality disorder. If dysphoria is the default mood, anger[21] is the default affect in personality disorder. Here, we borrow from Kernberg (2015), who recently provided an insightful analysis of anger and aggression in fragmented personality. Massive negative representations make the individual predisposed toward experiencing others as persecutory and/or

21. Called "rage" when one has low or no power to control it.

rejecting. The experience is easily activated by negative stimulation in interactions, which put the patient in a chronically assumed role of a victim. Such a fixed persecutor-victim relationship leads to anger and aggression which the patient, by the mechanism of projective identification, attributes to others. In order to maintain the omnipotent power position and sense of control, the patient (victim) seeks conflicts with others (persecutors), and eventually becomes the victimizer. In short, an individual with fragmented personality is prone to anger and aggression, usually impulsive-affective outbursts, which further cement the polarized inner world and perpetuate the psychopathology of personality disorder.

Personality disorder is experienced intrapersonally but requires fantasy and even more so interpersonal stage to execute its compensatory role. The vital need of interpersonal stage may explain why trait-aggression sometimes alternates with helpless dependency: the dynamics reflects a frustrating stalemate between the need for inner organization and inability to achieve it without the supporting roles of selfobjects who define and maintain the patient's sense of self. [22] Active conflict seeking reflects the patient's attempts to change others into supporting his or her (the patient's) inner needs (aka "alloplastic adaptation"). Because of projective identification, the patient feels equally aggressive towards own self and towards the recipient of projected aggression during such conflicts. "I was furious at myself for being in a position to need anything from that horrible person," a patient once said. Such trait aggression maintains and fortifies personality fragmentation into "black- or-white" units of experience, making aggression a perpetuating mechanism in all variants of personality disorder, fearful, impulsive, and aloof alike. Aggression here does not refer to a heritable disposition or a drive (these would act as trait vulnerability) but arises as a consequence of fragmented personality and a (mis)perceived threat to self, which explains its ubiquitous presence and perpetuating effects in all variants of personality disorder.

Impulsive-affective aggression. Aggressive outbursts are usually impulsive, hostile, and accusatory, in response to a real or more frequently misattributed provocation (rejection, snub, or slight), accompanied by intense affect states of rage or fear. In the polarized inner world of the patient, negative stimulation (frustration, fear, perceived provocation) easily activates negative self- and object images and negative affect states (rage, anger, leading to aggressive behavior), which easily spin out of control, facing no serious opposition from hypofunctional cognitive

22. Another way is omnipotent fantasy as in the schizoid variant of personality disorder but not sufficient for patients with other variants.

processes (the mentioned amygdala hijack). The act of impulsive aggression is not gain oriented but is an end unto itself, aimed to destroy or correct the perceived provocation, which is a threat to the precarious inner compensation. Volatile interpersonal conflicts are the main avenue for the patient to coerce others to assume supporting roles. Violence is generally rare excepting the antisocial variant. Because of subeffective prefrontal control, the patient fears his or her own sadistic aggression and its destructive consequences. Internally, excessive affects can collapse the splitting mechanism, annihilate the positive fragments (figuratively, psychological death), and increase the risk of psychological disintegration, in some instances leading to psychosis and self-harm, among other serious consequences.

Predatory aggression. This type of aggression is variably referred to in the literature as predatory, premeditated, planned, organized, controlled, gain-oriented, and instrumental. The predator disguises his or her intentions, chooses a vulnerable target, and strategizes the attack, which is typically *not* a response to an immediate threat or provocation. It is called "instrumental" because it is driven by the expectation of reinforcement following the behavior, whether primary and/or secondary reinforcers (sex, money, property, etc.). Being a means to an end, predatory aggression requires effective impulse control and executive function. In humans, it is thought to be orchestrated by higher cortical systems and less driven by the hypothalamic and limbic structures in comparison to impulsive-affective aggression.

Career predatory aggression is rare with validly diagnosed personality disorder. These individuals usually have poor executive function, frequent erratic moods, and unstable goals and relationships—not the best set of features for successful predation. It can be occasional with schizoid and paranoid variants, and some antisocial personalities with schizoid traits. Sexual predation, either driven by sexual fantasies (frequently with compulsive features) or due to lack of sexual opportunity in the context of social isolation (prisons), is seen with schizoid and antisocial-schizoid variants. Some variants, notably paranoid and antisocial, manifest a mixture of impulsive-affective and controlled-planned aggression—"mixed aggression" (treatment is discussed in Chapter 5).

Rare with bona fide personality disorder, career predation is common as a self-approved social strategy by individuals with an egotistic character and an unprincipled system of moral values, but no profound personality fragmentation. Hence, we refer to it as "character disorder" to capture the pathology of social behavior which is not associated with a deep personality pathology of personality disorder but reflects one's adaptive strategy by choice, whether intuitive of deliberate, to get ahead by preying on others. Importantly, neural circuits underlying escalated predatory violence and moral decision-making largely overlap (Miczek et al., 2007; Raine and Yang, 2006). To improve public, forensic, and scientific classification of antisociality, we advocate that the concept of character disorder be reinstated as a diagnosis, to capture not only career criminal predators, as discussed, but also a spectrum of other repulsive or obnoxious social behaviors (arrogant, selfish, haughty, inconsiderate, entitled, Machiavellistic, greedy people) in the context of statistically integrated personality but underdeveloped prosociality (character) and egocentric morality ("if it benefits me, it's moral to do").

Emotional detachment and social disinterest. Emotional detachment, reserved and aloof emotions, emotional poverty, and disinterest in social relations are most frequently observed with schizoid, paranoid, anankastic, and antisocial individuals with prominent schizoid traits. The schizoid variant epitomizes emotional detachment and social disinterest. The defining features are social disinterest (referring to a peculiar lack of desire to have social contacts or sexual experiences), preference for a solitary lifestyle and activities ("loners"), indifference to praise or criticism, flattened emotions (negative and positive), excessive daydreaming (autistic fantasy), and excessive introspection. In contrast to other variants, these individuals are not conflict seeking, do not actively disturb the environment, keep to themselves, and rarely break laws or engage in risky behaviors. This variant is both experienced and expressed intrapersonally, as a form of unilateral adaptation. The individual appears to have withdrawn from the bilateral social world into the autistic world of fantasy and daydreaming, with full control over mental events, which is instrumental in organizing internal fragments. It is the pattern of such globally hypoactive temperament combined with personality fragmentation and compensatory withdrawal into fantasy that we consider a bona fide schizoid personality disorder. The main trait vulnerability is low social RD (social detachment), coupled with low NS (stoicism, low impulsivity), low HA (low sensitivity to fear), and low PE (indolence, lack of ambition). The neurobiology of detachment is discussed with mechanism-based pharmacotherapy of low social RD.

Some authors argue that schizoid is not a bona fide personality disorder but a member of the Schizophrenia spectrum. In our opinion, the controversy is fueled by incorrect diagnosis, rather than the invalidity of the schizoid variant. When properly diagnosed, this variant is equally frequent (~0.5%) in the general population and among the relatives of patients with Schizophrenia (Maier et al., 1994), questioning its genetic link with the latter. On the other hand, we all carry common genetic polymorphisms implicated in Schizophrenia. Those with a high genetic load but who do not reach the illness threshold may express social disinterest, emotional flattening, or detachment. These individuals certainly manifest genetic schizoid or schizophreniform features, but not schizoid personality disorder.

Cognitive distortions, dissociative phenomena, and psychotic symptoms. Psychosis is not continuous with normalcy. It follows a discontinuous distribution on the continuous liability scale, the latter determined by polygenes combined with epigenetic factors (Svrakic et al., 2013). In contrast, nonpsychotic cognitive distortions and odd beliefs are continuous in the general population, and follow a positively skewed normal distribution. Common superstitions (e.g., rituals for good luck and against bad luck) reflect elements of primary process ("magical") thinking, that is, denoting a fallacious attribution of causal relationships between actions and events. The severity varies from fleeting and mild to persistent and strong. The latter are held with conviction but not with delusional inflexibility. At its extreme and under stress, such magical thinking may reach the level of frank delusions seen in psychoses.

Individuals with any variant of personality disorder can more or less transiently regress to the psychotic level of mental functioning, especially those with a family history of psychosis and when they are under stress (hence the label "brief reactive" psychoses). The intensity of stress-related destructive anger or apprehension may erode the precarious stability of the mind achieved through the compensatory self, perhaps by overriding the splitting mechanism, thereby opening the floodgates for the primary process to impair reality testing. The concept of primary process refers to nonlinear, often nonverbal thinking. It employs concrete symbolization, condensation, and displacement, resulting in disregard for logical connections, contradictions, and realities. Patients with a latent psychotic potential may experience such reactive regressions to the psychotic level rather frequently.

Here belong dissociative phenomena of depersonalization and derealization, frequently co-occurring, and defined as disconnection in the experience of self and the outside world, respectively. Dissociation can be thought of as "thinking and perceiving without feeling." It is thought to be the mind's way of dealing with distress that threatens its integrity, such as tension, apprehension, boredom, panic, conflictuous motivations, among others. The experience is described as dreamlike or surreal, accompanied by a sense of blurred borders with the outside world, interrupted continuity in the sense of self (feeling divorced from one's own personal self), a distorted perception of time, and interference with mindfulness. Usually, there is no notable memory disturbances and reality testing remains intact. The experience can be mild or severely disturbing, at times crippling, stirring up a profound fear of disintegration. More pathological (persistent, severe) forms are classified as "dissociative disorders" in DSM-5, as persistent or recurrent depersonalization and/or derealization, dissociative amnesia, or dissociated identity. Short-lived experiences of depersonalization are common in the general population (~20% annual prevalence), and are in fact the third most common psychological symptom after anxiety and depression (Simeon, 2004). Mild depersonalization and derealization can happen to anyone who is experiencing anxiety or stress, but it can be chronic and/or recurrent in individuals who have experienced childhood interpersonal trauma (stress, neglect, abuse), who have DSM borderline personality disorder (meaning personality disorder in general), and who suffer from chronic anxiety (panic disorder, OCD, GAD), migraine, sleep deprivation, jet lag, or temporal lobe epilepsy, among others. This vitiation of the perception-emotion-cognition union appears to arise from widespread alterations in metabolic activity in the sensory association cortex, or dysfunctional hyperactivation of PFCx, perhaps the default network, resulting in inhibition of limbic responses to aversive stimuli or experiences. Autonomic blunting and hypothalamic-pituitary-adrenal axis dysregulation have also been reported (Simeon, 2004). *Déjà vu* and *jamais vu*, frequently mistaken as dissociative phenomena, are actually reflective of dysfunctional memory, not dissociation.

Chronic and mainly subpsychotic ("soft") cognitive distortions observed in personality disorder fall into two broad categories:

1. Symptoms of *loose (undisciplined) cognitive functioning* are rooted in the fragmented infrastructure of the mind and reflect a strong presence of the primary process, dominated by wishes, conflicts, affects, and fantasy (Auchincloss and Samberg, 2012), all of which are frequent in personality disorder. The operative phrase is "strong presence," not the mind controlled by the primary process, as in psychosis. The approximately even mixture of primary and secondary process (the latter based on logic, reality, and problem-solving) is distinctive for personality disorder. These individuals characteristically manifest limitations in reality testing both in terms of deficits in the subtle aspects of interpersonal functioning (Kernberg, 2015), and in their sense of self, filled with fantasies only vaguely recognized as wishful.
2. Symptoms of *biased cognitive functioning* arise from the unrealistic compensatory self which dictates subtype-specific cognitive distortions

and motivational priorities. A few selected examples include egocentric perception of reality (primarily defined through the prism of one's own needs, such as misattribution of admiration by narcissistic personalities), pervasive suspiciousness with paranoid personality ("no one is to be trusted"), sexualization of all interpersonal contacts with histrionic personality (control by seduction), behaviors revolving around pecking-order type dominance with antisocial personality (submissive to the stronger, ruthless to the weaker), or isolation into the fantasy world, "far from the maddening crowd" with schizoid personality, among others. Pharmacotherapy of these cognitive symptoms is discussed in Chapter 5.

INTERPERSONAL RELATIONS: A SCARRED, UNFORGIVING CHILD WITH A CONTINUING NEED FOR SELFOBJECTS

Literary all phenomenology, symptoms, and signs of personality disorder are on full display in interpersonal relationships. The latter represent one of the two stages for the compensatory self-image to operate; the other avenue is fantasy. As a step forward, both the DSM-5 alternative model and ICD-11 recognize the important role of interpersonal dysfunction in the diagnosis of personality disorder. As Kernberg (2015) noted, all peak affect states involve a relationship between self and others. Peak affect states, whether revengeful aggression or primitive idealization, are common with these individuals, placing others in the way of such stable instability in self and object images, which render interpersonal relations turbulent and incoherent. The phrase "I hate you, don't leave me" summarizes the dynamics, especially if amended by the expectation of unconditional approval. Limited cognitive regulation of mood and impulses causes great difficulties in interpersonal and/or partner relationships and life and work arrangements, most of which are disorganized, chaotic, transient, and poorly defined. Relationships are built quickly and intensely, and broken up with the same pace and intensity, swing between idealization, anger, and detachment, always at the brink of a collapse (this is also a major obstacle in establishing and maintaining a relationship with the therapist). Relationships are impoverished insofar they revolve around a few juvenile themes (e.g., acceptance-abandonment, support-betrayal) for years after the relationship is established. We discuss a selection of interpersonal features next; others are discussed throughout the book.

Why do people with personality disorder not learn from previous interpersonal fiascos but keep repeating the same interpersonal patterns over and over, despite isolation, dislike, and (even) ridicule? The dynamics is, we believe, rooted in the underlying fragmented personality: these individuals have "unfinished business" with selfobjects (in terms of unfinished personality integration), with little capacity to deal with actual objects. Each variant of personality disorder is characterized by a general interpersonal dysfunction best summarized as a need for enduring selfobject-type approval in a unilateral manner. Outside of the one-way and intense relationship with selfobjects, the connection with other people is weak and ill defined. Interpersonal actions and interactions primarily concern the psychological state of the individual, while external adaptation is of secondary importance with very little actual social learning. Active seeking of interpersonal conflicts is intended to change others' reactions to one's own misconduct as the way to manage stress (alloplastic adaptation) or to coerce them to follow the expected synopsis for the supporting cast (i.e., to become selfobjects who define, support-maintain, and reinforce the patient's compensatory self). In Kohut's (1971;1977) terms, the patient has never transmuted selfobjects into a cohesive independent self but rather as an adult continues to need others to be selfobjects to help define and organize his or her inner world. As a result, control of others increases the stability of the patient's own mind. Those who are not engaged as selfobjects, and to an even greater extent those who express even minor criticism, are seen as conducting malicious and personal attacks. Even compliant selfobjects are seen through their function as "mirrors" or "idols," not as independent human beings. Inflammatory interpersonal conflicts are the main way to address "provocations" (usually misperceived) fueled by the associated intense negative emotions, rage in particular, which further sabotage the already suboptimal cortical influence on the patient's own behavior. "The lack of affective integration maintains the primitivity of negative affects, and fosters impulsivity in order to deal with unavoidable negative experiences" (Kernberg, 2015, p. 7). The negativistic-dependent and anankastic variants of personality disorder seek conflicts through passive rather than active aggression.

Selfishness, exploitation, manipulation, unreliable reciprocation, and similar misuse of others are interpersonal features shared by all variants of personality disorder. The motivations vary, from vengefulness, entitlement, and grandiosity to outright immorality, among others. Interpersonal immorality uniquely distinguishes personality disorder from other types of nonpsychotic psychopathology and psychoses. Due to poorly integrated, unprincipled moral values, these patients do not recognize the effects of their own immorality on others ("moral blindness") and have difficulties in appreciating genuine moral principles in others ("moral cynicism"). Other interpersonal aspects of immorality are mock ethics (leaving a false impression of morality) and pathological lying (leaving a false impression of success and stability).

Each variant of personality disorder demonstrates its own specific style of interpersonal deviance. The shared affect state is revengeful anger, manifested as omnipotent fantasies of control and frequently as overt aggression. Accordingly, each variant shows a significant association with vindictiveness, distrust and suspiciousness of others, and decreased concern about the needs or safety of others. All of these rather extraordinary features are accompanied by minimal personal distress, suggestive of ego-syntonicism, as reported in a recent meta-analysis (Wilson et al., 2017). Other aspects of interpersonal relations are stylistically molded by the particular compensatory self-image. The latter defines one's style of interaction as a means to maintain inner organization. The schizoid, paranoid, and callous antisocial variants of personality disorder are characterized by social coldness and disinterest, lack of empathy, low intimacy, and occasional crime, with antisocial and paranoid variants tending to be more vindictive and domineering than the schizoid variant. With the domineering, exhibitionistic, and intrusive variants (antisocial, narcissistic, histrionic), the distinguishing features are grandiosity and social coldness (narcissistic and antisocial), or sexualization of all relationships, theatricality, and rush into intimacy (histrionic). Reticence, rigidity, and perfectionism characterize interpersonal relationships of the anankastic variant, while a domineering, passively aggressive dependency characterize the negativistic-dependent variant. A detailed meta-analysis of interpersonal traits and their variation across relationship domains (parent-child, family, peer, romantic) is reported in Wilson et al. (2017).

An informative study examined interpersonal profiles of "borderline" (i.e., fragmented) individuals using the interpersonal circumplex model (Wright et al., 2013). Borderline symptoms were associated with general interpersonal distress with heterogeneous interpersonal styles trending toward non-assertiveness, with only modest prototypicality. Latent class analysis revealed that within this global pattern there were six subgroups with distinct profiles: nonassertive, avoidant, exploitable (extreme and moderate), intrusive, and vindictive (Wright et al., 2013). The authors conclude that individuals with borderline pathology comprise an interpersonally heterogeneous group with several distinctive styles, roughly corresponding to individual adaptive styles of schizoid, dependent, histrionic, narcissistic, paranoid, and antisocial variants. These results, we believe, support the concept of fragmented personality as the totipotent ancestor modifiable into a number of compensatory self-images, each with a respective behavioral and interpersonal style, as discussed next.

INDIVIDUAL VARIANTS OF PERSONALITY DISORDER: THE SEVEN FACES OF FRAGMENTED PERSONALITY

We describe seven clinical variants of personality disorder as distinct but in fact usually overlapping (mixed) adaptive styles arising from the compensatory self-image: schizoid, paranoid, antisocial, narcissistic, histrionic, negativistic-dependent, and anankastic. The relatively distinct behavioral and phenomenological façade stands in contrast to the shared fragmentation cutting across these variants. They all show, albeit in the background of the dominant image, an inconsistent sense of self, incoherent identity, fragile self-esteem, sense of inauthenticity, feelings of inferiority, emptiness and boredom, anger and aggression, lack of genuine interest, dysphoria, paranoid fears, among other shared features. Official systems largely ignore this covert shared dimension between the variants.

Behavioral *adaptation* and personality *disorder* are fundamentally different concepts. An adaptive style can be observed along the entire spectrum of mental health and disorder: a completely healthy and a profoundly fragmented personality may have a similar adaptive style (Table 2.3). Adaptive styles summarize the content (the what) of someone's functioning. Normalcy or psychopathology are not decided by adaptive styles but by the underlying degree of integration of personality ("no mind fragmentation, no personality disorder"). In everyday clinical diagnosis, at the minimum, identity coherence, reality testing, defense mechanisms, and interpersonal relations are used to assess this degree. The seven adaptive variants, each with its official DSM-5 label and polythetic criteria (total number with a minimum for diagnosis) are described in Table 2.3. The DSM criteria have been validated as clinical descriptors of pervasive maladaptive styles. The criteria are better conceptualized as a dimension quantifying the pervasiveness of behavior ("more is worse"). Their number of criteria as a cut-off for the diagnosis is completely arbitrary. In Table 2.3 both official and colloquial terms for each style of adaptation are used. Colloquialisms are positive connotations for traditional diagnostic categories and more natural descriptions of personality (Joines and Stewart, 2002), here used to imply healthy adaptive styles.

Table 2.3 ADAPTIVE STYLES AND DSM-5 CRITERIA FOR PERSONALITY DISORDER VARIANTS

Personality Adaptation	Personality Disorder
Common general features: **identity**: integrated, historically coherent **defense mechanisms**: higher order, mature and neurotic (centered around suppression and repression) **reality testing**: intact **object relations**: whole **interpersonal relations**: stable and/or ambivalent **social adaptation**: functional (auto and alloplastic)	*Common general features*: **identity**: diffuse, historically incoherent **defense mechanisms:** lower order, mostly immature (centered around splitting) **reality testing**: mainly preserved but with limitations (under stress, in subtle aspects of interpersonal functioning) **object relations**: partial (fragmented) **interpersonal relations**: subserving inner organization **social adaptation**: maladapted, alloplastic (conflict-prone)
Colloquial names	***Classical nosology*** **DSM-5 Cluster A:** ***odd, eccentric***
BRILLIANT SKEPTIC Cautious, seeks control, highly analytical and perceptive: the clearest, sharpest, most detailed thinker of all, seldom misses anything; authoritative, ambitious and competitive; skeptical, tends to anticipate but not convinced of malicious motivations of others; hypervigilant, alert and keeps on top of things; likes to be in charge; bright, highly sensitive; avoids confiding but can be close to few friends and partners; strives to be perfect and strong. *Areas of difficulty*: may be grandiose ("knows it all") and rigid in thinking patterns ("my way or highway"); may be hyper-critical and blaming of others but retracts rapidly in important relationships; hypersensitive, believes in subjective assessments without checking them; fear of getting too close in relationships; wants to be informed to avoid being vulnerable; tends to be jealous and envious of others; attacks when scared.	**DSM-5 PARANOID PD** **(6 criteria, 4 minimum for diagnosis):** 1. suspects, without sufficient basis, that others are exploiting, harming, or deceiving him/her; 2. preoccupation with unjustified doubts about the loyalty or trustworthiness of friends or associates; 3. reluctance to confide in others because of unwarranted fear that the information will be used maliciously against him/her; 4. reads hidden demeaning or threatening meanings into benign remarks or events; persistently bears grudges, i.e., is unforgiving of insults, injuries, or slights; 5. perceives attacks on his/her character or reputation that are not apparent to others and is quick to react angrily or to counterattack; 6. has recurrent suspicions, without justification, regarding fidelity of spouse or sexual partner.

(*continued*)

Table 2.3 CONTINUED

Personality Adaptation	Personality Disorder
CREATIVE DAYDREAMER Highly sensitive, shy, kind, and supportive of others; comfortable with solitude, prefers solitary activities and one-to-one relationships when can relate in-depth; eccentric, spiritual; rare initiative for social relationships but accepts invitations by friends to participate; creative and deep thinker; tries to be strong and stoical ("does not have needs"), shows reduced emotional expression but reacts to praise and approval *Areas of difficulty*: can be seen as aloof , "idle" daydreaming in the world of fantasies; reduced verbal communication; keeps low profile; avoids making demands as these may mean closeness; ignores own needs until stressed; withdraws when criticized (hence may overlook important aspects of reality).	**DSM-5 SCHIZOID PD** **(7 criteria, 4 minimum for diagnosis)** 1. neither wants nor likes close relationships, counting being part of a family; 2. almost constantly picks introverted activities; 3.little if any, thought in engaging in any sexual experiences; 4. seldom derives pleasure from any activities; 5. has no close friends other than immediate relatives; 6. appears apathetic to the admiration or disapproval of others; - 7. emotional coldness, detachment, or flattened affectivity.
Colloquial names	*Classical nosology* **DSM-5 Cluster C:** ***fearful***
RESPONSIBLE WORKAHOLIC Responsible, conscientious, reliable; mostly respected for reliability and punctuality; hard-working and usually successful in career; scrupulous, meticulous, neat; conforming to rules; values control and order; strives to be perfect; strict moral standards; over-adapted. *Areas of difficulty*: difficulty enjoying what is accomplished; rarely relaxes, plays, and has fun; strict conscience makes him or her own worst critic; may feel anxious and guilty; wants very much close relationships but can be critical and/or passive-aggressive when others don`t meet his or her high standards.	**DSM-5 O-C PD (ANANKASTIC)** **(8 criteria, 4 minimum for diagnosis)** 1. preoccupation with details, rules, lists, order, organization, or schedule to the extent that the major point of the activity is lost; 2. perfectionism that interferes with task completion; 3. excessive devotion to work and productivity to the exclusion of pleasure and interpersonal relationships; 4. over-conscientiousness, scrupulousness, and inflexibility about matters of morality, ethics, or values; 5. inability to discard worn-out or worthless objects (hoarding); 6. inability to delegate tasks or to work with others unless they submit exactly to his/her her way of doing things; 7. rigidity and stubbornness; 8. miserly spending style toward both self and others (money is viewed as something to be hoarded for future catastrophes or unreasonable reluctance to allow others to do things)

Table 2.3 CONTINUED

Personality Adaptation	Personality Disorder
NEGATIVISTIC FOLLOWER	**DSM-5 DEPENDENT PD** **(8 criteria, 5 minimum for diagnosis)**
Pacific temperament, helpful, cooperative and agreeable frequently at own expense; Pollyanna cognitive style but lacks confidence to be fully independent; seeks a capable person for support, tends to feel inferior, inadequate, less efficient or capable than others; prefers to be a follower not a leader; worries about losing support; if angry, expresses passive aggression (complains, pouting); indecisive, rarely forms firm standings in controversial themes *Areas of difficulty*: strong expectation of nurturance/protection may make others feel they are not doing enough (uneasy relationships); despite talents frequent underachiever due to difficulty to separate from the nurturing selfobject; pouts after perceived lack of nurturance, anxious outside comfort zone; has a hard time asking directly what he or she wanted; attracts attention in negative ways (helplessness, neediness, pouting)	1. difficulty making routine decisions without input, reassurance, and advice from others; 2. requires others to assume responsibilities which he/she should be attending to; 3. fear of disagreeing with others and risking disapproval; 4. difficulty starting projects without support from others; 5. excessive need to obtain nurturance and support from others, even allowing other to impose themselves rather than risk rejection or disapproval; 6. feels vulnerable and helpless when alone; 7. desperately seeks another relationship when one ends; 8. unrealistic preoccupation with being left alone and unable to care for him/herself. *Note: passive-aggressive traits are pronounced in the dependent variant of personality disorder. Accordingly, we define the negativistic-dependent variant. These individuals have a fused identity with their selfobject, expect to be nurtured/protected and express passive aggression when not, i.e., when face own helplessness*
Colloquial names	**Classical nosology** **DSM-5 Cluster B: dramatic**
OVER-REACTING ENTHUSIAST Enthusiastic, active, fun, and enjoyable to be around; high energy and very imaginative, cares for appearance; enjoys relating to people and helping them feel good; loves to be center of attention; tends to please others; very dramatic, with accentuated emotional reactivity; fast in behavior and speech, impatient.	**DSM-5 HISTRIONIC PD** **(7 criteria, 5 minimum for diagnosis)** 1. attention-seeking, self-dramatization, theatricality, exaggerated expression of emotion; 2. inappropriate sexual seductiveness; 3. rapidly shifting and shallow expression of emotions; 4. physical appearance used to draw attention to self;

(*continued*)

Table 2.3 CONTINUED

Personality Adaptation	Personality Disorder
OVER-REACTING ENTHUSIAST *Areas of difficulty*: may escalate feelings when upset; tends to hide justified anger or dissent for concern of hurting other people, moves away from difficult situations rather than trying to find a solution; excessive attention seeking, may become interpersonally seductive; may be seen as self-centred and vain.	**DSM-5 HISTRIONIC PD** 5. speech is excessively impressionistic and lacking in detail; - 6. suggestibility, 7. relationships seen as more intimate than they actually are.
SELF-ABSORBED CHARMER Charming, verbose, exhibitionistic (showing off), can be highly successful in career; acts as if he/she is perfect, capable, and has no problems or can solve any problem easily; sense of self-importance or specialness; hypersensitive to failures to which he/she responds with shame but may recover quickly; carefully disguises deficient empathy and low-self esteem; can be a successful artist, fund raiser, actor, etc. *Areas of difficulty:* self-absorbed (difficulty accepting he/she is not the center of the universe, and that other people`s feelings and needs have to be taken into consideration along with his/her); feels defective when vulnerable, if not special and unique; may fake empathy as socially desirable.	**DSM-5 NARCISSISTIC PD** **(9 criteria, 5 minimum for diagnosis)** 1. grandiose sense of self-importance; 2. fantasies of unlimited success, power, brilliance, beauty, or ideal love; 3. self-perception of being "special"; 4. need for constant and excessive admiration; 5. sense of entitlement; 6. exploitative of others to achieve personal gain; 7. lack of empathy; 8. intense envy; 9. arrogant and haughty demeanor
ADVENTUROUS MANIPULATOR Charismatic risk taker; loves action and risky excitements; effective agitator to start new movements; dresses to shock, seduce, or impress; tries to outdare those around; invests a lot of energy in attempt to dominate and control, to be tough; can be a successful explorer, fundraiser, salesman, frequently becomes entrepreneur, soldier, political leader, field journalist, police officer, etc.	**DSM-5 ANTISOCIAL PD** **(7 criteria, 3 minimum for diagnosis)** 1. failure to conform to social and legal norms (behavior grounds for arrest); 2. deception (lying, use of aliases, or conning); 3. impulsivity or failure to plan ahead; 4. irritability and aggressiveness; 5. reckless disregard for safety of self or others;

Table 2.3 CONTINUED

Personality Adaptation	Personality Disorder
ADVENTUROUS MANIPULATOR	**DSM-5 ANTISOCIAL PD**
Areas of difficulty: tends to manipulate and take advantage of others; ignores or excludes rules (the ends justify the means); may intimidate others to gain advantage; can disregard rights of others; can be impulsive, selfish, egocentric; lack of empathy not perceived as a problem; has difficult time with intimacy (avoids being "soft"), is afraid to trust and is "commitment phobic" (abandons before he/she can be abandoned), can be close only when in full control.	6. consistent irresponsibility (failure to sustain consistent work or honor financial obligations); 7. lack of remorse; - **at least 18 years old;** - **evidence of conduct disorder with onset before age 15 years.**

PD = personality disorder; DSM-5 = *Diagnostic and Statistical Manual of Mental Disorders* (fifth ed.; APA, 2013).

Personality disorder is defined not by adaptive styles, not by personality traits, and not even by the intensity of these traits but by the fragmented level of functioning compensated for by a defensive self-image, maintained externally by selfobjects and internally by fantasy. Adaptive styles can be thought of as "horizontal diagnoses" that helps determine the variant of personality disorder (*what* a person thinks, feels, or brings into a relationship). In social contexts, adaptive styles are "delivered" by character traits: raw and self-serving in the context of immature character, measured and sublimated in the context of mature character. As described in Chapter 3, levels of functioning are assessed for "vertical diagnosis" (*how* a person feels, thinks, relates in the relationship): the same adaptive style will have different qualities at different levels of mental functioning (from casual and flexible to vitally needed to psychologically survive). Vertical diagnosis determines the depth of treatment, which must be reconstructive, not simply reparative, for the deep fragmentation of personality disorder. Horizontal diagnosis determines the way of treatment (how to approach the patient).

No style of adaptation presents as pure but is instead uniquely interwoven with other styles. One style is usually dominant (primary), while secondary, even tertiary styles serve as modulators that nevertheless influence treatment planning. For example, histrionic-anankastic adaptation is similar yet importantly different from histrionic-antisocial adaptation, with the histrionic style being primary in both. Millon et al. (2009; Millon's Clinical Multiaxial Inventory) describe a detailed phenomenology of dozens of combinations of adaptive styles, configured as trios of common styles, helpful for clinical systematization of subtle individual variations. By doing so, Millon et al. have stratified averages almost to the point of being specific for individual cases, in accord with recent trends of personalized evidence-based approaches. Joines and Stewart (2002) further qualify adaptive styles vis-à-vis their function: at least one style for "survival" (e.g., under stress) and one for "presentation" (to fulfill expectations), thereby adding another dimension to individualized diagnosis. In summary, seven discernible adaptive styles are defined based on the primary style which dominates the combination, rather than being prototypes.

Adaptive styles may include any combination of behavior patterns. The common combinations are antisocial and paranoid (As+Pa), antisocial and narcissistic (As+Na), narcissistic and histrionic (Na+Hi), narcissistic and anankastic (Na+An), schizoid and anankastic (Sc+An), anankastic and histrionic (An+Hi), and negativistic-dependent and histrionic (N/D+Hi), among others. The most frequent are combinations within the same cluster; somewhat less frequent but not rare are intercluster combinations, such as narcissistic and anankastic (Na+An).

Next we present five vignettes of de-identified[23] patients that illustrate that one's adaptive style is most commonly a mixture of prototypes as well as the duality of the self-experience of these individuals.

De-identified vignettes: the phenomenology of the dual self and mixed adaptive styles. The following vignettes illustrate the phenomenology and adaptive styles of individuals with fragmented personality, the way they see and experience themselves and the way they present socially. These are real people, but here we only report heavily modified excerpts to illustrate the duality of the self-image and mixed adaptive styles in personality disorder. Quotation marks indicate the exact original words used by the patient.

1. **A Lonely Princess**
   (schizoid-negativistic/dependent variant of fragmented personality)
   Self-reported symptoms: persistent dysphoria, cutting skin to "release tension," multiple fears, of crowds, streets, people; isolated and

23. De-identification means that the person's identity cannot be connected with information.

disinterested socially, can't find a steady romantic partner; "idling in life and school".

Compensatory self-image: lonely princess: righteous victim, "misunderstood" princess, unjustly left behind but actually better than others:"others have gotten what belongs to me," passive aggressive towards others (gossip, procrastination), feels dignified in her loneliness by choice.

Real self: feels deprived and victimized, inferior, envy, suicidal thoughts; guarded, critical of everyone but appreciates positive feedback; dissatisfied, bashful, and reticent; revengeful but scared of own anger.

2. **A Tamed Shrew**
(histrionic-narcissistic variant of fragmented personality)

Self-reported symptoms: obese (50 lbs above ideal weight), now with asthma; "My boyfriends do not stay for long, break up with me one after another"; "I might be too direct in my expectations"; "I don't know what to think about my family, friends . . . they are all actually distant." "I do so much for everyone, but get so little in return"; "I am unhappy".

Compensatory self-image: omnipotent rescuer (of everything and everyone): the dominant façade is joyful communicability, highly competitive, tries hard to leave the impression of a very strong, "can-do" person who always feels "fantastic," energetic; fakes closeness to put herself in a position to seduce and rescue, uncritical toward her own objective capacities.

Real self: angry at everyone, feels horrified inside "like the Munch's 'Scream,'" feels as if she was "sitting naked on a slab of ice, stuck to the frozen surface, can't get up . . . would leave half of my body behind," strong but subliminal feeling of inferiority.

3. **A Prince on a White Horse**
(narcissistic-antisocial variant of fragmented personality)

Self-reported symptoms: "auto-sabotaging"; always late, "people think of me as unreliable," although successful unsure of his decisions, relationships; craves closeness but highly promiscuous; now concerned that some work-related unethical decisions (softly illegal) could get him in trouble.

Compensatory self-image: the prince of greatness: handsome, arrogant, boastful, flashy, seductive womanizer, professionally successful (manages a big, rich company), strives for perfection but undermines self with professionally and legally questionable decisions, manipulative, takes pride in his ability to cheat: " Nietzsche said that scruples only slow you down".

Real self: a little boy: second-guesses all decisions, needs someone to lead him, feels like a "little boy fretful of being sent to the quiet corner" for doing something wrong, bored and empty when nothing "special" is happening.

4. **A Queen of the Night**
   (paranoid-anankastic variant of fragmented personality)
   Self-reported symptoms: dysphoria, "shaken by her imminent divorce", disarray in the family ("I am unable to control it"), damaged interpersonal relationships due to her "moodiness", hostile work environment (the patient sees all as the fault of others).
   Compensatory self- image: righteous persecutor: projects the image of a domineering, angry, serious ("hates jokes"), and annoyed "knows-it-all," verbally authoritarian, categorical, aggressive comments, strong need for control. Typical interpersonal pattern: goes hard after people for minor omissions, then "forgives" them grudgingly.
   Real self: poor victim: depressed, lonely, unhappy, distrustful, tries hard to put everything in order, suspicious of friends and family, unsure of their real motives (vital need: closeness and trust).
5. **A Heroic Rescuer**
   (histrionic-narcissistic variant of fragmented personality)
   Self-reported symptoms: multiple somatic symptoms, oscillating moods - "my mood changes constantly from elated to worried," highly anxious most of the time—feels false, fake; "I am inefficient at work, in school," although generally considered to be talented (collateral information).
   Compensatory self-image: heroic rescuer: joyful, charming, wide smile, goes out of his way to help everyone, active, full of ideas and initiatives, emotionally appears worm and engaged, views himself as "energetic motivator".
   Real self: an angry sulky victim: deeply unhappy, passive, "I am falling apart inside"; "it feels like a huge boulder is rolling inside that's going to kill me"; self-absorbed into worries about own psychological safety.

CLINICAL VARIANTS OF PERSONALITY DISORDER ARE MORE ALIKE THAN DIFFERENT

Despite efforts to classify personality disorder into distinct symptomatic categories (ICD, DSM) or using the severity criterion (as more or less severe) (Kernberg), individual clinical variants are fundamentally more alike than different. Although behavior styles differ between the individual variants, the most frequent presentation is mixed, as discussed. More importantly, the functional dynamics and phenomenology, both critical for a precise diagnosis, are shared. All true cases of personality disorder are of *high severity*, with predominantly partial object relations, fragmented subsystems of personality, split-off real self, and compensatory deviance. Without these characteristics the diagnosis of personality disorder is not warranted in the first place. Some quantitative variation is expected, however. In all nature, quantitative variations in the expression of a phenotype are not entitized, because a more fundamental principle for classification is used, as Darwin powerfully showed. With personality disorder, that fundamental principle is a fragmented personality, which underlies an enduring, pervasive, frequent, and predominant pattern of mental dysfunction, referred to as "fragmented level of functioning," intrinsically a severe psychopathology. Individual differences among those who predominantly function at the fragmented level do not exceed one-fourth of a standard deviation (15% variation), thus staying within the range of severe. Those who manifest partial object relations, primitive defenses, or incoherences in identity, but in a sporadic, temporary, or selective manner, do not warrant the diagnosis of personality disorder, as discussed.

Our early research (Divac-Jovanovic et al., 1993) showed that different stylistic variants of personality disorder share a common denominator: patients with a valid DSM-III diagnosis of personality disorder (all subtypes) were found to share high scores on the "borderline dimension," a measure of severity in the Millon's Clinical Multiaxial Inventory (the 1987 version). Moreover, the borderline dimension distinguished patients with any personality disorder (those who made the DSM-III cut-off) from those who did not make the cut-off for that particular subtype but had similar behavior styles ("controls with matching behavior styles"). This result was our first to indicate that "borderline" may be better conceptualized as a dimension shared by all subtypes rather than itself a subtype of personality disorder. This shared core dimension makes clinical variants of personality disorder more fundamentally alike than different in terms of *developmental dynamics* (early developmental deficit followed by active pathological growth), *phenomenology* (the "stable instability"), *psychodynamics* (partial object relations, immature defenses, the characteristic "duality" of the self, incoherent identity), and *interpersonal relationships* (turbulent, unstable and oscillating, subserving inner organization at the expense of social adaptation).

ON SOME CONTROVERSIAL ISSUES

Decriminalizing antisocial personality disorder. Antisocial personality disorder is widely viewed as synonymous for illegal and/or criminal behaviors, but in fact these are *optional* features which are neither necessary nor specific for the diagnosis. More important for the diagnosis are the features indicative of profound personality pathology (fragmented personality). Accordingly, Hare's (1996) widely used psychopathy checklist (PCL), the best available diagnostic tool for antisocial personality disorder, includes one underlying factor of personality pathology (corresponding to the DSM "borderline" personality with affective, behavioral, and interpersonal instability) and three factors of behavioral symptoms: (i) arrogant and deceitful interpersonal style (superficial charm, inflated sense of self-worth, pathological lying, and conning-manipulative); (ii) deficient affective experience (lack of remorse or guilt, shallow affect, callousness, lack of empathy, failure to accept responsibility for own actions); and (iii) impulsive and irresponsible behavioral style (need for stimulation, proneness to boredom, irresponsibility, impulsivity, parasitic lifestyle, lack of realistic long-term goals). In brief, the PCL captures a profound personality pathology behind the three correlated antisocial dimensions, summarized as narcissism, lack of empathy, and impulsivity, respectively. Criminal behavior is *optional*, and is neither diagnostic of nor specific to antisocial personality disorder.

"Psychopathy" and "sociopathy" (Greek "*psykhe*" for "mind," Latin "*socius*" for a tribe or a city; in both Greek "*pathos*" for suffering) have been replaced with the term "antisocial personality disorder." This seems appropriate for the concept of psychopathy[24] ("suffering of the mind") but not for the concept of sociopathy ("suffering of the society"). The defining feature of sociopathy is violation of social norms, a far more prevalent occurrence than antisocial personality disorder. The majority of transgressions are in fact performed by people who do not meet the criteria for personality disorder but manifest a character-based and self-approved antisocial/criminal adaptive strategy, as discussed next.

What is not a personality disorder: character disorder—an abandoned but useful concept. The concept of character disorder, eliminated by both the WHO and the APA as "stigmatizing", is useful both clinically and forensically. Individuals engage in violence and victimization of others for a host of reasons. The concept of character disorder helps differentiate antisocial

24. Psychopathy as conceptualized by Hare (1996) is equivalent with antisocial personality disorder, a compensatory albeit antisocial solution for the fragmented personality core.

personality disorder (formerly "psychopaths") from career criminals with no appreciable personality fragmentation (formerly "sociopaths"). It also helps distinguish any variant of personality disorder from a number of other abusive character traits, for example, habitually selfish, violent, egotistic, greedy, parasitic, predatory, and exploitative individuals, among many others. As noted, character is partly rooted in internal models of behavior developed with caregivers (thus not involving volition and deliberation) and is partly formed by a choice of adaptive strategies during adolescence or young adulthood. The choice of antisociality is made based on one's assessment, whether calculated or intuitive, of the most effective ways to ensure personal success and/or obtain resources (to get ahead) without necessarily committing to observing the social norms (i.e., to get along). In short, antisociality here is self-approved as adaptive strategy. Popular concepts of character imply self-made psychological features, suggesting that individuals with character disorder somehow willfully opted to be deviant. With what was said previously, this is to an extent true.

Social predation: career predators. As discussed, human career predators combine elements of classical predation (disguised intention, premeditation, vulnerable targets) with elements of offensive aggression (seizure of resources with or without violence). Such mixed aggression is accompanied by more or less significant cardiovascular and emotional arousal and adrenaline rush. In other words, career social predators are not necessarily cold-blooded but are able to keep emotions in check by cognitive control, with the assistance of a notably high IQ and consummate executive function (Ishikawa et al., 2001; Bate et al., 2014). Such executive ability enables them to maintain heightened awareness and focus while blocking other sensory information and controlling autonomic arousal, which all contribute to the effectiveness of predation; hence the label "controlled" aggression in contrast to impulsive affective outbursts of antisocial personality disorder (although a subgroup of the latter may engage in controlled predation as well).

Comparative analysis of immorality and criminality: not all crime is created equal. Antisocial and immoral behaviors fall in to three main categories with some overlap between them but retaining relatively distinct origins within the categories, namely dynamics, phenomenology, and manifestations (Table 2.4).

As seen in Table 2.4, the listed variables are diverse, ranging from the degree of personality integration to colloquial labels. The first column analyzes individuals whose immorality and/or criminality occur in the context of antisocial personality disorder. The next two columns describe antisocial characters, individuals with an integrated personality core but

Table 2.4 COMPARATIVE ANALYSIS OF IMMORALITY[A] AND ANTISOCIAL BEHAVIORS

Nosology → Variable ↓	Antisocial Personality Disorder antisociality as Modus Vivendi [b]	Character Disorder antisociality as Modus Operandi [c]	Character Disorder antisociality as Modus Imperandi[d]
	←overlapping etiology, phenomenology, and behaviors→		
Personality core	**Fragmented (polarized elementary units)**	**Normatively healthy (integrated elementary units)**	**Normatively healthy (integrated elementary units)**
Etiology	**Disposition to excessive affects ± Abuse/neglect/trauma** (early developmental defect)	**Heritable impulsivity** + **family/subculture of violence** (early onset—early learning)	**Plan and premeditation** + **family/subculture of afluenza** (late onset—adult strategy)
Underlying dynamics	**Compensatory solution** (psychological survival via deviance)	**Adopted adaptive strategy** (reward-reinforced aggression)	**Calculated lifestyle choice** (entitlement-permitted aggression)
Type of AS behavior	**Nonviolent + violent conflicts** (crime optional)	**Violent + nonviolent crime** ("blue-collar")	**Nonviolent crime** ("white-collar")
Type of aggression	**Affective:** (mis)perceived provocation interpersonal conflicts	**Mixed**: **(affective and predatory)** interpersonal outbursts + premeditated crime	**Predatory:** premeditated crime, low signaling of intention, vulnerable targets
Colloquial label	**Conflict-seeking bullies** ("losers of crime")	**Street criminals** ("proletariat of crime")	**Office criminals** ("elite of crime")
Specific sensitivities	Hypersensitivity to rejection	Hypersensitivity to authority	Hypersensitivity to commonness

Nosology → Variable ↓	Antisocial Personality Disorder antisociality as Modus Vivendi	Character Disorder antisociality as Modus Operandi	Character Disorder antisociality as Modus Imperandi
Acquired morality ("social norms")	**Permissive (self-serving):** reinforcing internal stability	**Permissive (overt):** antisociality as public image	**Permissive (masked):** Fake public image of reciprocity
Biological morality	**Dormant** ("strangers" to altruism)	**Developed and abandoned** ("deserters" of altruism)	**Developed and deformed** ("cheaters" of altruism)
Objectives	**Self-interest (egotism):**	**Self-interest (egotism):**	**Self-interest (egotism + greed):**
Gain	Psychological gain (organization of inner world)	Material gain (crime-based livelihood)	Material + psychobiological gain (wealth, alpha type social dominance)
EF	**Impaired EF** (developmental hypofrontality)	**Impaired EF** (subcortical impulsivity)	**Strong EF** (effective cognitive control)
Autonomic reactivity to stress— fear	**High** (panic prone)	**Decreased** (learned or natural born)	**Normal or High** (well controlled by IQ)
Treatment	Reconstructive psychotherapy Mechanism-based pharmacotherapy Legal	CBT (anger management) Legal	Legal (no effective therapy)
In a nutshell	**Immorality of the weak**	**Immorality of the ignorant**	**Immorality of the arrogant**

PD = personality disorder; CBT = cognitive behavioral therapy; WM = working memory; EF = executive function; AS = antisocial; HR = heart rate. [a]Immorality: ignoring existing knowledge of right versus wrong; amorality: no knowledge of right vs wrong (extremely rare). [b] Modus vivendi: method of living. [c] Modus operandi: method of operating. [d] Modus imperandi: method of power and influence.

who have learned or chosen crime as an adaptive strategy. These are further classified as "successful" (colloquially white-collar) and "unsuccessful" (colloquially blue-collar) criminals. Next and in Table 2.4 we compare the three groups based on a combination of scientific evidence and anecdotal observations.

Successful and unsuccessful criminals: the elite and the proletariat of crime. In the psychological literature, "successful" criminals are said to abuse the law for personal gain but are able to evade punishment, sometimes for decades, with many likely evading detection altogether.[25] These individuals distort the basic principle of universal morality into "what applies to others does not apply to me" and in so doing defy the fundamental premise of civilization: namely, that the group would be equally beneficial for all members who follow the rules and the principle of reciprocity. The attitude is frequently found within the affluenza subculture of high social status and wealth (e.g., some politicians, tycoons, bankers, financial managers, among others). The antisocial elite engages in nonviolent crimes in an informed and premeditated manner. The gain is both material (wealth) and psychobiological (power, influence), hence the label "modus imperandi" (Table 2.4). Their biological roots of morality (reciprocity, empathy) appear normal in childhood, and their higher intelligence might have protected them from crime early on but not from late-onset, white-collar predation, hence the label "cheaters of altruism" (Table 2.4). Accordingly, Stevens et al. (2012) outline a mediated model in which the positive relationship between successful criminals and unethical decision-making is explained through the process of moral disengagement, defined as a cognitive orientation that facilitates unethical choice. In what has become a clichéd form of dissimulation, most successful career predators eventually engage in philanthropy and charity. The generosity, as Chomsky (2000) notes, perpetuates the belief by which greed and accumulation of wealth are always justified, because the resources ultimately "trickle down" to the benefit of others, namely the victims of predation. Creating an impression of morality can become an end in itself, as it is a manipulative way of ensuring one-way benefit, while remaining disguised (an element of classical predation). This is the essence of white-collar crime: the individual poses as moral and publicly condemns immorality of others, all the while committing irrevocable harm to unsuspecting victims (e.g., Bernard "Bernie" Madoff).

25. The literature on the subject uses the term "psychopaths" widely associated with antisocial personality disorder (which implies a profound personality pathology and a diagnosis for which crime is neither necessary nor specific). We use the term "criminal" and alternatively could have used the term "criminal characters" for crime committer as a self-approved and deliberate choice.

The "unsuccessful" career criminals also violate the basic principle of universal morality but follow a less glamorous course in life. Their antisociality typically involves high impulsivity and is cultivated (learned) in subculture, poverty, and/or family. These individuals usually have no intrinsic disdain for others but violate them nevertheless, treating their victims as fair-game "prey" more than "low life." The latter is seen with affluent predators. Their biological roots of morality (reciprocity, empathy) also appear normal in childhood[26] but are abandoned early on and thus not further cultivated trough positive identifications, earning them the label "deserters of altruism" (Table 2.4). They engage in early and hands-on blue-collar crime against either a person or property (theft, physical violence, extortion, drug cartels) as their chosen way of livelihood (hence the label "modus operandi") (Table 2.4). Some may accumulate wealth (e.g., Pablo Escobar, the Medellin drug cartel boss) and may become well-regarded in their local communities as they may come to be seen as generous and protective, perhaps also in an attempt to justify their own crimes by giving to the poor. Despite this generous, as it were, Robin Hood persona, blue-collar criminals can be tyrannical to competitors in crime. In comparison to the carefully planned white-collar fraud, blue-collar crime is easier to detect and punish, hence these individuals spend a large portion of their lives imprisoned. Even if they rise to become some of the richest individuals in the world, they are rarely able to shed the public perception of them as blue collar criminals, hence the label "proletariat of crime" (Table 2.4).

White-collar and blue-collar criminals share many characteristics, for example, permissive morality, selfishness, sense of entitlement, among others, but successful criminals tend to have a better executive function and a higher autonomic reaction to anticipated stress (Ishikawa et al., 2001). High intelligence (high IQ) has been shown to facilitate the regulation of emotional responses to evocative images in individuals with high levels of antisociality, a feature that could facilitate their remaining undetected or "successful" (Bate et al., 2014) hence the labels "elite of crime," "corporate psychopaths," or "office criminals." These cognitive features also may explain why so many successful criminals may achieve high social status, power, and influence. In contrast, "unsuccessful" criminals tend to have poorer executive function and decreased autonomic reactivity to anticipated stress, making them more likely to commit crime on an impulse (hence the labels "proletariat of crime" and "street criminals"), perhaps also explaining their usually lower socioeconomic status and significant prison time. The difference between the two is not simply in their absolute

26. Except in callous prepubescent antisocial boys.

IQ or general cognitive dysfunction but, as Ishikawa et al. (2001) report, appears to be associated with "complex integration of higher cognitive and executive-type skills used on the task" (p. 430), or, figuratively, it takes some talent to be successful in crime. Surprisingly, the difference in executive function was less responsible for apprehending unsuccessful criminal psychopaths (they had a comparable executive function to the controls), than it is in helping successful criminals to evade detection (Ishikawa et al., 2001). In a very loose sense, we label these two antisocial character types as "immorality of the rich and arrogant" and "immorality of the poor and ignorant," respectively (Table 2.4). In both instances, the level of mental functioning is not fragmented (we may even venture to call it normal); their biological roots of morality appear intact, but their acquired character traits and moral norms have either not been internalized (juvenile-onset, blue-collar criminals typically take pride in their immorality) or have been distorted (late-onset, white-collar criminals typically try to disguise their immorality by projecting an image of reciprocity and care). For both, material gains are the ultimate objective. Both types are far more frequent than antisocial personality disorder proper.

Antisocial personality disorder: immorality of the weak. How is the immorality of the ignorant and the arrogant different from the immorality seen in individuals with antisocial personality disorder? All three groups know right from wrong, which none has truly internalized; all have permissive morality, lack remorse, possess a sense of entitlement, and commit crime. The difference rests in the fragmented personality found in individuals with antisocial personality disorder. The latter do not deliberately choose their antisocial lifestyle, which is here a nonconscious developmental outcome that compensates for inner fragmentation and keeps the person psychologically together. Of course, the argument can be made that as adults they did not deliberately reject the antisocial lifestyle or replace it with one that is more prosocial, either through a self-initiated effort or in therapy. Notwithstanding, underneath the antisocial façade, the person is left feeling empty, bored, and artificial, as depicted in Hare's (1996) PCL. Antisocial personality disorder becomes recognizable (but not diagnosable) at about six to seven years of age, by manifesting itself in conduct problems which are the defining self-concept of the child ("conduct disorder") who also has numerous other emotional and interpersonal precursor symptoms. Together, this is suggestive of general and early personality pathology (reviewed in Bozukluklarının et al., 2015). Nonviolent aspects of antisociality, both emotional (lack of remorse or guilt) and/or interpersonal (exploitation, manipulation, entitlement, selfishness, Machiavellianism), are not unique to the antisocial variant but shared by all variants of personality disorder. It is the outbursts of affective aggression with violence and occasional crime that are unique to this variant, although they are not necessarily decisive for the diagnosis. In short, this "immorality of the weak" is essentially different from calculated white-collar and blue-collar crime: in the former, the gain is primarily psychological (i.e., organization of the inner world) and only secondarily materialistic. Psychological testing, Hare's checklist, and a careful clinical interview provide valuable information which reveals the personality structure underlying manifest behaviors. The distinction between character-based and personality disorder–based crime carries treatment implications. Antisocial personality disorder may benefit from biomedical interventions and psychotherapy, but such interventions are rarely beneficial for predators who commit crimes by choice and premeditation. Once a criminal act has occurred, the transgressor is responsible before the law. Even the psychopathology of fragmentation does not exculpate a person from legal responsibility, since people are found to be responsible for both conscious and nonconscious motives in the eyes of the law.

Personality disorder: a misnomer for maladaptation? Official nomenclatures identify mental disorders by their dominant symptoms (e.g., anxiety disorder, depressive disorders), according to the prominent dysfunction (e.g., sleeping or eating disorders), with respect to the hypothesized underlying psychopathology (e.g., the word "Schizophrenia," rooted in Greek, means "splitting of the mind"), or according to their clinical course (e.g., bipolar disorder with alternating phases of euphoria and depression). Personality disorder is the only nosological entity that places the total personality, that is, the individually unique configuration of the mind, into the focus of the diagnosis instead of depicting its functions involved in maladaptation. Hence, the term "personality disorder" actually means "mind disorder." It is the least specific in all of psychiatry and psychology as it is applies to all disorders of the mind (aka "mental disorders").

As noted, fragmented personality may have its roots in innate biogenetic factors and/or early environmental factors—most frequently in both. With this in mind, we have suggested (Svrakic et al., 2009) replacing the term "personality disorder" with the term "adaptation disorder." The former term is overly general (applicable to all mental disorders), nihilistic (has the reputation of irreversibility), blaming (the common perception is that the person him/herself is responsible for the failure to adapt), and stigmatizing (carries with it the profound implication of immorality). The term "adaptation disorder" distributes the "responsibility" for maladaptation evenly, between the individual and the environment, is less stigmatizing (depicts adaptation as a function of personality), conveys optimism (these patients can mature), and is more acceptable to the patient (who finds it easier to improve adaptation than to restructure personality, although the later certainly involves the former).

Personality disorder may never cause a health care crisis . . . and this is bad news for the patients. Personality disorder is a serious diagnosis but not an irreversible one. Both brain and mind dysfunction can be corrected with expertise and time. Developed Western societies have accepted the substantive reality of the disorder, but less so its seriousness, and still less the requirement for the time and resources needed for expert treatment. It appears that the disorder has not alarmed the United States health care system to the point of crisis, which is usually a necessary event before an organized reaction to a problem can be mobilized (e.g., recent opioid crisis prompted numerous prescribing regulations and treatment facilitation). It is not certain that personality disorder shall ever have such a strong impact. Its prevalence appears to be saturated at 10% to 15% in the general population, and not all of these people really *have* to be treated; it is simply preferable. The United States health care system, academic centers, and the society in general, although scientifically and artistically curious about the syndrome, are not yet ready to define professional paths and allocate resources to educate expert clinicians, as discussed later. Given a slim prospect that a health care crisis will force a strategy change toward personality disorder, society could decide to wait out the disorder—to wait for it to disappear. Is this realistic? Perhaps. It could happen when and if human civilization evolves into the swarm society of the future, as discussed. Still, is this the right thing to do? Perhaps from a dry pragmatic standpoint, but certainly not an ethical approach because it violates the basic principle of civilization as a consensual bidirectional relationship in which the individual willingly surrenders many aspects of his or her own personal interests in favor of the group. In in return, the group helps him or her deal with the dangers posed by the forces of nature, other human beings (e.g., crime), and/or disease or injury through organized systems of health care. The increasing awareness of the real, albeit reversible, brain pathology of personality disorder may become a tie-breaker here, even in the absence of a full-blown health care crisis.

The current stalemate in health care for these patients is tridirectional: most patients are reluctant to seek help, most clinicians go through the motions and at least "see" these patients with low expectations, and most insurance companies try to avoid paying at every point in the process whenever possible. It is not simply about money, however. The problem is that individuals with personality disorder are not seen as victims by the public but rather as bullies. The media and unfortunately some professionals treat ordinary criminality, character deviance, and personality disorder as if they were one and the same. We try in this book to correct this misconception. The real disability in individuals with personality disorder is for the most part not immediately obvious. It primarily affects their quality of mental life (poor), their functionality within families (poor), and their capacity for good-enough parenting (low), all rather invisible to others. It is the visible effects that impress others the most, particularly unpredictable and immoral interpersonal relationships, unhealthy work environments filled with conflicts and litigation, violations of the law, addictions, to name just a few among many others. In contrast to individuals with character disorder, who ultimately self- approve their own behavior, we posit here that individuals with personality disorder are victims by origination, who later come to be seen as victimizers by virtue of the very healing process that helps them survive from a psychological standpoint. Behind this aggressive façade there is a wounded child in every one of them, even the antisocial ones. They are victimized by bad genes and bad parenting, whether coupled or not with psychological trauma, and are likely to pass the same features, both genetic and behavioral, onto their offspring.

Most psychiatry programs train residents to use the DSM categorical model of personality disorder, as a medical decision or "case" versus "no case" paradigm based on descriptive criteria, which is inadequate because it overlooks the dynamisms which are essential for the diagnosis. The alternative DSM-5 model is much better conceptually, although it is far from ideal as discussed earlier. If the public is ever to take personality disorder more seriously, responsible diagnosing is imperative. Casual labeling of every loud, confrontational, demanding, or malingering individual as a person with a "personality disorder" only harms its cause. To begin with, we at the very least call for a mandated curriculum in in-depth personality assessment to assist all clinicians in training to treat individuals with mental problems as well as, ideally, for a fellowship in personality pathology that would cover diagnosis and management of personality disorder. This seems especially important now given that Axis II has been eliminated from the DSM-5, an unfortunate decision likely to further blur the boundaries between personality traits, spectra disorders, illness diatheses, and circumscribed neuropathological processes. At the same time, without the mandate to assess personality on Axis II, the frequency of such assessment in daily practice is likely to decrease, thus further distancing the clinician from the subject of his or her interest and diagnosis: namely, the mind of the patient.

CHAPTER 3

Dynamic Nosology and Clinical Assessment of Fragmented Personality

PERSONALIZED, CONTEXT- AND TIME-SENSITIVE DIAGNOSIS OF PERSONALITY DISORDER

Back in 1993, we were invited to a meeting devoted to borderline personality disorder in Lago di Garda, Italy. The two-day conference resulted in the publication of a monograph *II disturbo borderline di personalita: Prospettive sulla diagnosi* (Borderline Personality Disorder: Perspectives on Diagnosis) edited by C. Maffei (1993). Particularly illuminating was the opening statement made by one of the participants who said: "When therapists say personality disorder, they mean borderline." At the time, the colleague's insight that an important concept such as borderline personality could actually be a shared feature common to all subtypes of personality disorder was an avant-garde understanding of the syndrome, then widely conceptualized as 12 discrete categories. Yet, the observation matched our clinical observations and research results. We have long argued that a specific and pervasive mental dysfunction represents a common characteristic cutting across all clinical variants of personality disorder (Divac-Jovanovic et al., 1993). At the time we called the dysfunction a "borderline" level of functioning, but over time we have adopted the term "fragmented" instead: it is person-centered and focuses on fragmentation, that is, lack of integration within a person, which is the essential feature of personality disorder shared by all its variants. As a version of this idea, Kernberg (1975) distinguishes less severe and more severe variants of personality disorder, the more severe sharing "borderline personality organization," a poorly integrated personality structure with partial object relations and primitive defense mechanisms. We contend that all bona fide cases of personality disorder are severe (characterized as they are by fragmented personality) and that nonsevere cases (not fragmented or transiently fragmented) with excessive personality traits or social problems should not be classified as personality disorder in the first place.

Diagnosis of personality disorder is based on three main sources: (i) characteristic *intrapersonal* indicators, notably an inconsistent sense of self, diffuse identity, character traits which subserve self-image at the expense of social adaptiation, unprincipled morality, and immature defense mechanisms; (ii) characteristic *interpersonal* indicators, such as oscillating, intense, and fractuous interpersonal relationships, which maintain one's self-image rather than facilitate his or her interpersonal communication; and (iii) characteristic *behavior* indicators, observed as coexisting contradictory behaviors which alternate (one-or-the other) in the here-and-now. Frequently misdiagnosed as having a personality disorder are individuals who are functionally adapted but with pronounced behavior traits (e.g., very adventurous, theatrical, or shy people, among others). Also frequently misdiagnosed are individuals with self-approved deviant character traits but without inner fragmentation of personality (e.g., habitually violent, arrogant, manipulative, or suspicious people), and finally individuals with rigid characters, armor-plated by neurotic defense mechanisms (e.g., extreme stubbornness or scrupulousness, aka "neurotic characters"). Differential diagnosis also includes affective disorders, especially treatment-refractory depression, bipolar II disorder, and psychotic disorders, the latter because brief psychotic episodes may happen under stress in patients with fragmented personality.

LEVEL OF FUNCTIONING: THE VERTICAL DIAGNOSIS OF PERSONALITY DISORDER

Adaptive flexibility of the mind, accepted as a fact by general consensus, requires that its component subsystems and functions must also be flexible and semi-stable, one of the central points in our model of personality disorder. As discussed in Chapter 1, we define the mind as a semi-stable configuration of mental faculties (cognition, motivation, emotion) canonically self-organized into partially overlapping and interacting subsystems or modules (temperament, the sense of self, identity, moral values, and character), each as a specific adaptive contribution to the mind as a whole, whether dealing with the inner or the outside world. Individuals vary with respect to the degree of integration or pathology of object relations, referred to as levels of mental functioning. The concept is critical to bear in mind as it is necessary to establish in-depth the observable behaviors and symptoms required to make the diagnosis ("vertical diagnosis"). The concept was pioneered by one of us (MDJ) (Divac-Jovanovic and Tatar-Radojkovic, 1987) and as a more or less revised and operationalized version, nowadays is used in the *Psychodynamic Diagnostic Manual* (PDM Task Force, 2006) and the *Operationalized Psychodynamic Diagnosis* (OPD Task Force, 2008), and it has been proposed for the *Diagnostic and Statistical Manual of Mental Disorders* (fifth edition [DSM-5]; American Psychiatric Association, 2013) alternative model. A level of mental functioning is rooted in the quality of internalized object relations as the substrate of the mind formed during the first one to two years of life, and is reflected in the degree of integration and adaptive effectiveness of the mind as a whole along with its subsystems. The four main levels are normal (healthy), neurotic, fragmented, and psychotic, in descending order of mental integration, cohesion of the subsystems, interpersonal relations, and functional adaptability. Each level is enduring rather than fixed and does not contain firm boundaries with respect to the other levels. The levels can be thought of as the "how" of one's mind, i.e., the balance, consistency, accuracy, and cognitive sophistication of feelings, thoughts, and motivations about self and others. As biogenetic dispositions to temperament define the affective biases of internalized object relations, the how of the mind is "seasoned" by the affective overtone of temperament (fearfulness, detachment, persistence, or anger). Recently, the DSM-5 alternative model introduced the concept of levels of mental functioning as indicators of health (no impairment) and psychopathology (some, moderate, severe, and extreme impairment), and defines the levels as a continuum based on the degree of impairment in both self and interpersonal functioning.

Fragmented mental functioning is specific to personality disorder and is characterized by alternating polarized dyads, "all-or-nothing" or "either/or" extremes of the mind. It is the core impairment shared by all individual variants, regardless of the behavior façade: the self-image is inconsistent, personal goals are vague and changing, identity is incoherent, and temperament frequently "hijacks" the mind, leading to poor self-regulation of mood. In the interpersonal sphere, one's capacity for intimacy and empathy is low, character and moral values are impoverished and mainly subserve internal needs ("psychological gain") at the expense of social adaptation, relationships oscillate between ecstatic over-involvements (idealizations) and angry conflicts (devaluations). In such a patchy and dysfunctional inner world, conflicts are hardly worked out internally but are resolved mainly in the interpersonal sphere (OPD Task Force, 2008). Hence, personality disorder is said to be lived internally (internal maladaptation) but is expressed interpersonally (external maladaptation). The levels of functioning are not sharply delineated but instead overlap, usually with the neighboring levels, except for the fragmented level which may overlap with all of them (Fig. 3.1).

Our concept of levels of functioning, as dynamic, flexible, and potentially reversible, stands in contrast to the static concepts of personality organization and borderline personality disorder, as defined by Kernberg (1975) and the DSM, respectively. Important, albeit subtle differences characterize Kernberg's concepts of "borderline personality organization" and our concept of "fragmented level of functioning": the former describes a hypothetical structure, a presumably static and rather stable stage of development, whereas our concept captures the clinical reality that individuals may, as it were, move between the levels of mental functioning in both time and context. There exist, we believe, no real structures in the mind, just a continuously moving substrate, consisting of object relations as structural-functional dualities, dynamically self-configuring into semi-stable subsystems, as discussed. The shifts among the levels may be frequent and fast, or can sometimes be so slow to leave the impression of constancy. The actual level of personality functioning can be determined based on i) intrapsychic, ii) interpersonal, and iii) behavioral parameters, whether longitudinal (history), cross-sectional (therapeutic relationship, psychological tests), self-described, or through collateral information, as discussed later in this chapter.

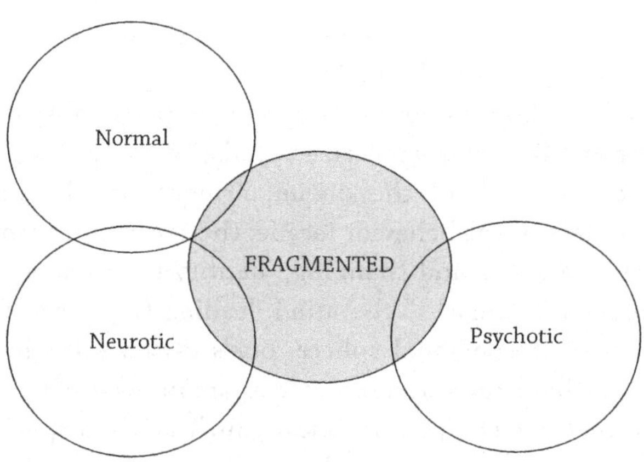

Figure 3.1 Schematic illustration of the overlapping levels of mental functioning (the size of overlap illustrates the likelihood/frequency of interlevel shifts). Only fragmented personality can function at all levels.

Does the mind really move around its levels of functioning? We would answer "by all means and to a sizable extent." Reflecting the dynamic nature and a variable degree of integration of object relations coexisting in everyone, no level of mental functioning is fixed *ipso facto*. Nonetheless, everyone has his or her usual level, a segment that he or she commonly occupies on the vertical axis of psychopathology-to-health (ranging from psychotic, via fragmented, neurotic, to normalcy). Some individuals are more and some less anchored at a level, but most can more or less temporarily and more or less frequently rise or descend to a higher or lower level of functioning, with partial or complete reversibility. The latter has been well documented by clinical psychotherapists. One of the notable example is the paranoid-schizoid and depressive position described by Melanie Klein (1952) who proposed a mental position theory instead of a stage theory due to the reversible nature of the positions. She observed shifts occurring over a lifetime from partial object relations (paranoid-schizoid position) to whole object relations (depressive position) and vice versa, in response to stress, loss, or personal crises and the resolutions thereof. As hinted earlier, the excursions usually occur between neighboring levels of functioning, except for individuals with fragmented personality, who can function at all four levels. The likelihood, frequency, and duration of the periods of regression or progression among the levels depend on (i) the degree of personality integration (at the healthy level, regression is least frequent and of shortest duration and vice versa), (ii) context (internal or external stress can render the mind suboptimal for the given circumstances, leading to regression), and (iii) external structure (structured environments are stabilizing, fostering organization and protecting against regressions and vice versa). The question is: what is the level of functioning of individuals with personality disorder? In the model we propose, it is *predominantly* fragmented.

Vertical diagnosis of personality disorder is based on the typical or usual level of functioning, that is, on the duration, pervasiveness, and frequency of periods of fragmented functioning versus other levels. Depending on the outside context or progress in therapy, these individuals can more or less transiently and more or less *en masse*[1] function at the neurotic level, occasionally even at the healthy level while conversely they may briefly regress to the level of psychosis. In other words, the fragmented level of functioning is common yet reversible

1. Circumscribed regressions and improvements are also observed, limited to a particular self-image or a relationship (e.g., the mentioned selective splitting in a romantic relationship).

with personality disorder, frequently quite enduring, and is decisive for the diagnosis. Moreover, vertical diagnosis helps determine the type, depth, and duration of treatment, from supportive to reconstructive psychotherapy with more or less substantial use of medication. Horizontal diagnosis, that is, the diagnosis of one's dominant maladaptive behavior style, yields information related to a person-centered strategy in psychotherapy, as different styles call for different priorities, therapeutic sequencing, ports of entry (feelings, behavior, thinking), and goals in therapy. The described dynamic approach to diagnosis captures the flexibility of the mind, its self-reorganizing capacity in the face of changing conditions (positive or negative, internal and/or external), and champions the positive connotation associated with change, in contrast to the widespread therapeutic nihilism about severe personality pathology.

What is the advantage of such flexibility in mental functioning? Among many others, it provides a *range of operating alternatives* to the mind, rendering it adaptable to any type of change in internal or external conditions, destabilizing and stabilizing alike. This reversibility can be thought of as an adaptive advantage capitalizing on the mind's imperfections (i.e., both primitive and mature options are available), which allow more (less) mature mental functioning in stable (destabilizing) internal or external conditions or, figuratively, mental progressions (regressions). It is our belief that such a broad range of operating alternatives is in fact optimal from the standpoint of the mind's homeostasis in order to master whatever adaptive challenge is before the person. For example, we have observed that splitting can operate in just one area of functioning, in this particular patient with his romantic partner ("partial splitting") as an adaptive albeit regressive solution for the stressful relationship. This emphasizes the need for a personalized, contextual, and flexible diagnostic system sensitive to fluctuations in mental functioning in both time and context. Our dimensional and dynamic approach to the diagnosis of personality disorder, centered as it is on the concept of fragmented level of functioning, accomplishes this goal.

Personality disorder: a diagnosis that goes in and out of remaining diagnosable. The previous discussion of reversibility applies to personality disorder as well, which is not a fixed, lifelong diagnosis. Its psychopathology peaks in early adulthood and fluctuates through the next several decades, with some variants showing stable, spontaneous improvement by middle age, notably impulsive and eccentric variants but not so much paranoid-antisocial and anxious variants (the latter can often worsen with age). McGlashan et al. (2005) reported that many diagnostic criteria for personality disorder remit after two years, with at least 25% of patients remitting vis-à-vis the most persistent criteria while the less stable criteria disappeared completely. After a two-year follow-up, it was found that 50% to 60% of patients diagnosed with personality disorder at enrollment no longer fulfilled the required number of criteria (Grilo et al., 2004). Even outside formal treatment, at least some spontaneous inner integration may frequently occur. For example, individuals with fragmented personality may have moral values at a higher level than expected given the severity of their personality pathology. One explanation for the paradox may be that positive environmental influences later in life lead to subsequent positive introjections or identifications, thereby improving the integrity of the person's moral values (Kernberg, 1975). Such spontaneous integration ("late bloomers") applies to other subsystems of the mind as well, for example the self, character, identity—even excessive temperament tends to improve with time, although this applies more to novelty seeking and social reward dependence than it does to persistence and fearfulness. With this in mind, personality disorder is best conceptualized as a dynamic and semi-stable, subfunctional but compensatory configuration of the mind. It reflects the mind's nonconscious homeostatic maneuver to organize, stabilize, and psychologically survive. The disorder can change insofar it is influenced by accumulated life experience, the positive influence of others, deliberate effort, or, most reliably, expert therapy.

Differentiating the fragmentation spectrum: partial, transient, masked, and proper. In our practical work, we distinguish fragmented personality proper versus a number of partial and pseudo conditions with elements of fragmented functioning. Also described is masked but real fragmentation, in the context of a major mental illness or super-directive external structure, as in these cases the diagnosis of personality disorder can be missed.

Partial fragmentation refers to patterns of emotions, thoughts, motivations, or interpersonal behavior that are suggestive of fragmented personality but are selective, infrequent, low intensity, and nonpervasive. Such partial fragmentation can be thought of as a marker of instability in a variety of normal and neurotic adaptive styles. We call it "partial" because of its limited pervasiveness within one's internal space. It can affect one area of functioning (e.g., interpersonal), where shifts between idealization and devaluation may be occurring only within a specific type of interpersonal relationship, usually but not exclusively with a romantic partner. In other relationships (e.g., at work) the same person if not exactly mature can at least stably refrain from interpersonal conflicts. We emphasize that partial fragmentation is not indicative of personality disorder but may occur at the neurotic and psychotic levels of functioning as well. Moreover, it can occasionally be observed in normal individuals in ultra-demanding relationships or situations. These clinical observations support the idea of a continuity of psychopathology without clear cut-off points between the "normal" and the "pathological."

Pseudo or transient fragmentation refers to a temporary regression to fragmented functioning in individuals with otherwise well integrated personality. Such regression is typically caused by a trigger, frequently high stress, a severe personal crisis, or an episode of mental illness. Here, the mind appears unable to handle the situation by its usual defense mechanisms, but regresses to a lower level of functioning, a nonconscious homeostatic maneuver. For example, signs and symptoms of fragmentation may suddenly appear during an episode of major depression and disappear after the episode remits (Lečić-Toševski and Divac-Jovanovic, 1989). Such transient fragmentation in the context of major depression might explain the high co-occurrence of false positive personality disorder in cross-sectional studies, leaving the mis-impression of "depressive personality disorder." Inversely, an early mood disorder, with an insidious onset, chronic course, and progressive severity, may lead to a misdiagnosis of personality disorder in young adults (Skodol et al., 1999). Here, the early onset and the chronicity of depression coupled with irrational behaviors (overactivity, irritability, addictions, among others) may mislead the clinician to diagnose a personality disorder instead.

Masked fragmentation refers to a situation whereby an episode of mental illness (such as major depression), a highly structured environment (such as cults, advocacy groups), or an existential threat (war) may improve the fragmented level of functioning beyond clinical recognition as personality disorder ("masked fragmentation"). One of us (MDJ), an experienced therapist, did not recognize a profoundly fragmented personality masked by a dramatic episode of major depression in one of her patients during their first encounter. I (MDJ) was about to close the psychotherapy of depression, only to realize that the treatment was in fact just beginning: once the depression remitted, the psychopathology of fragmented personality penetrated the therapeutic scene with vengeance. Another patient of ours (MDJ) with fragmented personality reported that she felt improved during the NATO bombing of Serbia in 1999. "Everything was so uncertain . . . so iffy, obscure, unpredictable . . . exactly how I usually feel." Indeed, she functioned her best during the war period: she was determined and much better organized, and was even the only employee regularly showing up for work. This paradox can be explained by several mechanisms: by a phenomenon of "psychological distraction" when terrifying external circumstances downgrade the importance of internal struggles; by self-preservation instincts, when the horror of existential threats enables a person to resort to every available capacity and resource to survive both psychologically and physically; or by the (temporary) easing of envy, otherwise a powerful destabilizer of mental functioning, as the surrounding environment and the lives of others for once do not seem to be any more enviable than one's own.

Fragmented personality proper refers to the fragmented substrate of the mind pathognomonic of personality disorder. The above distinctions are clinically relevant because they reduce the potential for diagnostic and treatment errors.

ADAPTIVE STYLES: THE HORIZONTAL DIAGNOSIS OF PERSONALITY DISORDER

People at any level of mental functioning manifest a characteristic adaptive style, the "what" of feelings, thoughts, and social behaviors—or figuratively the thematic priorities of the mind. As noted earlier, adaptive styles are rooted mostly in the *content* of early models of behavior around four to five years of age. For example the content of control and trust in paranoid-flavored families, guilt in anxious families, perfectionism in obsessive families, or admiration and exhibitionism in narcissistic families, among many other dominant themes in early relationships. These early contents are further molded by the child's temperament and, further down the road, by character traits and moral values, as well as externally by local culture, largely but not exclusively without choice or planning. Different maladaptive styles can also be thought of as variant-specific modi operandi of the underlying fragmented personality, namely the means by which it maintains its internal compensation through social interactions, figuratively "same problem, different acts" (as discussed, this compensation is in part also maintained in fantasy). The stylistic aspects of maladaptive behavior, a total of seven, help to clinically differentiate the variants of fragmented personality, as it were its diverse "faces" (although the most frequent presentation is mixed). This we call horizontal diagnosis, and it is informative insofar as it helps us plan the course and sequence of therapy, therapeutic goals, priority of themes, and ports of entry (e.g., feelings or behaviors) most likely to reach the patient's important issues. Adaptive styles are assessed through behavioral and phenomenological indicators (e.g., clinical interviewing and direct observation) and/or with one of the numerous multidimensional personality questionnaires (e.g., Cloninger, 1987; Millon et al., 2009).

DYNAMIC NOSOLOGY OF PERSONALITY DISORDER: 3D DIAGNOSTIC SPACE FOR PERSONALIZED DIAGNOSIS

Our system of dynamic personalized diagnostics defines a tridimensional diagnostic space in which each individual is uniquely and flexibly positioned. The coordinates cross-match the person's dominant adaptive patterns (the "style" or horizontal diagnosis) with his or her current level of functioning (the "depth" or vertical diagnosis) at a point in space and time (Fig. 3.2). Levels of functioning are both dynamic and reversible, and styles of adaptation not only overlap but also combine, thus creating a vast number of presentations, only one of which fits the person in question at the given time and within the given context.

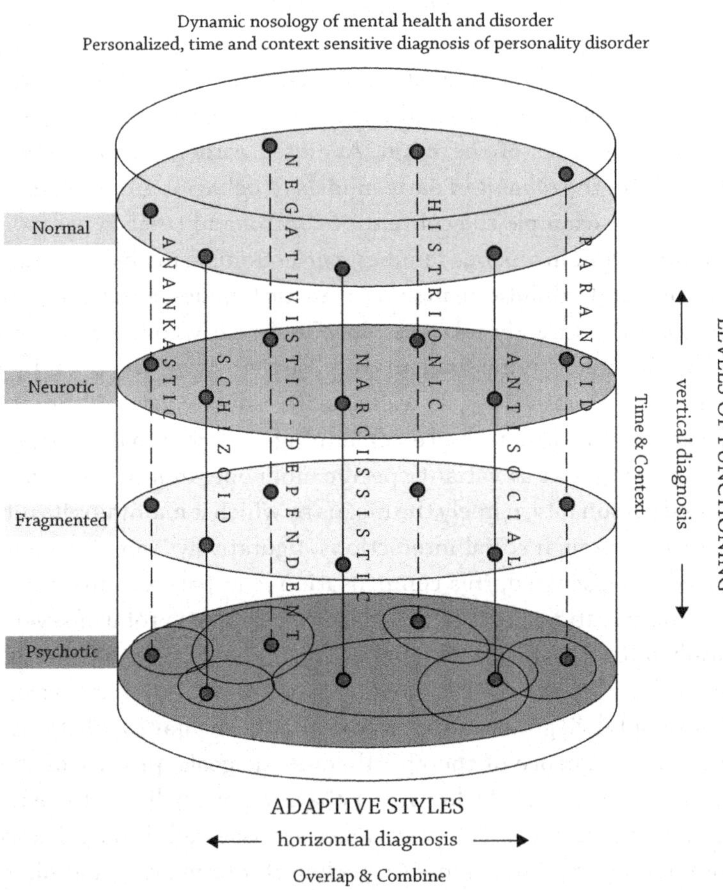

Figure 3.2 Dynamic nosology of mental health and disorder. Ovals are inserted to illustrate the most frequent combinations/overlap of adaptive styles (used with permission from the Taylor & Francis Group, UK).

The person's position in the diagnostic space is relatively stable but not fixed, as it may and often does change. As shown in Figure 3.2, any style of adaptation can appear at any of the levels of functioning: for example, a histrionic style at the normal level involves histrionic traits, a variant of health, and a charming, playfully seductive, sociable, joyful person. At the neurotic level of hysteriform type neurosis, the same behaviors may be seen but with an intensified need for acceptance sought through social seductiveness, also stirring some guilt. At the fragmented level, now veritable histrionic personality disorder, the same style is intensified by conspicuous theatrical manners, mood swings between worthlessness and exaltation, need to control others because of projected guilt, surprising islets of transient but genuine empathy, the mental position of a "righteous victim," and demanding, loud, and/or promiscuous behaviors. Our model provides a highly individualized assessment and offers a personalized diagnosis given a large number of possible configurations of adaptive styles cross-matched with the levels of functioning at a specific point in time and within the specific context. The model pioneers a *dynamic nosology* of mental health and disorders, sensitive to fluctuations in mental functioning, in contrast to the static classifications of the DSM or the ICD or other concepts of psychopathology. With our system, clinicians can monitor the individual as he or she moves around in the diagnostic space, that is, progresses or regresses whether in therapy or spontaneously in life. Such personalized assessment is highly relevant to the psychotherapeutic process and treatment planning.

COMBINING CROSS-SECTION AND HISTORY: INTRAPERSONAL, INTERPERSONAL, AND BEHAVIORAL ASSESSMENT OF PERSONALITY DISORDER

Modern clinical psychology views psychopathological phenomena as related to personality as a whole, that is, in the context of its overall organization (intrapersonal view) and functioning (interpersonal and behavioral views). These diagnostic pathways include a transversal dimension (the here and now) and a longitudinal dimension (history), the latter as self-reported and/or through collateral information. Determining the relationship between personality and psychopathology is a complex process that involves differentiation between normal personality and personality disorder (the "normalcy-pathology" dilemma), differentiation of personality disorder from other mental disorders (the "trait–state" dilemma), as well as the nature of interaction between personality disorder and other mental disorders (the "comorbidity" dilemma; Dzamonja Ignjatovic, 1999). These complementary perspectives are combined into a more comprehensive diagnostic framework of personality. To avoid the misleading safety of symptom-centered diagnosis, a frequent place of refuge in clinical psychiatry, psychologists have historically tried to relate the observed symptoms to relevant aspects of personality, for example, to early life experiences, behavior traits, defense mechanisms, cognitive functioning, personal goals and motives, as well as to the actual situation of the individual.

Current relational models of psychological assessment, or, as some call it, "collaborative psychodiagnostics," shift the focus from intrapsychic (intrapersonal) to relational (interpersonal) and from formal testing to naturalistic techniques, such as clinical interviewing. This shift reflects the postulate that the most important information about personality can be inferred from its relations. However, both formal and naturalistic assessment search for latent intrapsychic processes underlying visible behaviors and symptoms. There have been commendable attempts to define criteria for interpersonal diagnosis of intrapersonal psychopathology, such as primitive defense mechanisms and identity diffusion, among others (Clarkin et al., 2007; Divac-Jovanovic and Tatar-Radojkovic, 1987).

Interpersonal (relational) assessment of personality disorder focuses on relations with others, capacity for mentalization, self-regulation of mood, and type and intensity of emotions provoked in others, among other features. *Behavioral* assessment includes habitual behavior patterns that mediate adaptation to the external environment (character and moral values), as well as careless or high-risk behaviors (e.g., addictions), and self-destructive activities, among others (all of which are observed in the here-and-now or obtained via a reliable collateral informant). *Intrapersonal* assessment focuses on defense mechanisms, the sense of self, identity, and reality testing, among others. This division of these diagnostic paths is rather pedantic, as they are frequently interdependent and interwoven. Since behavior and interpersonal relationships are mainly rooted in the intrapersonal dynamics, the latter carries the highest weight of the diagnosis.

INTERPERSONAL ASSESSMENT OF FRAGMENTED PERSONALITY: RELATIONAL DIAGNOSTICS

Relational diagnosis provides an immediate insight into the type of patterns that explain how the patient's relates to others in real life, as these (the patterns) are recreated with the therapist from the very first meeting. What patients bring into their relationships with others (including the therapists) is amenable to assessment in real time. The main interpersonal phenomenon suggestive of fragmented personality is the therapist's emotional reactions, whether they reflect countertransference proper[2] or spontaneous reactions to the patient's psychopathology (diagnostic countertransference). In addition to these here-and-now data, relational diagnosis can draw from the history of the patient's interpersonal relationships, through self-report and/or collateral information. Fragmented personality is suggested whenever interpersonal relations follow a repetitive pattern whereby others are expected to define and maintain the patient's sense of self (selfobjects) in what is supposed to be an adult relationship. This is observed as an insatiable one-way relationship, awaiting yet demanding, with frantic efforts to avoid abandonment which would mean weakening the roots of self-image. The patient's lack of empathy, low capacity for mentalization, and difficulty adapting to other people and/or communicating in a way that shows understanding of others' emotional signals (aka closed system) result in numerous breaks in romantic relationships, friendships, and families, with frequent misunderstanding arising on both sides. These patterns are highly indicative of personality disorder.

In what becomes an important clue in relational diagnostics, individuals with personality disorder create a rather specific first impression, a puzzling combination of contradictory features, which are readily expressed even in superficial contacts: humility and arrogance, openness and inhibition, theatricality and shyness, intimacy and aloofness, suspiciousness and naivety, among many others. With patients who manage to stir up the therapist's emotions to high intensity during the first contact, one should immediately think of the possibility of fragmented personality. With such patients, therapy starts from the first contact, before the diagnostic process is fully finished. Since these patients frequently rush into transference already during the initial contact, therapists are actually conducting assessment and therapy simultaneously, relying on the naturalistic methods of biographical information, interview, and observation of behavior and transactions; they must also monitor their own affective resonance with the

2. Originally defined as a result of the patient's influence on the therapist's nonconscious feelings toward objects of the past projected onto the patient. Per modern definition, countertransference includes "all of the analyst's emotional responses to the patient," some from his own inner life and some induced by the patient (Auchincloss and Samberg, 2012). These two aspects are also called personal countertransference (close to the original concept) and diagnostic countertransference (i.e., the therapist's emotional responses that indicate the nature of the patient's psychopathology), although both aspects are used in diagnosis.

patient. So many characteristic phenomena indicative of the fragmented personality are manifest in the therapeutic relationship that psychological testing frequently merely confirms what was clinically obvious all along.

Additional relational indicators of fragmentation include rapid shifts between the position of victim and persecutor, idealization and devaluation, and especially chain redefinitions of the content of communication (Divac-Jovanovic and Tatar-Radojkovic, 1987), among others. The concept of chain redefinition refers to the nonconscious tendency of the patient to evade dealing with problems by giving the therapist the "run around" by redefining questions: "yes, but" and the like, and/or questioning the meaning of simple concepts: the question "Have you ever loved someone"? is answered by "What is love"? To an individual with fragmented personality, the presence of another person who is there to help, but is in control, is threatening. When someone is "good" to the patient, he or she readily sees this as a "prelude to abuse," so he or she may shift from fearful to guarded and arrogant, which in part explains high drop-out rates in therapy.

Occasionally, direct communication with the patient may reveal very little of significance despite a rich history of problematic relationships. Yet, after the testing is completed, the protocol is flooded with signs of psychopathology. Whenever the patient reveals conspicuously little in direct early contact, it is recommended to administer the testing early. This is especially helpful in distinguishing fragmented personality proper from the aforementioned sporadic fragmentation found in normal individuals, transient decompensation in mood disorders ("pseudo-fragmentation"), and to rule out incipient Schizophrenia.

BEHAVIORAL ASSESSMENT: WHEN THE HERE-AND-NOW TELLS THE STORY

Behavioral assessment of personality disorder includes observation in the here and now, which basically means monitoring the priorities in the content brought to sessions as well as actual behavior during the sessions, both those related and unrelated to transference. Historical aspects of behavior are assessed based on self-reported and collateral-reported history as well as on behavior-ratings based on standardized scales, such as the Temperament and Character Inventory (TCI) or Millon's Clinical Multiaxial Inventory (MCMI) and other multidimensional tests. In the here and now, behavioral markers suggestive of personality fragmentation include coexisting contradictory polarizations (mentioned earlier), which may appear bizarre to the observer while the patient follows each pole with natural emotional resonance and conviction, as if the other did not exist for them at all. The patient tends to either exaggerate or minimize his or her behavior only to be set straight by a collateral informant who may reveal the true extent of behaviors as well as the patient's lack of insight (blind spots). It is not unusual for self-report and collateral information to portray the same behavior or relationship in a diametrically opposite direction; for example, the husband describes his wife as dissatisfied and angry from the beginning of their marriage, while she, surprised, claims the opposite.

Since character reflects habitual behavior patterns that optimize one's social adaptation, character is mostly expressed through social behavior. Character traits, as defined by Cloninger et al. (1993), operationalize the quality of personality integration (self-directedness [SD]) and the quality of social adaptation (cooperativeness [CO]), a conceptual oversight with no impact on the reliability of research, as discussed. A low product score on these two traits (SD × CO) reliably establishes the probability that the test-taker may have a personality disorder. The traits capture multiple behavioral indicators of fragmented personality. These are related to (i) low SD or self-insufficiency (operationalized as reduced capacity for self-reliance with more or less pronounced dependence on others, a passive-reactive mindset, weak sense of personal responsibility, counterproductive or nonproductive habits vis-à-vis long-term goals, among others) or (ii) low CO or self-serving interpersonal attitudes and moral poverty(operationalized as intolerance, entitlement, insensitivity and lack of compassion, envy, selfishness, among others).

Together these two traits (SD and CO) encompass the all-important dyad of personality disorder: a poorly integrated self and maladapted social relations, the latter includes egotistic character and impoverishment moral values. Affects and impulsive behaviors are poorly controlled by cognitive functions, which in fact are so heavily influenced by temperament that they reliably differentiate the DSM clusters: low RD differentiates cluster A (aloof, disinterested), high NS cluster B (impulsive, dramatic), and high HA cluster C (fearful). Although not pathognomonic, this "reflexiveness" (rather than reflectiveness) aids the diagnosis. As mentioned, low scores on SD and CO correlate with immature defense mechanisms as measured by the Defense Style Questionnaire (DSQ) and vice versa (Mulder et al., 1996). The result provides suggestive evidence that poorly developed SD combined with low CO likely reflects an underlying immature personality structure (low SD) and its ripple effect into interpersonal relations (low CO), shared by all clinical variants of personality disorder. In the Mulder et al. study, SD was twice as good a predictor of immature defenses compared to CO (r = −0.44 vs. −0.22, respectively) and showed a higher negative correlation with these defenses (r = −0.54 vs. −0.45, respectively), supporting the interpretation that the "caseness" (or personality disorder) is primarily associated with a poorly integrated self (low SD) and only secondarily with maladaptive interpersonal relations (low CO). In our model, low SD would be considered for the in depth, vertical diagnosis while low CO captures the horizontal diagnosis of adaptive styles, as discussed.

INTRAPERSONAL ASSESSMENT OF PERSONALITY DISORDER: A CLOSER LOOK AT THE BATTLEFIELD

Intrapersonal diagnostics searches for the underlying in-depth processes that influence the phenomenology and symptoms of personality disorder. It involves naturalistic and psychometric methods. The naturalistic approach refers to structured clinical interviewing, of which one of the best is the mentioned Structured Interview for Personality Organization (STIPO) designed to assess "borderline personality organization" as defined by Kernberg (1975; Clarkin, et al., 2007a). The STIPO covers the following dimensions of personality: identity, quality of object relations, primitive defenses, coping and rigidity, aggression, and moral values. The second (psychometric) approach includes projective tests and personality questionnaires as well as, optimally, a test of defense mechanisms and identity disturbance. Next we discuss the assessment of the most important intrapersonal parameters regarding personality disorder: identity and the sense of self, defense mechanisms, and reality testing.

Assessment of identity integration and self-cohesion. The degree of identity integration follows spectrally from good to moderate, diffuse, and confused. Integrated and moderately integrated identity are both observed in healthy and neurotic individuals; identity diffusion is pathognomonic of personality disorder, and identity confusion of psychosis. Identity diffusion is the final common pathway of partial object relations, failed individuation and the related lack of self- and object constancy, and other psychological deficits as described earlier. Such inner disarray gives rise to diffuse identity, an incoherent autobiographical narrative of the self (an incoherent "who of me") also affecting one's ability to reliably relate to others as well as to project into his or her own future (unreliable prospection). This incoherence is clinically recognized as mental discontinuity (frequent and extreme variations in self-perception), lack of authenticity (tendency to pretend, to engage in "as if" behaviors and feelings), tendency to imitate others (psychological "mimicry"), defective body schema, and ambivalent sexual identity, among other features. Shedler and Western (PDM Task Force, 2006, p. 583) provide a useful operationalization of identity diffusion:

- lack of a stable sense of who she/he is (e.g., attitudes, values, goals and feelings about self seem unstable and ever-changing);
- appears to experience the past as a series of disjointed or disconnected events; has difficulty giving a coherent account of his/her life story;
- is prone to painful feelings of emptiness (e.g., may feel lost, bereft, abjectly alone when in the presence of others, etc.);
- seems unable to settle into, or sustain commitment to, identity-defining life roles (e.g., career, occupation, lifestyle, etc.);
- tends to identify with admired others to an exaggerated degree, taking on their attitudes, mannerisms, etc. (drawn into the "orbit" of a strong or charismatic personality);
- sense of identity revolves around a "cause," movement, or label (e.g., adult child of alcoholic, adult survivor, environmentalist, born-again Christian, etc.); may be drawn to extreme or all-encompassing belief systems;
- tends to feel she/he is not her/his true self with others; may feel false or fraudulent;
- has a deep sense of inner badness; sees self as damaged, evil, or rotten to the core (whether consciously or nonconsciously).

In everyday practice, identity diffusion, a critically important indicator of personality disorder, is usually assessed based on the clinician's impression during the few initial interviews. The short but reliable 35-item Identity Disturbance Questionnaire (IDQ) helps to objectivize the impressions about cohesion versus diffusion with minimal inference (Wilkinson-Ryan and Westen, 2000). On the IDQ, individuals with fragmented personality manifest high *role absorption*, as they tend to submerge themselves in, or define themselves in terms of, a specific role, cause, or unusual group (all external organizing factors). The second aspect is called *painful incoherence* and reflects the patients' subjective experience and concern about the lack of coherence. The third aspect, *inconsistency*, captures objective manifestations of incoherence which are not associated with distress. The fourth aspect is *lack of commitment* to jobs or values and the like. In a study of individuals with borderline personality disorder, those with other personality disorder, and those with no personality disorder, Wilkinson-Ryan and Westen report an important finding: identity disturbance distinguishes "borderline" (fragmented) patients from subjects with no personality disorder but does not distinguish "borderline personality disorder" from other variants of personality disorder. This finding supports our position that all clinical variants of personality disorder share a fragmented core, which is implicated by identity diffusion as detailed in this study.

Assessment of defense mechanisms in personality disorder: polarized reality is easier to handle. Defense mechanisms are nonconscious psychological distortions of reality employed automatically to guard against a painful or disturbing (unacceptable) inner state (Auchincloss and Samberg, 2012). Ultimately, a defense mechanism serves to protect the established image of oneself, whether the self is mature, immature, or neurotic. Although any thought, emotion, or behavior can serve as a psychological defense, a person is characterized by his or her commonly used set of mechanisms which are automatically activated in stressful situations or personal crisis. This is also known as a defense style, which is a revealing characteristic of the quality of personality integration (Auchincloss and Samberg, 2012). As Vaillant (1992) observed, the function of defense mechanisms is to alleviate stress and facilitate adjustment, and to do all this without undergoing energy-consuming major internal perturbations. It is already evident that economy is an important advantage of defense mechanisms. Protective effects of mature defense mechanisms are manifold. First, they keep affects within tolerable boundaries during sudden changes in emotional life, for example, after sudden loss of a significant object, perceived threat to self-esteem, or increase in intimacy or dependency in close relationships. Second, they help re-establish the disturbed homeostasis—by deferring (suppression) or rechanneling (sublimation) the abruptly intensified biological impulses, for example, anxiety associated with the rising libido in puberty. Third, they help to buy the time needed to integrate the abrupt changes into the self-image that cannot be instantaneously integrated, for example, during puberty or after major surgery. Fourth, they help the person process unresolved conflicts with significant people (living or dead) from whom he or she cannot fully separate. In contrast to these positive effects of mature defenses, persistent and dominant neurotic or immature defense mechanisms can have serious negative consequences in reality perception (repression and dyadic polarization of reality, respectively), as discussed next.

Defense mechanisms can be organized according to the degree of maturity (or developmental level), also shown in Table 3.1. The classification is primarily didactic. Anyone, depending on the circumstances, may use mechanisms from different levels:

Table 3.1 DEFENSE MECHANISMS LEVELS I THROUGH IV: PSYCHOTIC, IMMATURE, NEUROTIC, MATURE

Level I Psychotic (Centered Around Dissociation)	Level II Immature (Primitive) (Centered Around Splitting)	Level III Neurotic (Centered Around Repression)	Level IV Mature (Centered Around Suppression)
MODUS OPERANDI: Deny Reality and Impulses	MODUS OPERANDI: Polarize Reality and Impulses	MODUS OPERANDI: Hide Reality and Impulses	MODUS OPERANDI: Beautify / Postpone Reality and Impulses
Delusional projection, psychotic negation, psychotic regression	Projection, acting out, primitive phantasy, denial, primitive idealization and devaluation, projective identification, hypochondriasis, passive aggression	Displacement, reactive formation, isolation, intellectualization, rationalization, undoing, negation, somatization, passive aggression	(Pseudo)altruism[a], humor, anticipation, sublimation

[a] The prefix "pseudo" for altruism is used to differentiate between altruism as a defense mechanism (here not fully authentic since it is instrumental in the person's defense against anxiety or psychological pain) and "proper" altruism (directed toward the well-being of others and not serving the altruistic person at all).

Level I (most immature)—psychotic defense mechanisms (centered around[3] dissociation): delusional projection, psychotic negation, deep regression

Level II—immature (or primitive) defense mechanisms (centered around splitting): projection, acting out, primitive phantasy, devaluation, primitive idealization, projective identification, hypochondriasis, passive aggression, denial

Level III—neurotic defense mechanisms (centered around repression): displacement, reactive formation, isolation, intellectualization, rationalization, undoing, negation, somatization

Level IV (healthiest)—mature defense mechanisms (centered around suppression): (pseudo)altruism, humor, anticipation, sublimation.

3. The phrase "centered around" is used to emphasize that four mechanisms (dissociation, splitting, repression, and suppression) are central in each of their respective groups. These four mechanisms create the stage for other mechanisms in the group to operate: for example, the mechanism of splitting polarizes reality, setting up an environment for idealization-devaluation, projection, denial, and other mechanisms in the group to operate; the mechanism of repression sets the stage for displacement, reactive formation, and rationalization, and so on.

The same types of psychological dangers may be handled by different types of defense mechanisms. Which mechanism is employed depends on the adaptive fitness of the mind in the given context and at the actual moment. As a simple rule, a decreasingly fit mind resorts to more severe distortions of reality to protect itself and vice versa. As discussed in Chapter 1, the general network of cognition represents sensory information, affects, and memories at all levels of consciousness, including the nonconscious working memory, at the level of which, we believe, defense mechanisms operate. From here, these nonconscious mechanisms can protect the current equilibrium of the conscious mind (i.e., current level of mental functioning) from the disruptive impact of psychological dangers. The process involves automatic homeostatic adjustments occurring below the level of decision-making or strategy planning. Mature defense mechanisms either suppress reality (here a painful or unacceptable inner state of which individuals are aware but push aside), sublimate reality (whereby people turn its negative energy into a positive motivation on another front), or beautify reality (whereby individuals use humor and anticipation of better times) to make it more bearable. A conflict-ridden neurotic person represses the disturbing reality and/or impulses, pushing them out of full awareness, so that he or she does not have to face it. The fragmented personality relies on primitive mechanisms (centered around splitting) which divide reality into contradictory dyads, creating an unrealistic but simpler world to grasp and handle, one extreme at the time. When diagnosed in an adult, these mechanisms are highly suggestive of personality disorder. Differential diagnosis of one's defensive style is based on the predominance of certain defense mechanisms employed. With increasing cognitive capacities during development, some defenses are used only very early (splitting, denial) to be abandoned later, while others (humor, anticipation) appear for the first time later in development, at a higher level of cognitive organization. The risk of reverting to earlier, more immature defenses is always present, especially under stress or crisis, a well-known regressive phenomenon further illustrating the dynamic and reversible nature of the mind.

What are immature defense mechanisms and how are they diagnosed? Immature or primitive defenses appear early in life as a crude but effective way to deal with fundamental early anxieties about self and objects. Their pathological persistence into adulthood is widely considered to be indicative of severe personality pathology. However, we concur with Willick (1983) that all kinds of defenses may be used by people with all types of disorders, so the diagnosis should not be based solely on one's defense style but also on identity integration and reality testing, as discussed in this chapter.

Immature defense mechanisms are diagnosed using (i) *biographical information* (assessment of life events involving impulsive behavior, mood swings, and intense and unstable interpersonal relationships, among others), (ii) *psychological testing* (manifestations of splitting on projective tests, self-report questionnaires like the Inventory of Mechanisms of Defense (iMOD), (iii) *interpersonal contact* (the patient "rushes" into transference, oscillates between idealization and devaluation, assuming by turns the role of a victim and a persecutor, and uses chain redefinitions in transactions, among others), and (iv) *phenomenology* (the inner experience of diffuse identity and unclear boundaries, confused descriptions of self and an equally confused portrayal of significant objects, as well as inability to define one's own feelings, among others). Note that the assessment of defense mechanisms and identity uses the same methods and relies on the same information, illustrative of the functional overlap between these constructs.

Given the high correlation between defense mechanisms and levels of personality functioning, description and assessment of immature defenses characteristic of fragmented personality are discussed in more detail below.

Splitting: the precondition for other primitive defenses. In Chapter 2, we referred to splitting as a "barrier to growth but a hero of psychological survival." This is true of personality disorder but not of normal development, where splitting actually facilitates early growth. In early development, it is a normal mechanism which allows the brain and mind to organize around positive introjections of love and care while keeping them at a safe distance from threatening negative experiences. Such normal early division within the mind is a function of the brain's anatomy (positive and negative affects associated with early experiences are processed separately and at the time still neurally immature prefrontal cortex). Splitting later may become a purely mental defensive maneuver in the context of neutrally mature prefrontal networks, as discussed. In personality disorder, developing amidst a massive influx of negative experiences, whether created by biological biases or adverse environment, splitting persists as a protection of the positive personality core. Its continuing use could reflect the continuing hypofrontality, that is, slow to develop networks of cognition in the context of stress. Alternatively, its persistence could represent a homeostatic issue of mind economy wherein less energy is required to keep contradictory affects and impulses apart than to repress the negative ones into the nonconsciousness; splitting this way becomes more economical than repression. It is also more pathological than repression as it maintains an unrealistic, polarized perception of the self and the external world.

Phenomenologically, splitting refers to the tendency to see oneself and others as either "entirely good" or "entirely bad" in a way that is equally unrealistically all positive or all negative. Triumphant one day, the patient becomes a failure the next, his or her heroes readily become traitors, and vice versa. Splitting diminishes one's capacity to register the intermediate values of reality ("grey" areas) between the two extremes. Consequently, it turns into an obstacle to the development of ambivalence, the next step in normal development toward individuation. In adults with personality disorder, splitting serves as a defense against ambivalence, as a merger of good-with-bad could overpower the splitting and annihilate positive experiences, which would become a sort of mental implosion of the self.

In contact with the patient, splitting is manifested through unpredictability and inconsistency in discourse, leaving the interlocutor either surprised or confused. In practice, it is recognized through a number of operationalized manifestations that are relatively easy to diagnose (OPD Task Force, 2008):

1. Alternating experience of contradictory feelings or thoughts, with preserved memory of both, while the patient remains unaffected by their striking inconsistency; in other words, the patient is neither able to account for these contradictions nor resolve them, so his or her thinking and motives impress as unclear.
2. Very low motivation on the part of the patient to engage in resolving contradictory experiences (the typical explanation is "not interested");
3. A tendency to unrealistically idealize certain persons and see them as perfect and without any flaws and unrealistically devalue others as completely bad and devoid of any positive qualities whatsoever (these mutually exclusive views can quickly turn into their opposites);
4. A tendency to stir conflicts in one's surroundings by describing the same situation differently to different people, or differently to the same people at different times.

In addition to these direct manifestations, splitting can be assessed using projective tests. Here it is manifested as contradictory, oppositely affectively charged and poorly formed perceptions, conspicuous verbalization with preserved final control, sudden shifts in the quality of interpretations, and so on. Other clinical manifestations which can be useful to diagnose splitting include a diminished capacity to experience ambivalence, wild oscillations in self-esteem, self-intensifying affect states, erratic decision-making, and ego-syntonic aggression and impulsivity (which are recognized by the patient but seen as "justified" and without any feelings of guilt). Characteristically, aggression is ego-syntonic during the acting-out episode but becomes ego-dystonic after the episode.

Projective identification: from mediating mind development to maintaining its fragmentation. This applies to all primitive defenses but the most by far to splitting and projective identification. As discussed, projective identification is pivotal for the first reflections of the self in early interactions: it contributes to the formation of the internal world, helps self-object differentiation, and influences how every adult experiences the outside world. If persists beyond the early phases of mind development, it becomes one of the most primitive and most typical mechanisms used by individuals functioning at the fragmented level in their close relationships. We borrow from Ogden (1979) to address this mechanism. In a schematic way it can be thought of as a primitive form of projection: an unbearable part of the self (threatening fantasy, emotion, impulse) is projected into another person (lover, partner, or therapist) taking over the recipient from within. Then there is pressure—real emotional and behavioral pressure—exerted via the interpersonal interaction such that the recipient of the projection experiences pressure to think, feel, and behave in a manner congruent with the projected fantasy. Finally, the projected feelings, after being psychologically processed by the recipient, are reinternalized ("recovered") by the projector as safer than they were originally. In simple projection, which does not blur the boundary between two people, the projector gets rid of the projected material and feels psychologically separate from the object. In projective identification, one feels profoundly connected with the object, the boundary is blurred, and the recipient experiences the emotions equivalent to those contained in the projected bad part, which would otherwise be alien to him or her. If angry, the person makes others feel and behave as though they were angry; in the therapeutic setting, the therapist might become uncharacteristically cruel or insensitive. The blurring is achieved by shifting nonconscious emotions and fantasy (the patient) which are experienced as conscious by the recipient (the therapist). The recipient of the projection may experience a loss of identity and insight as he or she is caught up in and manipulated by the projector's fantasy (Laing, 1969).

Since threatening ("bad") parts of oneself are projected most frequently, persons using projective identification usually see others as bad, unreliable, or immoral, and these same others begin to feel that same way about themselves. In everyday relationships, wherein the recipient does not contain, analyze, and process the projection but behaves by its dictate, projective identification can become a self-fulfilling prophecy, wherein others treat the person exactly the way he or she fears to be treated in the first place. Of note, some argue that every projection includes parts of the self and that the individual always maintains some contact with that projected part; in other words, that projection and projective identification are very close, if not the same. Our discussion outlines fundamental differences between the two mechanisms, although there can be no doubt that a part of one's self, usually a bad part, is contained in every simple projection.

Projective identification is a complex defense as it bridges the intrapsychic and the interpersonal domains. Nonconscious motives for projective identification include the need to rid the self of unwanted experience, to control the object from the inside, to avoid separation, and to communicate a state of mind (Auchincloss and Samberg, 2012). An interesting model of projective identification was provided by Ogden (1979) describing the four functions of projective identification: as a defense mechanism, a mode of communication, an object relationship, and a path leading to psychological change.

In therapy, projective identification becomes more than just a defense mechanism; it becomes a therapeutic tool through the analysis of both countertransference proper and natural emotional reactions in the here and now (diagnostic countertransference). With these patients, the former (countertransference proper) inevitably includes nonconscious emotions towards the worst of the past bad objects, whereas spontaneous reactions are strikingly uncharacteristic of the therapist (morally judging, anger, retaliation, among others). The therapist should be able to recognize, analyze, contain, and process the projected material and thereby enable the patient to re-introject his or her own contents in a modified (safer, acceptable) form and ultimately transform his or her internal world. An important therapeutic element of this process lies in the patient's realization that neither he or she nor the therapist were "destroyed" in the process, the therapist by the projection and the patient by the re-introjection of (transformed) negative affects. In other words, everyone "survived." In practice, the re-introjection phase of the content originally projected on the therapist is often neglected. For example, after projecting their hostility onto the therapist, patients can feel better because of this "detoxification" effect. An unexperienced therapist may end the therapy here ("the patient is better"). However, the therapy should have been continued until the patient re-introjects the projected hostility, which the therapist is able to tolerate and process into a milder, more balanced affect thereby "presenting" it for re-introjection as balanced interactive reality. Projective identification is a delicate mutual process, and its proper processing is vitally important to what is usually referred to as "corrective emotional experience" in psychotherapy. In everyday life, another source of "processed" re-introjection of negative affects and self-images that carries a healing property is within a relationship with an unconditionally loving mature partner, a rare but fortunate milieu for the fragmented partner.

There is also the phenomenon of positive projective identification (Bion, 1959; Klein, 1952) when the patient projects and deposits positive identifications and healthy aspects of him/herself into the therapist. This is a form of projection for "safe keeping," which mobilizes in the therapist the feelings of interest and optimism about saving the patient. In this way, the patient's good representation of the therapist is not just the reflection of acceptance, kindness, or the help received but also the result of projective identification. The mutually positive experience is gradually being re-introjected by the patient in the course of therapy. In contrast to negative projective identification, typical of the paranoid schizoid position or fragmented personality, positive projective identification is more characteristic of the higher level of functioning (depressive position or whole object relations) where the good projected part secures a relation with the world endowed with goodness (reviewed in Auchincloss and Samberg, 2012). Accordingly, Bion cogently distinguished between pathological and normal projective identification: the former is characterized by hatred and violence, omnipotent control, and reality distortion and the latter by the effort to communicate one's state of mind by inserting it into the mind of another, as what commonly happens in relationships involving love.

Projective identification is mainly diagnosed directly, within the context of the therapeutic relationship, rather than by specific tests. The diagnosis involves analyses of transactions, personal and diagnostic countertransference, and the therapist's emotional resonance in the therapeutic relationship and obviously requires expert training.

Passive aggression: a normal, neurotic, or immature defense? Passive aggression, a defense mechanism typical of neuroses, is fairly common in personality disorder and occasionally occurs in healthy individuals. The mechanism can be figuratively described as "silent feuding": resistance to fulfill others' expectations, negativism, sarcasm, cynicism, deliberate inefficiency or procrastination, and tendency to demoralize others or spoil their enjoyment, among other manifestations. Personality disorder is known for interpersonal conflicts, but a significant portion of these patients also manifest passive aggression, especially toward people of authority, here reflecting their struggle for control. Millon (2000) describes individuals who use passive aggression as follows:

> Some people just seem unsure of which way to turn in life. Ever ambivalent, individuals who use passive aggression vacillate between uneasy feelings of

> dependence and an equally uneasy desire for self-assertion. Simultaneously needy and independent, they agree to conform to requests for performance, but nevertheless have strong issues with authority and resent external control. Inevitably, they feel misunderstood, unappreciated, and disillusioned. As their discontent deepens, they begin to find fault with the way others treat them and engage in indirect or passive forms of behavioral and emotional protest. (pp. 548–549)

Passive aggression is a defense against acts of rage which are feared because they could destroy the loved object (in neurosis) or the selfobject and thus own self (in personality disorder). The relationship between ambivalence and passive aggression may help explain its globality, as the mechanism is seen with healthy individuals, neurotic characters, and personality disorder alike. Ambivalence means the coexistence of both loving *and* hateful feelings toward the same object. It is suggestive of a higher, neurotic level of functioning, where the mechanism of repression has replaced the mechanism of splitting. The latter was a barrier to ambivalence, not the cause of it. Indeed, the fragmented personality is characterized by a strong, but not total, intolerance of ambivalence. These patients employ denial and splitting (either love *or* hate) to prevent their psychologically dangerous merger into love *and* hate, as this could lead to mental implosion, as discussed. The emergence of passive aggression in therapy is a manifestation of progress, a step towards but at the same time a defense against ambivalence, which is unattainable as it could mean overriding the splitting with the danger of destruction. The word "progress" refers to behavioral progress, as passive aggression now replaces acts of aggression, but not progress in integration. In neurosis, passive aggression arises from deep ambivalence and serves to express repressed aggression while protecting the loved object. Reflecting their different dynamics, individuals with personality disorder respond to confrontation of passive aggression by further extremizing their aggressive position, while neurotic individuals are caught by surprise and retract apologetically. As a transient phenomenon, mature individuals may show passive aggression as the lesser of two evils in situations when the person they love stirs their anger. In a loose sense, a healthy person loves, a neurotic person loves and hates, personality disorder hates, while psychotic individuals neither love nor hate.

Other immature defenses, both derived from and centered around splitting, are employed by persons functioning at the fragmented level. These include *denial, withdrawal into phantasy, primitive idealization and devaluation, acting out, somatization.* These are not as pathognomonic for personality disorder as splitting and projective identification, and can be manifested by neurotic individuals as well, albeit less frequently and less pervasively.

Is there a passive aggressive personality disorder? We use Millon's (2000) concept of passive aggressive personality disorder (negativistic, as he calls it), one of the most elaborated, to address the question. Millon describes negativistic personality disorder through functional (i.e., behavior) and structural (i.e., intrapersonal) domains. With minor modifications, the four functional domains include:

1. *Expressive behaviors—resentful* (resists fulfilling expectancies of others, frequently exhibiting procrastination; inefficient and obstinate as well as contrary and irksome behaviors; reveals gratification in demoralizing and undermining the pleasures and aspirations of others);
2. *Interpersonal conduct—contrary* (assumes conflicting and changing roles in social relationships, particularly dependent and contrite acquiescence and assertive and hostile independence; conveys envy and pique toward those more fortunate, as well as actively concurrent or sequentially obstructive and intolerant of others, expressing either negative or incompatible attitudes);
3. *Cognitive style—skepticism* (cynical, doubting, and untrusting; approaches positive events with disbelief and future possibilities with pessimism, anger, and trepidation; has a misanthropic view of life; is whining and grumbling, voicing disdain and caustic comments toward those experiencing good fortune);
4. *Defective regulatory control—displacement* (discharges anger and other troublesome emotions either precipitously or by employing nonconscious maneuvers to shift them from their instigator to settings or persons of lesser significance; vents disapproval by substitute or passive means, such as acting inept or perplexed, or behaving in a forgetful or indolent manner.

The four structural domains (trait-like) of negativistic personality disorder, as defined by Millon, are:

1. a *discontented self-image* (sees self as misunderstood, luckless, unappreciated, jinxed, and demeaned by others; recognizes being characteristically embittered, disgruntled, and disillusioned with life);
2. *vacillating object-relations* (internalized representations of the past constitute a complex of countervailing relationships, setting in motion contradictory feelings, conflicting inclinations, and incompatible memories);
3. *divergent morphologic organization* (a clear division in the pattern of morphologic structures such that coping and defensive maneuvers are often

directed toward incompatible goals, leaving major conflicts unresolved and full psychic cohesion often impossible by virtue of the fact that fulfillment of one drive or need inevitably nullifies or reverses another;
4. *irritable mood* (frequently touchy, temperamental, and peevish, followed in turn by sullen and moody withdrawal; is often petulant and impatient; unreasonably scorns those in authority and reports being annoyed easily or frustrated by many).

These features, both functional and structural, described for passive-aggressive (negativistic) personality, are invariably observed with all other variants of personality disorder, thus they are not specific enough to entitize passive-aggressive personality disorder.[4] However, negativistic, passive-aggressive traits are integral to the negativistic-dependent variant of personality disorder, as described.

Assessment of reality testing: a polarized mind creates a polarized world. External reality is defined as everything that exists independently from human volition and outside the mind or what is consensually agreed upon to be actually "out there" (Auchincloss and Samberg, 2012). Personal reality of one's relationships and one's actual self-image (as believed to be seen by others) always includes subjectivity which in most cases falls within the range of normal quantitative variation of subjective distortions. Reality testing is defined as the capacity to differentiate between subjective experience and outer reality or, roughly, between internal and external reality. It is preserved for the most part in persons functioning at the fragmented level, however the qualifier "for the most part" is needed to indicate that it can be transiently and partially impaired under certain conditions. These individuals may experience significant inconsistencies between their inner experiences and the outer reality of the situation, especially when under stress or emotionally upset, sometimes to the point of developing overvalued ideas and/or delusional thinking ("brief reactive psychosis"). Partially impaired reality testing is one of the consequences of a blurred, but generally established, mental boundary with the outside world in personality disorder. The co-presence of the primary and secondary process explains the partial blurring but not a full breach of the boundary. As noted, these individuals characteristically have limitations in reality testing, both in terms of their sense of self being saturated with autistic wishful fantasies, and as deficits in subtle aspects of interpersonal functioning (Kernberg, 2015) which may be observed as misinterpreting

4. The disorder was eliminated in the DSM system in the mid-1990s.

a relationship, feeling confounded by it, or being unsure what to make of them (here, impaired reality testing overlaps with difficulties in mentalization).

Although their reality *testing* is for the most part intact, persons functioning at the fragmented level may have impaired *sense* of reality,[5] known as the dissociative phenomena of derealization and depersonalization (described in Chapter 2). To complicate things further, these individuals typically gauge reality through their own "gut feeling of reality" ("I feel he is a bad person") rather than through cognitive analysis of reality. Such gut "feeling" for reality goes beyond a healthy intuition (in contrast to intuition, it has high impact on actual behavior), because it usually reflects the patient's reliance on affective "assessment" (their strong side) rather than rational analysis (their weak side), giving rise to idiosyncratic decisions, as well as relationships and behaviors that are perplexing to others. Reality testing and latent psychotic potential are best assessed by projective tests, particularly the Rorschach Inkblot Test (the Rorschach).

Additional diagnostic indices: lack of object constancy, pathology of attachment, deficient mentalization. Object constancy, attachment pattern, the sense of self, and capacity for mentalization all emerge early in development and are critical for self-regulation of mood, capacity for empathy, spontaneous and deliberate mentation, attention, and mature interpersonal relations. They are also important indicators of personality disorder.

As discussed, *object constancy* is a developmental milestone enabling the individual to preserve a stable internal representation of an object in the face of complex or contradictory emotions experienced toward that object; for example, positive feelings toward a loved object in the face of disappointment and negative feelings toward an object in the face of whatever contradictory positive experiences may arise at the moment (Auchincloss and Samberg, 2102). Object constancy arises from whole object relations and the lack of it results from partial object relations, and is thus indicative of personality disorder. Here, polarized units of experience are split off and do not cross-talk to neutralize each other. For this reason positive and negative stimulation easily activate corresponding positive and negative self- and object images and their associated affects. Such self- and object instability in part explains poor self-regulation of affect states and turbulent interpersonal relations. Object constancy is assessed based on biographical information about interpersonal relationships and in the therapeutic

5. Sense of reality is defined as experiencing what is happening as real, not imaginary.

setting, through transference. Persons who lack object constancy may tend to cling to others with pseudo-empathy: they care about others only insofar as it maintains the appearance of a two-way relationship, while they are actually horrified at the prospect of losing the object, who provides attention, affection, support, and/or concrete help. Abandonment sensitivity, a related but a deeper phenomenon, involves the fear of losing the selfobject who defines and maintains the sense of self. These patients do not tolerate separation, which means in their experience being left helpless against the world. For example, a patient of mine (MDJ) showed catastrophic expectations about my health during periods when therapy was paused because of my vacation ("I thought something happened to you") or during my common cold ("I was afraid it was something serious"). We understood both statements more as an expression of her fear of losing the therapist (both as support and as selfobject) and anger, expressed as passive-aggression, because of the break, rather than her own genuine concern for my well-being. The latent message "I hate you, don't leave me" so aptly reflects the quality and nature of interpersonal relations frequently seen with individuals with personality disorder.

Attachment theories have contributed to the understanding of personality disorder by explaining the specific affective bonds of these patients. They can show the whole spectrum of pathological attachment patterns, primarily the disorganized-disoriented but also the anxious-ambivalent and anxious-avoidant type pasterns. Some patients show different attachment patterns in different contexts; for example, they may be anxious-ambivalent in most relationships but with the romantic partner they "fall apart" and regress to the disorganized-disoriented pattern. Attachment patterns are assessed based on self-reported biographical information about interpersonal relationships, frequently at the forefront of the patient's concerns, as well as in the therapeutic setting. Numerous psychometric self-report tests are also available to assess attachment.

Mentalization refers to the capacity to understand one's own behavior and the behavior of others as a reflection of authentic and meaningful mental states, beliefs, desires, feelings, morals, and memories. Capacity for mentalization arises from whole object relations and secure attachment; the lack of it is rooted in partial object relations, with emotional and mental fragmentation, lack of object constancy, and disorganized-disoriented attachment, all being characteristic of personality disorder. Hence, these patients have significant mentalization problems, for example, limited capacity to implicitly and explicitly interpret themselves and others in terms of subjective states and mental processes. The inherent uncertainty of mentalization[6] is accentuated in fragmented personalities, mostly related to the characteristic lack of distance toward one's own assumptions, which makes the patient unlikely to check the reality of his or her assumptions, thereby further pathologizing interpersonal relationships. Four types of mentalization deficits have been described in personality disorder:

1. Inability to imagine the internal world of others and the lack of insight into one's own internal states (bewilderment or confusion about both);
2. Blurry awareness of the difference between the external and internal reality (aka the "omnipotence of subjectivity") and "psychic equivalence" (equating mental states and physical reality), which here converge with partially impaired reality testing;
3. Difficulties in separating fantasy from reality (e.g., "hyperactive mentalizing") as shown in delusional ideas about their relationships; and
4. Concrete (literal) thinking (understanding behaviors exclusively as a function of physical limitations and/or overtly detectable goals, or conviction that thoughts and feelings can only be changed through actions; Dimitrijevic, 2011).

The described difficulties in self-perception and mentalization represent one of the key factors involved in influencing a person's motivation, whether willingness or resistance, to enter psychotherapy and engage in a demanding therapeutic relationship. Defective capacity for mentalization and its assessment in fragmented individuals is particularly well elaborated in mentalization-based treatment (MBT) within the framework of contemporary relational psychoanalysis (Bateman and Fonagy, 2004). Capacity for mentalization is clinically assessed by naturalistic (interview) and projective techniques. MBT is described in detail in Chapter 4.

PSYCHOLOGICAL TESTS IN THE DIAGNOSIS OF PERSONALITY DISORDER

The fragmented level of functioning may overlap with all other levels, hence the importance of objectivized psychological exploration. Psychological testing involves a comparative cross-analysis of data obtained with different

6. One can never be certain what others actually feel or think but can only infer based on empathy or external clues.

test protocols. During the entire process of crafting the working diagnosis, test results are compared and then combined in order to be interpreted in the context of history, biographical information, current situation, and data obtained from direct contact with the patient. Tests increase the objectivity of the assessment but are not necessary when STIPO or similar structured interviews are used by an expert. We summarize a selection of psychometric tests as follows: at the minimum, the battery should include one projective test (preferably the Rorschach and/or Thematic Apperception Test [TAT]), a personality questionnaire (preferably the MCMI or the TCI), a test of defense mechanisms (preferably the iMOD;[7] Ignjatovic-Dzamonja and Divac-Jovanovic, 2014), and an identity test (preferably the IDQ; Wilkinson-Ryan and Westen, 2010). An intelligence test (preferably the Wechsler Adult Intelligence Scale [WAIS]) may be of importance but only secondarily. It is mainly used in order to provide a qualitative comparison of performance on structured (e.g., WAIS) versus nonstructured tests (e.g., TAT).

Of the many available personality questionnaires, we find the MCMI[8] and the TCI the most informative for the clinical-behavioral diagnosis and differential diagnosis of personality disorder, with MCMI also providing information relevant to the in-depth diagnosis and psychotherapy. The MCMI provides information about three relevant diagnostic planes: personality, its level of functioning, and its clinical syndromes. The protocol is interpreted by comparing the results on all three planes. The MCMI is used to differentiate normalcy versus pathology and within the latter neurotic versus personality disorder versus psychotic. The severity of personality pathology is assessed on the C scale, titled "borderline" as well as on the Paranoid (P) and Schizotypal (S) scale. As noted, in prior research (Divac-Jovanovic et al., 1993) the "borderline" C scale reliably distinguished individuals with personality disorder from healthy controls with matching behavior styles. High scores on the three severity scales reliably predict the fragmented level of personality functioning (personality disorder) provided that the scores on the scales capturing more severe syndromes (i.e., scales for major depression [SS], thought disorder [CC], and delusional disorder [PP]) are not increased, in which case depression and psychosis are further explored. The MCMI personality trait scales (narcissistic, histrionic, compulsive, schizoid,

7. The iMOD test is provided in the appendix to this book.

8. Here we discuss MCMI-III (published in 1994). The new MCMI-IV (published in 2015) includes a normative update, new and updated test items, changes to remain aligned to the DSM-5, an updated set of Grossman Facet Scales, the addition of critical responses, and the addition of the Turbulent Personality Scale. Each behavior is now described with three levels of personality functioning: (i) normal style: generally adaptive personality patterns; (ii) abnormal traits/type: moderately maladaptive personality attributes; and (iii) clinical disorder: likelihood of greater personality dysfunction.

among others) depict normal adaptive styles, provided that the scores on the severity scales are not increased, especially the borderline C scale, in which case the diagnosis of a corresponding variant of personality disorder is made. Clearly, a person can have high scores on the personality trait scales and not have a personality disorder, just a specific adaptive style. Finally, fragmented personality can manifest a "floating profile", i.e., significant increases on all or most scales for personality traits. The MCMI allows for dimensional diagnosis and captures mixed forms of personality disorder.

The TCI (Cloninger et al., 1993) is used for self-report of character traits, operationalized for easy identification and understanding. Low character scores, especially low SD, are correlated with immature defense mechanisms and are thus highly predictable of personality disorder. Low scores on the CO scale are suggestive of social maladaptation. Temperament scores are useful for differential diagnosis of adaptive styles, each a unique configuration of temperament traits (arranged in eight quartets—as shown in Table 2.1). Such a high level of stratification (resolution) personalizes the diagnosis to some extent. As noted, the inclusion of SD, an operationalized measure of personality integration, as a character trait together with CO, a measure of social adaptation, and with ST, a measure of spirituality, does not hinder the TCI's diagnostic reliability and validity, because the two scales (SD, CO) cover the two most important and highly correlated aspects of the diagnosis: intra- and interpersonal. The same approach, combining self- and its attendant interpersonal pathology is employed in the new DSM-5 alternative model and ICD 11, as discussed.

Projective tests (Rorschach, TAT) can offer powerful diagnostic hints about the fragmented level of functioning, particularly by providing indicators of the splitting mechanism "at work." On the Rorschach, these indicators may be either formal (quantitative), substantive (content related, qualitative), or both. With respect to the content, the most important indicators of splitting and, indirectly, personality disorder pathology are excessive verbalization (fabulized combinations, arbitrary responses, chain-like confabulations, etc.) and rapid successions of opposite affectively charged responses (one remarkably positive, the next remarkably negative for the same inkblot). All of these indicators point to the splitting mechanism and are highly suggestive of the borderline level of functioning, as it was called at the time of this study (Divac-Jovanovic, 1979). Similarly, the manifestations of splitting on the TAT are seen as shifting between oppositely affectively charged contents in thematic analysis. The way the story is constructed and especially the characteristics the patient attributes to the main character on the TAT test may reveal identification models and the quality of identity integration. Helpful diagnostic insights can be gained from the Machover Draw-A-Person Test (drawing of a human figure). Within the context of diagnosing fragmented personality, this test serves as a counterpoint (a contrapuntal) to other tests: poor quality of drawing within an otherwise normal performance on other tests is suggestive of personality fragmentation and vice versa. The test, a simple, unstructured drawing of a human figure, explores the deepest layers of personality, even more so than the Rorschach test, because it is fully nonverbal. As such, it is an important clue with respect to profound psychopathology which frequently becomes a tie-breaker in the generally minutiose differential diagnosis of personality disorder versus psychoses and neuroses, especially early in the course of therapy/diagnosis, when the Machover test is usually applied.

Cross-analysis of protocols on the administered tests provides a relatively reliable hypothesis about the dominant level of functioning. Since patients with personality disorder are unstable in many areas, they are equally "unstable" in their productivity on tests and can produce very rich or very poor content as well as both normal and pathological protocols. Sometimes no diagnostically relevant data are obtained even after applying a complete battery of tests (the so-called empty protocol), in contrast to the wealth of information collected in immediate contact with that patient or collaterally. Incidentally, the predictive validity of naturalistic techniques is often superior to that of psychometric tests, which (the latter) frequently have a relatively high percentage of false positives. In contrast, naturalistic interviews may yield an occasional false negative but very rarely if ever false positive results. Retesting is therefore recommended within six months to a year.

Differential diagnosis by psychological tests: a summary. Typical test patterns of persons functioning at the fragmented level can be summarized as follows: a rather normal reasoning, communication style, and verbalization are observed in highly structured test situations, such as the WAIS test; on unstructured, projective tests these individuals demonstrate deviant reasoning and peculiar thought processes and verbalization. Interestingly, on projective tests, these patients may show far more conspicuous responses, saturated with primary process, than psychotic individuals. There are several reasons for this paradox. First, unstructured situations facilitate projections of latent, fragmented, and unintegrated internal contents. Second, the primary process is no stranger to fragmented individuals, and they are not traumatized by it but rather they express it without distress or feeling threatened. Finally, the mechanism of splitting, which is here "in charge," lets the nonconscious materials to freely float around without threatening the rest of one's personality.

Differentiation of personality disorder from psychosis early in treatment is one of the most important tasks for clinicians, as treatment planning and prognosis greatly differ. Persons with personality disorder develop tolerance to and accept without much distress their own inconsistencies, controversies, and low rationality (e.g., their primary process). They manifest a particularly deviant content on projective tests, while persons in the initial stages of psychosis can have relatively inconspicuous protocols on projective tests (in psychosis, restrictive control of thought and emotions may be their last defense against psychotic decompensation). The paradox that the more severely disordered show "healthier" test results is explained by the inverse relationship between the degree of external structure and manifest aberrance. Due to the weak and poorly defined internal direction, persons at the fragmented level of functioning are exceptionally dependent on external direction: they function "normally" when the external situation provides reliable feedback and instructions for behavior which thus places minimal pressure on their capacity to interpret external cues. Without the fortification provided by an external structure, their latent psychotic potential becomes more evident, which may explain more psychopathology on projective rather than on structured tests. In contrast, persons with psychosis express pathological content openly but they project less on projective tests. It should be noted that at the most severe end of the fragmented spectrum individuals with personality disorder can be disorganized, paranoid, and emotionally unstable to the extent that they may appear and actually become psychotic, especially during intense emotional reactions and stress (brief reactive psychoses). However, after a short period of therapy or even spontaneously with the resolution of the emotional stressor, they can recover and begin to produce signs and symptoms of personality disorder while at the same time their psychotic symptoms abate.

With the neurotic level of functioning, differentiation from personality disorder is less demanding. In terms of the fundamental psychodynamic diagnostic triad (i.e., identity-defense mechanisms-reality testing), the neurotic level of functioning is characterized by an integrated identity, neurotic defense mechanisms (centered around repression), and fully preserved reality testing (without transitory psychotic regressions as seen with personality disorder). This is illustrated in Table 3.2.

On psychological tests, individuals functioning at the neurotic level show a balanced quality of responses on structured and unstructured tests, in contrast to those at the fragmented level who manifest a decrement in the quality of responses with decreasing degree of structure on tests. Mental boundaries in fragmented individuals are more permeable to the primary process, which (the primary process) these individuals manifest on projective tests much more readily than is found to be the case with persons functioning at the neurotic or normal level as well as with those with incipient psychosis. However, on the more structured intelligence tests, individuals with neurosis may underperform as a result of coexisting anxiety. This does not mean that psychotic and fragmented patients do not

Table 3.2 DIFFERENTIAL DIAGNOSTIC TRIAD: IDENTITY, DEFENSE MECHANISMS, REALITY TESTING AND RESPECTIVE ADAPTIVE PATTERNS

Level of Functioning / Area of Functioning	Normal	Neurotic	Fragmented (All Variants of Personality Disorder)	Psychotic
Identity	**Integrated**	**Integrated**	**Diffuse**	**Confused**
Defense Mechanisms	**Mature** (suppression)	**Neurotic** (repression)	**Immature** (splitting)	**Pathological** (dissociation)
Reality Testing	**Intact**	**Intact**	**Partially Impaired**	**Impaired**
Adaptive Pattern	**Flexibility**	**Rigidity**	**Polarization**	**Disorganization**

experience anxiety in test situations, it is simply to say that they manifest anxiety in different ways.

MENTAL PROFILES AT DIFFERENT LEVELS OF PERSONALITY FUNCTIONING: THE FLEXIBLE, THE RIGID, THE POLARIZED, AND THE POROUS

The healthy level of personality functioning is characterized by a functional adaptation to both internal and external environments. In the narrow sense, functional adaptation is any adaptation that helps an organism to survive. In a wider socio-psychological sense, the term refers to bilateral benefits, a win-win scenario for both the person and the people who surround him or her. Faced with challenges of problems, functionally adapted individuals are capable of including others who are willing to help and also become better able to adjust their own behavior and ask others to adjust theirs (flexible coping—a healthy mixture of alloplasticity and autoplasticity). They are capable of two-way cooperation in order to realize their own potential or satisfy their own needs, while at the same time not stirring up relationship pathology or standing in the way of others. On the contrary, they are spontaneously helpful (they lack envy) and may be inspirational to many because of their sincerity, compassion, composure, and principled fairness. At this level, individuals commonly engage in the so-called extended-self activities beyond one's narrow personal interest for the common good. They may employ neurotic or immature defense mechanisms during short periods. In reaction to stress or during personal crises (e.g., midlife crisis, divorce, or health crisis), they can manifest problems in adaptation (transient isolation, impulsivity, or dissociation), sometimes amounting to a full-blown adjustment disorder, as one of the mildest forms of maladaptive reactions to acute problems common in healthy individuals.

The neurotic level of functioning is characterized by relative rigidity in adaptation due to inflexible defense mechanisms which limit both the number and the effectiveness of coping strategies available to handle stress or changes in the social context. These individuals' repressed problems are reflected in particular themes within their style of adaptation, for example, the histrionic style typically involves themes of gender role, partner relations, and sexuality, the anankastic style revolves around problems of control, and so on. Neurotic defenses are concerned only with the particular rather than all relationships (e.g., only in the context of the relationship with the opposite sex or authority), in contrast to the pervasive primitive defenses seen in individuals with personality disorder. Outside these problem areas, neurotic persons may have adequate relationships, a good work history, and effective affect regulation and tolerance. They are able to successfully incorporate the help of others, although they may distort the contact by viewing themselves or others through the prism of dependence or guilt. Neurotic psychopathology is defined as conflict based, in contrast to the deficit-based pathology of personality disorder. Conflict-based pathology implies intentionality; that is, symptoms have objectives, meaning, and purpose, and defenses against anxiety include repression and disguising. At this level, identity is integrated, defense mechanisms are centered around repression, objects are whole even if relationships are ambivalent, and reality testing is intact, as it is with healthy individuals. In contrast, the deficit-based pathology of personality disorder shows no purposefulness and the mind is not defending itself against anxiety but rather against disintegration. The conflict versus deficit dilemma in the orientation of psychopathology implies certain differences in the therapeutic approach to patients at different levels of functioning. In persons with neurotic disorders, therapy is concerned with *hidden meanings* (the uncovering and interpretation of repressed contents); therapy of persons with fragmented personality with *missing meanings* and attempts to help the patient accept, affirm, and express real experiences versus the make-believe experiences of the dictatorial pathological self; and therapy of persons with psychosis with *common meanings* which are needed in order to recover reality testing.

At the fragmented level, the self-object boundary is established, so that the person can separate his or her own mind from that of others, which contrasts with what is seen in psychosis. However, the experience is unrealistically polarized ("black or white") and unstable, alternating between these extremes. The same holds true for emotions, alternating between elation and devastation. The capacity for introspection and self-correction is low. As noted, the problems of personality disorder reflect a developmental deficit, or a failure to integrate personality and its subsystems into effective adaptive functions. Deficits relate to problems with hypofrontality reflected as poor cognitive control of behavior and self-regulation of mood, low capacity for empathy and mentalization, among others. The fragmented internal world is perpetuated by the operation of splitting and its related primitive defenses: the more frequent and dominant the splitting, the more severe the personality pathology. In summary, object relations are partial, defense mechanisms are immature, identity is diffuse, and reality testing is preserved, albeit with occasional subtle impairments (Table 3.2).

It is important to keep in mind that psychotic level of functioning versus psychosis (e.g., Schizophrenia), are not synonyms insofar that the former may occur without the profoundly disorganized brain structure of psychosis. In contrast to all of the previous levels, the psychotic level of mental functioning is characterized by both concrete and overly generalized thinking, overwhelming episodes of anxiety stirred by the irruptions of primary process, impaired reality testing (i.e., thought disorder resulting in delusional or referential thinking), and confused or conflicting identity (alternatives collide and implode). The main defense mechanism is psychotic dissociation. At the psychotic level, individuals do not differentiate between self and others (porous self-object boundary), and they attribute their own feelings and thoughts to others and vice versa, with poor insight. As a specific feature, interactions with others are "tangential" in order to avoid the interpersonal differentiation that a deeper contact would create. Such differentiation may create grounds for a conflict which is perceived by a delusional person as potentially life-threatening. Individuals with the most severe forms of personality fragmentation may occasionally also experience reality distortions and may impute their own thoughts or feelings to others. Examples include erotomania (i.e., being convinced that a well-known person is reciprocating love despite evidence to the contrary), "hearing voices" coming not from an external source (as is the case in a psychotic disorder) but from within oneself and recognizing them as familiar (e.g., an angry parent's voice). The difference is that impaired reality testing is transient with fragmented individuals (lasting anywhere from several hours to several days) and long-standing at the psychotic level (weeks, months). The latter is also much more profound and pervasive.

CHAPTER 4

Psychotherapy of Personality Disorder

Personality disorder is experienced as *ego-syntonic*. These individuals typically see their symptoms as inseparable from who they are, leaving them convinced that the symptoms should not and cannot be changed, and thus they rarely seek help on their own initiative. They may accept treatment at the insistence of others, usually partners, because problems tend to amplify in intimate relationships. Alternatively, they might seek help for comorbid depression, eating disorders, hypochondria, alcoholism, or drug abuse. Personality disorder is expressed as *alloplastic*. These individuals typically try to resolve stress by actively trying to change others through conflicts, rather than attempting to change their own attitudes and behavior. Such alloplasticity is facilitated by primitive defense mechanisms (denial and projection in particular), subtle limitations in reality testing in interpersonal relationships, and specific character and moral traits (selfishness, opportunism), which are slavishly engendered to meet the demands of internal organization, at the expense of social adaptation. As discussed, a deeply fragmented personality is organized into a compensatory but unrealistic self-image, brought into existence through fantasy and on the interpersonal stage. In therapy, the patient has first to abandon this pathological compensation and thus temporarily decrease his or her own adaptive fitness before developing more authentic and realistic subsystems of the mind. This is known as "U-shaped" developmental dynamics. The three characteristics (ego-syntony, alloplasticity, and the initial loss of adaptive fitness) not only explain why these patients hesitate to seek help but outline the difficulties clinicians can expect during psychotherapy.

Psychotherapy and pharmacotherapy: reaching root mechanisms from different directions. Reconstructive in-depth psychotherapy is the primary treatment for personality disorder. Its main tool is corrective emotional experience, a concept first introduced by Franz Alexander (1946): "The patient, in order to be helped, must undergo a corrective emotional experience suitable to repair the traumatic influence of previous experiences. It is of secondary importance whether this corrective experience takes place during treatment in the transference relationship, or parallel with the treatment in the daily life of the patient" (p. 66). Corrective emotional experience in fact refers to the development of balanced emotional-cognitive units of the mind which is achieved through a long-term relationship with a constant object (the therapist), under controlled conditions and within a safe therapeutic setting. This experience, in all likelihood as discussed later, engenders the maturation of the patient's prefrontal cognitive networks and higher order mental capacities: self- and object constancy, more effective executive function, better self-regulation of mood, capacity for mentalization, and empathy and prosocial emotions, all of which arise as personality is rebuilt from the ground up. On the road to corrective emotional experience, a number of strategies and tools are used, as will be discussed later in the chapter. Psychotherapy is usually combined with pharmacotherapy, which can also be in depth (mechanism based), tailored to target temperament traits as root neurobiological vulnerabilities for personality disorder.

It is a myth that pharmacotherapy only works at the biological and psychotherapy only at the psychological level. Empirical data show that dialectic behavior therapy and psychodynamic psychotherapy alter brain function in borderline patients (Lai et al., 2007; Schnell and Herpertz, 2007). Psychodynamic therapy has been shown to normalize prefrontal hypofunction and tone down overactive amygdala-hippocampus connectivity in panic disorder patients (Beutel et al., 2010). Modern technology (single-photon emission computed tomography [SPECT] and positron-emission tomography [PET] scans in particular) allows us to measure molecular level changes after psychotherapy. Using SPECT, Lehto et al. (2008) showed significant increases in midbrain serotonin transporter density during psychodynamic psychotherapy in patients with atypical depression (highly indicative of personality disorder) but not among patients with run-of-the-mill depression, perhaps suggestive of the more specific healing mechanism in personality pathology than in mood disorders. Using PET scanning, Karlsson et al. (2010) and Hirvonen et al. (2011), studied patients with major depression randomized to receive either short-term psychodynamic psychotherapy or fluoxetine. Clinical outcomes in both groups were similar in terms of response and remission rates. However, serotonin receptor expression in the relevant brain areas was increased only in the psychotherapy group. The fluoxetine group, but not the psychotherapy group, was associated with altered dopamine neurotransmission[1] in the lateral thalamus. The finding seems to suggest that the recovery process in major depressive disorder after psychotherapy is different from recovery after medication.

The above studies demonstrate that a spoken word, with substance of course, in the context of a trusted relationship has the power to change the brain structure. In contrast to random relational influences on the mind, which can be either healthy or unhealthy, psychotherapy is an environmental intervention that consistently trends in the *healthy direction,* and is thus capable of correcting not only the pathological impact of adverse past environments (E × E interaction) but also of excessive patterns of neurobiology (G × E interaction). The correction is both mental (e.g., balancing of cognitive-affective units of the mind), and structural (in the sense that it is hardwired in remodeled brain networks by epigenetic mechanisms). As noted by R. Berezin in *Psychology Today* (December 2017), "psychotherapy addresses the brain in the way it actually develops, matures and operates (i.e., through interactive experience), it mediates remodeling of brain networks based on the fundamental processes of activity-dependent neuroplasticity." Once the main disputer, modern neuroscience appears to not only have reached a détente but has even underscored fundamental psychoanalytic hypotheses. Most notably, neuroscience supports the existence of nonconscious working memory, a prefrontal cortex (PFCx) function that pulls information from the engramized autobiographical affects and memories which we believe results in what psychoanalysis calls "internalized object relations," as discussed in Chapter 1. Psychotherapy and pharmacotherapy are not interchangeable but rather complementary, each adding its specific strengths to the healing process. Medication is effective in stabilizing subcortical networks involved in instinctive social behaviors (i.e., affect states involved in fear, defensive and offensive aggression, sexual behavior, etc.), but less so in changing cognitive abstractions about oneself and the world, which are more amenable to change in psychotherapy. The complementarity of the two treatments comes from their different directions of activity: psychotherapy works *top-down,* relying on the corrective emotional experience and stable insights[2] to epigenetically modulate one's own neuromolecular mechanisms. In fact, it has been hypothesized,

1. Because [11C]raclopride competes with endogenous dopamine for binding to dopamine-2/dopamine-3 (D2/D3) receptors, its increased binding may reflect either dopamine decrease or increase in D2/D3 receptor affinity, in this case associated with fluoxetine therapy.

2. An insight is defined as an act of understanding the inner nature of things, carrying cognitive and emotional elements and a positive motivation to change behavior.

based on preliminary data from mostly animal studies, that epigenetically active medication (e.g., histone deacetylase inhibitors which open chromatin to transcription) might enhance the learning effects of psychotherapy. In contrast, pharmacotherapy works *bottom-up*, stirring changes in the neurochemical environment which initiate homeostatic optimizations and thereby moderate and/or modulate[3] brain networks and *ipso facto* their interactive patterns, attenuating in the process affective biases in mental faculties (thought, emotion, motivation) and promoting cognitive impartiality. Complex subjective phenomena, such as self- or emotional awareness, are most likely emerging properties; that is, they arise from sequential cognitive representations and rerepresentations of lower order sensory information and thus may not be amenable to a precise biological dissection at present. Precise pharmacotherapy of emerging properties may well be an unattainable utopia, but with respect to more biologically rooted subsystems of the mind, such as temperament, mechanism-based pharmacotherapy is a realistic goal. Here, a pathological equilibrium of a temperament trait, suddenly disturbed by a chemical, can be driven toward a healthier equilibrium via homeostatic optimization that resets the trait in question.

PSYCHOTHERAPY OF FRAGMENTED PERSONALITY: INTEGRATIVE AND TRANSTHEORETICAL TO MATCH THE MULTIDIMENSIONALITY OF THE PROBLEM

Literally every school of psychotherapy has formulated its own method of working with people with personality disorder based upon each school's understanding of the syndrome. Each of the leading paradigms approaches an individual with personality disorder from a different but sensible point of entry. Psychoanalysis begins with emotions, cognitive-behavioral paradigm with behavior, humanistic paradigms with thought, and systemic theories and relational psychoanalysis with relations. However, after decades of theorizing, research, and clinical results, it seems that psychotherapy of personality disorder has to be *transtheoretical* in its view of mental functioning (psychodynamically based but making use of behavioristic, cognitive, humanistic, relational, and systemic concepts), *integrative* with respect to method, and *eclectic* with respect to techniques in

3. A moderator variable influences the strength of a relationship between two other variables, a mediator explains the relationship between the two other variables, and a modifier variable changes the characteristics of the relationship between two other variables.

order to meet the uniquely multicausal and multidimensional nature of the syndrome. It appears indeed that personality disorder has reconciled different theories and schools of therapy: today, the transtheoretical approach to treatment unites the psychoanalytic methods of transference and countertransference analysis with methods of behavior correction and analysis of interpersonal patterns. Reading about the goals and principles of mentalization-based treatment today feels like reading a piece of transactional (TA) literature; similarly, when one analyzes the work within TA, it may have just as easily originated from psychoanalytic literature. Therapists working with personality disorder understand each other well, despite different theoretical views and distinctive jargon. Our (MDJ) supervision group made up of two therapists of analytical orientation, two transactional therapists and one systemic therapist, has been successfully working together for years. The group's ideological diversity has proven to be an asset in treatment planning, rather than a hindrance (Divac-Jovanovic et al., 2005). Between the two of us, one (DMS) is a clinical psychiatrist and personality disorder researcher who underwent four years of Lehr-psychoanalysis[4] during residency as part of the master's program in psychotherapy. The other (MDJ) is a clinical psychologist and has been a certified TA therapist and trainer in clinical practice for decades, with a PhD in projective test diagnostics of borderline states. Such a mixture of neuropsychiatry and psychology, biogenetic, humanistic and psychoanalytic education, clinical practice and research, was indubitably helpful in conceptualizing the model of mental health and disorder presented in this book. The psychotherapeutic approach to personality disorder is paradigmatic of modern trends toward transtheoretical integrative psychotherapy in much the same way the diagnosis of personality disorder is paradigmatic of the differential diagnosis in general.

It was recognized early that Freudian psychoanalysis had to be significantly adapted in order to be effective with these different and "difficult" patients. These adjectives refer not only to the sheer number of symptoms and urgencies patients bring with them into treatment but also the challenges they pose to the therapist. The most successful models that have arisen from these adaptations are transference-focused psychotherapy (TFP) developed by Kernberg and colleagues (2008); dialectical behavioral therapy (DBT) developed by Linehan (1993); the related schema-focused therapy (SFT; Young et al., 2003); and mentalization-based treatment (MBT) developed by Bateman and Fonagy (2004). We have developed

4. Psychoanalyzed for teaching purposes.

reconstructive interpersonal therapy (RIT), an integrative, transtheoretical approach drawing from the psychoanalytic and humanist traditions (Divac-Jovanovic and Radojkovic, 1987; Divac-Jovanovic and Svrakic, 2017). Each model is discussed in more detail in this chapter. Comparative analysis of these approaches reveals many shared fundamental aspects, most notably the general strategy, general principles, and general goals of therapy, as discussed throughout the chapter.

Transference-focused psychotherapy (TFP). Otto Kernberg and his colleagues were among the first to describe specific psychoanalytic therapy for patients with identity diffusion and severe personality disorder. TFP is a highly structured, modified psychodynamic treatment theoretically based on Kernberg's (1984) object relation model of borderline personality organization. The main strategy of TFP consists in reactivation of the patient's split-off internalized object relations which are then observed and interpreted in the transference in the here and now. TFP is conducted in face-to-face sessions two to three times a week. The focus is initially on the patient's external, affectively invested situations and only shifts to transference interpretation later on when the corresponding transference development clearly begins to occupy the center of the patient's present interaction with the therapist (per the TFP manual; Clarkin et al., 2006). Patients are asked to free-associate around the problems that brought them to treatment, while the therapist observes the reactivation of regressive, split-off object relations in the transference, thereby helping patients to both recognize them and identify the role of such polarized views in creating current difficulties in interactions. One important goal is for patients to understand their nonconscious motivation that keeps these contradictory dyads separate. Interpretative integration gradually leads to the bridging of the mutually dissociated segments of experience and consequently to the modulation of intense affects and resolution of identity diffusion. At this time, a patient's depressive reaction is possible as it may reflect the capacity to recognize his or her own aggression that was previously projected or experienced as dysphoria.

TFP uses the essential techniques of psychoanalysis (interpretation, transference analysis, and technical neutrality in a modified form) but also heavily relies on countertransference to analyze the patient's internalized object relations and internal experiences. The early phases of interpretation involve clarification (focused on the patient's subjective experiences) and confrontation (tactfully drawing attention to inconsistencies or contradictions in the patient's communication). TFP is always linked with analysis of the patient's real-life problems and thus in this respect differs from standard psychoanalysis. Countertransference is not communicated directly to the patient but is worked into transference interpretations, as the therapist actually utilizes countertransference in order to glean clarification of the transference. The therapist is required to remain tolerant to intensive countertransference evoked by severely regressive behavior and acting out in the transference. Departing from technical neutrality is considered only in situations where it is necessary to protect the boundaries of the treatment and/or the patient from self-harm. In our view, TFP has brought psychoanalysis closer to humanistic and relational therapies, because it relies more directly on the patient-therapist communication in the here-and-now, and thereby represents a powerful step toward modern integrative therapy. Our approach, RIT, draws from TFP but adds an existentialist focus and brings the process a step closer to a direct communication of the countertransference.

Dialectic-behavioral therapy (DBT). DBT belongs to the second- and third-wave cognitive-behavioral therapies (CBTs). It combines the cognitive-behavioral paradigm with mindfulness, a concept originating from Buddhism. In the 1990s, DBT was seen as a fresh approach to the treatment of "borderline"[5] disorder, a condition that was previously treated almost exclusively using the methods of psychoanalysis. DBT conceives of borderline pathology as resulting from a complex interaction of biological-constitutional factors (e.g., mood dysregulation), environmental factors (e.g., early trauma), and a social-environmental component, referred to as an "invalidating" environment (Linehan, 1993). In an invalidating early environment, the child's personal (emotional) experiences are responded to by the caretaker as if they were invalid or inappropriate, thereby leading to self-invalidation and a failure to learn how to communicate and/or regulate emotions. Since extreme emotions are taken more seriously than moderate emotions in such environments, the child communicates either by extreme behaviors or by noncommunication of emotions and behaviors altogether. In practice, DBT combines validation of affect states (by teaching skills to tolerate or avoid distress in order to reduce or eliminate painful emotions) and control (stopping) dangerous behaviors, particularly self-destructive and aggressive behaviors. The term *dialectic* refers to a synthesis (acceptance and change) of the opposites: accepting life as it is, not as it should be, emphasizing change despite reality, not because of it. The therapist accepts the patient as he or she is but at the same time accepts the fact that

5. We keep this term "borderline" personality in this section as originally used by Kernberg et al. (1975), Linehan (1993), and Bateman and Fonagy (2001), instead of our term "fragmented" personality, to preserve the accuracy of citations.

the patient has to change in order to achieve the goals of therapy which are also his or her (the patient's) goals. DBT techniques and strategies are geared toward balancing these two opposites (acceptance and change) and are divided into two groups. The *acceptance-oriented strategies* include (i) mindful awareness (or learning to observe, reflect, and describe emotional states while developing focused attention in the given moment) and (ii) stress tolerance (or learning how to tolerate situational frustration and suffering). Mindfulness, one of the central moderators of change in DBT, is thought to help the patients both to develop perspective and tolerate and regulate negative affective experiences without being overwhelmed by them. Incidentally, the concepts of mindfulness, mentalization, and integrated representation overlap conceptually (Levy et al., 2006). The second group of DBT therapeutic strategies, *change oriented,* involve regulation of emotions (or learning how to change the emotions one wants to change) and improved interpersonal communication skills and effectiveness (e.g., learning how to request what one wants and decline what one does not want while preserving self-respect as well as good relations with others). Incidentally, a very similar strategy is employed by TA (Divac-Jovanovic, 1986). Significantly lower dropout rates in comparison to psychodynamic therapies are reported for DBT. DBT has also proven to be successful in reducing suicide rates, self-injurious behavior, and harmful substance abuse (Linehan and Heard, 1999). These benefits are not limited to personality disorder but have also been documented in depression, posttraumatic stress disorder, and eating disorders as well. Other forms of CBTs have been effective in personality disorder, notably Beck's approach (Beck et al., 2004) and Young's schema therapy (Young et al., 2003); the latter combines elements of CBT, psychoanalytic object relations, attachment theory, and Gestalt therapy so is actually a major expansion of CBT.

Schema-focused therapy (SFT).[6] SFT is an integrative approach to the treatment of personality disorder that combines CBT and Gestalt methods with psychoanalytic and object relations theory into one unified model. It expands on CBT by placing more emphasis on the therapeutic relationship, affective experience, and the discussion of early life experiences. SFT is based on the deficit model of personality disorder and emphasizes the early context of inadequate parenting that (i) does not satisfy the core needs of a child (for safety, nurturance, protection, affection, acceptance, empathy, guidance, validation, among others), (ii) traumatizes or victimizes the child (domineering, abusive, and/ or critical parents), and/or (iii) is unbalanced (overprotection, overindulgent,

6. "Schema-focused emotive behavioral therapy" is a variant developed in Germany.

too much freedom without setting the limits), among others. Consequently, the child develops a schema (or schemata, plural for schema) defined as fixed and automatic biases, that is, patterns of negative thought, emotions, and self-defeating behavior, colloquially referred to as "lifetraps." Schema can be thought of as a mini subsystem of the preconceptual mind, a configuration of biased thoughts and related emotions born through early interactions that organize sensory information and the relationships between them into a specific negative view of oneself and the world. These in turn produce self-defeating behavior patterns (aka "coping styles") that emerge in specific contexts. The concept of schema is very similar to the TA concept of "frame of reference," which is defined as the structure of associated responses which integrates the various "ego-states"[7] in response to specific stimuli; it provides the individual with an overall perceptual, conceptual, affective and action set, which is used to define the self, other people and the world (Stewart and Joines, 1987). The core negative beliefs (the emotional core of a schema) most often are related to one's own unworthiness, unimportance, low ability, the impossibility of one being loved, one not deserving of love, and/or seeing oneself as a bad person who deserves severe punishment, among a host of others. A schema is a valid representation of early childhood experiences, is rather stable (even in the face of contradictory information), is perpetuated over the course of a lifetime, and is activated under respective conditions. SFT identifies 10 "schema modes" and defines these as mind states consisting of a cluster of schemas and coping styles activated by a specific life situation (similar to the concept of "scripts" in TA). For example, the "Angry Child" mode (episodes of feeling enraged, anxious, envious, jealous, frustrated, self-doubting, unsupported in ideas, and vulnerable) is triggered by feelings of victimization or bitterness, and is associated with the coping style of self-harm and seeking interpersonal conflicts that can lead to harm toward others (Young et al., 2003). In patients with personality disorder, schema modes are more pathological and rigid and may seem split off from the rest of the personality (Young et al., 2003), perhaps best thought of as split off real self fragments influenced by specific interactions involving negative self- and object-images.

In comparison to attachment, a developmentally earlier phenomenon capturing nonconscious internalized object relations "in action," schemata require a higher degree of mental and behavior organization. They are present in passive phenomenal consciousness ("knowing how it feels") but not in autonoetic self-awareness (not accessible to active introspection). This places the development of schemata between two and five years of age.

7. A consistent pattern of feeling, thinking, and experience directly related to a corresponding consistent pattern of behavior.

From here, the adherence to the schemata most frequently results in self-defeating coping styles (with no personality disorder) but can also coexist with a full-fledged personality disorder. Namely, if built upon partial object relations and sufficiently overwhelming, self-defeating schemata may require defensive omnipotent fantasies—revenge, beauty, ideal love, sexual attractiveness, among others, eventually developing into the corresponding variant of personality disorder.

The central idea of SFT is that maladaptive schemas can be corrected by reducing root emotional memories and by revising the cognitive patterns associated with them (known as "redecision" in TA). To this end, SFT uses strategies of cognitive exercises (listing pros and cons of a schema, testing the validity of a schema, or conducting a dialogue between the "schema side" and the "healthy side"), experiential and emotion-focused discussion (Gestalt therapy psychodrama techniques, such as the empty chair dialog, and imagery techniques), and expanded standard behavior techniques (such as role playing an interaction and then assigning the interaction as homework). SFT also relies on the basic healing components of the therapeutic relationship (Young et al., 2003). SFT is explicitly supportive: therapists spend extra time with patients and nurture them even to the point of holding patients physically in their arms. All as means toward the development of a secure attachment to the therapist, within the bounds of a professional relationship. Such "limited reparenting" is central to SFT, and aims to meet unmet core needs by providing the patient with the experiences that were missed in early childhood, such as connection, joy, mutuality, adequate limits, and autonomy. These therapeutic experiences provide an antidote to the damaging experiences that led to maladaptive schemas and modes (Young et al., 2003).

Mentalization-based treatment (MBT). MBT is a relatively new version of psychoanalytic psychotherapy for borderline conditions (Bateman and Fonagy, 2004). It focuses on increasing patients' capacity to recognize and interpret mental states in themselves and others, including the capacity for self-reflection on own internal mental states. As with other psychotherapies for personality disorder, MBT aims to reconstruct personality (the mind) into a realistic (integrated) sense of self and others. MBT draws from relational psychoanalysis and other related theories that understand the need for social relationships as rooted in neurobiology (social reward is now understood as one of the unlearned primary positive reinforcers), which is observable in children by the first year of age.

Mentalization, or, colloquially "psychological mindedness," refers to the capacity to understand the behavior of others as a reflection of their own mental state, beliefs, desires, feelings, morals, and memories ("authentic and meaningful"), to reflect upon one's own mental states, and to understand that one's own state of mind may influence the feelings and the behavior of others (MBT blurres the distinction between mentalization and theory of mind of others, which are indeed similar, although many authors distinguish the two). Mentalization is intrinsic to emotional regulation and conducive to productive social relationships (Auchincloss and Samberg, 2012). Capacity for mentalization is a developmental milestone normally accomplished by age three to five years, in tandem with self-awareness, theory of mind of others, prosocial emotions, and explicit motivations. Formation of this capacity requires either whole object relations and secure attachment in the separation-individuation process or a successful resolution of pre-existing partial object relations and attachment disturbance (Auchincloss and Samberg, 2012). As such, mentalization is necessary in order to understand and accept preconscious and nonconscious feelings as well as the motives driving one's own behavior and that of others. It consequently stabilizes the sense of self and facilitates engagement in fulfilling interpersonal relationships. To summarize, the capacity to understand mental processes in oneself and others is a complex cognitive-emotional phenomenon that arises from our biological roots (empathy, reciprocity, fairness, altruism) processed by the general network of cognition, PFCx in particular. Without prosocial emotions, the capacity to understand others is limited to dispassionate, lifeless intellectualization, much like the affect dissociation and dry intellectualization in obsessive-compulsive neurosis.

A poorly developed capacity for mentalization is one of the key consequences of pathological early development (disorganized attachment) and is a perpetuating factor for personality disorder. The goal of MBT is to help the patient make sense of incomprehensible feelings, express them more adequately in social interactions, and employ them effectively in interpersonal relationships, thus furthering the development of patients' sense of personal responsibility. The authors of MBT provide a detailed description of different forms of deficient mentalization in personality disorder, each arising from disorganized attachment, and leading to problems in affect regulation, attention, and self control.

In summary, MBT represents an interesting departure from classical psychoanalytic treatment of severe personality pathology, as is, in fact, the case with the entire field of relational psychoanalysis from which it is derived. MBT is primarily focused on conscious and preconscious processes even though it is presented in the literature as a variation of psychoanalytic therapy. SFT and relational psychoanalysis, including MBT, are similar to humanistic therapies, most notably to TA which pioneered integrative psychotherapy by combining psychoanalytical concepts with CBT techniques aiming to develop a practical, active, in-depth, and effective therapy for severe personality pathology. All of these modalities promote a position of nonassuming and "not knowing" (referring to the pre-existing knowledge of what is normal), flexibility with different personal narratives and perspectives, emphasize the importance of empathy as the key element of the therapeutic relationship, and support a practice model of honesty and openness in the relationship with the patient (the latter refers to therapists' ongoing review of their work and acknowledging mistakes).

CONSENSUS ON STRATEGIES, PROCESS, AND GOALS IN PSYCHOTHERAPY OF PERSONALITY DISORDER

Irrespective of its many modalities, psychotherapy is a unique process that always has requisite stages—a beginning, a course, and an end—regardless of the method used. In short, psychotherapy of personality disorder must first establish and maintain a therapeutic relationship with the patient based on trust and mutual confidence, then work through contents and processes with him or her at all levels of personality functioning, analyze achieved changes and encourage patients to practice them in real life, and finally work on separation to eventually terminate the process, although never completely (which is actually the patient's decision). The process is sometimes quick, sometimes slow, sometimes continuous, sometimes intermittent, sometimes brought to completion, sometimes not—but its essence remains the same, irrespective of the theoretical context, method, discourse, and paradigm. Of note, the recent expansion of virtual communication has propagated to psychotherapy as well ("tele-psychotherapy"). We believe that psychotherapy of personality disorder has to remain "analog," face-to-face in order to provide a natural stage for the corrective emotional experience involving all senses, much like in infancy.

Effective psychotherapy of personality disorder has to be creative, flexible, intensive, and transtheoretical. Both the fragmented substrate and the precariousness of the pathological compensation are in focus as interrelated, cause-and-consequence phenomena. To handle the specific psychodynamics of individuals with personality disorder, notably the underlying fragmentation and the continual risk of decompensation, psychotherapy is optimally reconstructive (or in depth, like psychoanalytic psychotherapy), but at the same time it has to be highly structured (similar to CBTs) while emphasizing an empathic relationship (like humanistic therapies). None of these modalities individually in their original form was able to fulfill these criteria at the same time. Humanistic and systemic therapies and relational psychoanalysis opened the space for a true synthesis of intrapsychic and interpersonal planes in the psychotherapeutic process. Existentialistic and interpersonal therapies, within the humanistic paradigm, were, by definition, eclectic and "free" to combine everything that was useful in achieving therapeutic change. This gave them the potential to integrate the three requirements (in depth, high structure, empathy) in both the theoretical and the practical sense (Dryden, 1996). Humanistic and systemic approaches were less focused on etiopathogenesis and more focused on "normalizing" psychopathology and recognizing the patient's strengths, who was seen as capable of changing (the influence of existentialism). The humanistic approach is thus often called the "third force" in psychology, after psychoanalysis and behaviorism (Maslow coined the term). In retrospect, the psychodynamic framework was a common root for the subsequent paradigms, with cognitive-behavioral and humanistic-relational discourse making later contributions, while together they are able to address all aspects of mental functioning that must be covered in psychotherapy.

Since every person undergoing therapy is unique, it is to the clinicians' advantage to have at his or her disposal an array of specific techniques and methods developed from different approaches. This will invariably enrich the experience of every therapist and patient engaged in psychotherapy. In the early phases of therapy, with turmoil (family friction, spouse threatening to leave, looming job termination, or interpersonal conflicts) and risky behaviors (impulsivity, self-harm, rage, substance use) that can incapacitate the patient, a directive approach (cognitive, behavioral, or both) and supportive techniques that build rapport and trust are not only helpful but also indicated. Direction and support are continued for patients who continue to be regressive and stressed out; protective therapeutic contracts are of vital importance here, such as antisuicidal, antiviolence, etc. When some stabilization of behavior and at least some control over situational stressors are achieved, less directive approaches are used. The latter involves long-term psychodynamic exploration of transference feelings and object relations, analysis of interpersonal transactions, and/or working on the development of mentalization, etc. During the closing phases of treatment, when the patient is now "living" his or her real self in real time, the approach can again revert to one that is more supportive and cognitive. The described sequence is important for a successful treatment of personality disorder.

Next we summarize the basic therapeutic strategy, process, and goals of psychotherapy of personality disorder around which we believe a relative consensus has been attained.

Psychotherapeutic *strategy* is based on the following premises:

- Therapy as a long-term strategy in all patient-therapist relationships, not only during the therapy sessions;
- Need for a stable therapeutic framework and highly structured therapeutic process (order and rules);

The active role of the therapist;
Clearly defined roles and responsibilities should be made explicit to the patient and the therapist;
Clear limits should be set and maintained;
Establishing behavior control on the part of the patient;
Defined hierarchy of priorities (at the top are suicidality and homicidality, then serious acting out in therapy and outside, dishonesty, concealing important events, trivializing the content of the sessions, breaking the therapeutic contract);
Flexible approach (readiness to depart from the "rules");
Therapeutic formats are combined (individual, group, and partner) according to the needs of the patient and the therapy process.

Elements of psychotherapeutic *process* include the following:

Developing a strong therapeutic alliance and setting up therapeutic contracts;
Intense involvement on the part of the therapist: creating a positive and supportive emotional setting; tolerance and control of intense transference, negative and positive, by the therapist;
Ongoing monitoring and utilization of countertransference and spontaneous, natural emotional resonance/reactions in the therapy;
Establishing a relationship between the patient's behaviors and feelings in the present;
Increasing the patient's awareness of his or her own emotional states as well as of those of others and interpreting them;
Blocking acting out and nongratification of self-destructive behaviors;
Focus, clarification, and interpretation in the "here and now;"
Protecting the patient's extreme sensitivity to separation;
Bridging: merging the split of polarized parts of self and objects.

Therapeutic *goals* involve the following:

Learning how to tolerate one's own fragmented self;
Internalization of emotional support (aka "good internal object");
Personality consolidation (integration) is achieved by helping the patient to develop representations of self and others that are multidimensional, cohesive, and integrated;
Reducing misrepresentations and distortions in social interactions;
Developing the capacity for self-reflection (self-observation, rational and critical thinking, insightfulness);

Developing ambivalence in the perceptions of self and others (with reduced need for "protection" via primitive defense mechanism);
Developing the capacity to assume the positions of others (empathy);
Recognition and understanding of one's own and others' motivations and feelings underlying behavior;
Understanding one's own dominant role in psychological "games" in communications and its (the role's) consequences in interpersonal relationships;
Accepting oneself and one's own negative feelings when one is not doing well;
Developing the capacity to tolerate uncertainty and pain;
Developing tolerance of separation and building the capacity to cope with it.

RECONSTRUCTIVE INTERPERSONAL THERAPY: OUR APPROACH TO PSYCHOTHERAPY OF PERSONALITY DISORDER

Introduction. Reconstructive interpersonal therapy (RIT), as we apply it in practice, combines intrapsychic and interpersonal discourse by using the analysis of interpersonal relationships to reconstruct internal personality structure (Divac-Jovanovic, 1986; Divac-Jovanovic and Svrakic, 2016; Divac-Jovanović and Svrakic, 2017). RIT is truly transtheoretical, as it integrates psychodynamic, existentialist-humanistic, and cognitive paradigms, thus moving closer to the idea of a multifocal approach, a model of choice in contemporary psychology and psychotherapy in general (Prochaska and Norcross, 2003). For this reason, an alternative name for this form of therapy could be "reconstructive transtheoretical therapy."

RIT outlines a *specific strategy* in the therapy of personality disorder. The therapy takes place (is active) from the very first encounter and in every contact with the patient, including periods between sessions, telephone calls, text messages, and so on. As personality fragmentation is pervasive (it affects all mental faculties and subsystems), so the therapy has to be just as pervasive: everything done with and about the patient is thus a part of therapy. These interim events may be just as important as the formal sessions, because the patient learns from the real, caring, and candid relationship as much as from the transference relationship, as in psychodynamic psychotherapy proper.

RIT's focus is, first, on nurturance of the therapeutic relationship and, second, on change. It is explicit in therapeutic contracts which activate the patient's responsibility (i.e., the cognitive aspects) at the very beginning of treatment (similar to existentialist psychotherapy). This approach places the patient in the role of a responsible participant who is required to master certain facts about psychology (similar to CBT). Similar to psychoanalysis, the spotlight is on the therapeutic relationship, transference-countertransference analysis, and on the unlimited capacity to contain all of the turbulent affective contents that may emerge. The ultimate goal is to develop corrective emotional experience, this time with a stable and supporting object (the therapist) who, in addition to confronting nonfunctional behavior, also and unequivocally encourages the patient to feel and think. The therapy also involves working on the patient's value system using the narrative approach,[8] and even including stories about the therapist's own experiences. In addition to serving as a projection screen, the therapist is also a real living being in the patient's life and is encouraged to show all feelings, positive and negative, including genuine caring about the patient (Novellino, 1984), always a powerful message. Such balanced exchanges of affection and acceptance, coupled with confrontation, bring therapy quite close to a natural relationship. RIT is flexible with regard to technical neutrality, control of the therapeutic process, and the therapist-patient hierarchy. Thus this approach is acceptable to patients who need to feel in control (e.g., rescheduling sessions to fit the patient's calendar, flexibility with tardiness and payments, etc.). Such initial flexibility reduces dropout rates throughout the process (Joines and Stewart, 2002).

Once patients feel understood and accepted as they are, regardless of how "bad" he or she was (the method of empathic transactions), the patient finds it easier to talk about feelings and to activate/ develop his or her true self in the relationship. The therapist must make it perfectly clear that everything can be talked about in the session, especially if it involves something critical to the therapeutic relationship. The rule that "everything that is not harmful is allowed" in psychotherapy captures the idea. Other rules are continually adapted and new ones set into place to customize the approach for the individual patient during different stages of therapy. The goal is to help the patient come to see him/herself in a realistic light and to learn how to tolerate negative reactions, disappointments, and failures. The therapist needs to be patient with regard to the emotional attitude of the basic "message" of these patients ("I hate you, don't leave me";

8. A narrative approach separates the person from the problem and encourages reliance on his or her own skills to reframe the problem.

Kreisman and Strauss, 1991) and be ready to find a way to "accept and love what he/she does not like." The therapist is advised to keep in mind the "wounded child" in the inner world of the patient regardless of his or hers acting-outs.

RIT: the basic principles and phases of psychotherapeutic work. RIT is transtheoretical insofar as it integrates humanistic and psychodynamic paradigms into a single psychotherapeutic *strategy* for the fragmented personality. Next the basic principles of RIT are described. Of note, the therapeutic steps follow chronologically in a sequence, but the manner in which they unfold is canonical: the beginning of each new step does not mean the end of the preceding one, which therefore remains active in parallel with the subsequent steps.

Attuning to the affective resonance with the patient. The therapist's consistent position is one of freely expressed empathy, active presence, and genuine interest, of neither assuming nor knowing beforehand (not relying on previous experience with similar stories), of close observation of verbal and nonverbal signs, and of unlimited containing, that is, giving the patient the opportunity to deposit all of his or her unaccepted feelings and impulses into the session. All of this is done in order to win the patient over to engage in therapy and then stay in it. From the start, the therapist expects a negative transference and is prepared to monitor countertransference in order to be able to better endure the demanding relationship.

Informing and contracting. The process and the theoretical framework of treatment are made known to the patient. In practice we inform patients about the basic principles of psychotherapy (e.g., confidentiality, transparency, the need for patience, the commonality of resistance, among others), about the philosophy of psychotherapy, both general and specific to RIT, and about what they themselves can do to make progress. *Therapeutic contracts* specify the desired change and are made by mutual agreement. Everything important to the patient, big or small, can be made a subject for contracting. Finalizing ("closing") the contract can take time before the desired change is mutually agreed upon. *Protective contracts* are made exclusively for behavior, to control acting out of any kind (which, if continued, would threaten the therapeutic process): antisuicidal, antihomicidal, and/or antipsychotic contracts. Early experience of control over oneself in therapy gives the patient an initial sense of success and reinforces positive motivation.

Analysis of the patient's ongoing relationships—transactions (including the therapeutic relationship). This principle involves inferring the patient's priorities from the contents he or she brings to sessions. Individuals with personality disorder "rush" into transference with the therapist or present outside relationships that are laden with transference dynamics. The transference is absorbed by the therapist in order to preserve the therapeutic relationship (later to be used as a tool). These patients usually first describe their turbulent interpersonal conflicts with important others (parents, colleagues, friends), which provides material for analysis during the early phases of therapy. Providing comfort and showing empathy for the patient's sense of injury or injustice must continue until all the conflictual relationships are exhausted (i.e., analyzed and interpreted). Work on the recognition of the repetitive patterns of interpersonal conflicts is then very slowly introduced.

Reparenting. The concept refers to the nurturing of the therapeutic relationship in order to ameliorate psychological deficits caused by neglectful, even abusive, parenting and thereby maximize corrective emotional experience. The latter goal, "developing a more realistic emotional experience" is explicitly shared with the patient. Reparenting involves providing protection, giving feedback, giving advice, and providing physical care (sometimes offering a meal or refreshments), teaching ethical principles, life coaching, and lifestyle analysis, among others. This phase extends throughout therapy and even after therapy (the therapist as "third parent").

Analysis of the transference relationship. Primary objects are gradually introduced into the process, and the patient's "here and now" feelings are linked with those in the "there and then." This is a major step as it leads to insights into one's own nonconscious motivation in present relationships, experiences, and behaviors. Following numerous conflicts with the therapist, boss, husband/wife, friend and so on, the patient begins to recognize not only the repetitive behavior patterns and attendant feelings (deconstructed in the analysis of "psychological" games, a TA concept) but also his or her unfulfilled genuine needs. At this stage in transference analysis, it is critical for the patient to recognize and adequately interpret his or her own real feelings towards self and others, first in the present and then in the past as well. The latter work also helps the patient to recognize and revise the symbiotic, selfobject nature of the conflict-prone relationships in the here-and-now.

Reframing. This principle refers to giving different meaning to a known content, to make a change in the frame of reference colloquially, or to look at things from another angle or another discourse. Reframing helps the patient work on accepting pain, loneliness, fear, and sadness, which then leads to decontamination of grandiosity about his or her feelings. This is a regressive stage which can last quite some time and even occasionally resurface, as discussed later in more detail.

Redecision. This principle refers to replacing early nonconscious conclusions and decisions about oneself, others, and the world with new or revised ones. It also involves analyzing one's options for fulfilling needs in different and healthier ways (i.e., other than self-defeating behaviors, or hurting others, or damaging relationships). Redecision also includes practicing new behaviors arising from new decisions with the support of the therapist (and the group where applicable). The possibility of self-sabotage, even returning to previous painful patterns of experience and behaviors are anticipated and shared with the patient, which becomes an effective way to preserve motivation (aka "feed forward" technique).

Open-ended therapy. The therapy with these patients does not actually end. The therapist remains available, mostly for consultation, support, and coaching, for as long as the patient needs, which may last for years, although at a much lower pace.

Next we elaborate on selected main principles at work in the therapeutic process when dealing with fragmented personality. We confine ourselves to a discussion of the basics only, as it is close to impossible to explain the nuances of the whole therapeutic process in full detail.

Affective resonance: a powerful diagnostic and therapeutic tool. It has been said that psychotherapy of persons with personality disorder involves two patients, not one (Searls, 1986). The therapist has the responsibility to see him or herself both as a clinician and as a patient who brings his or her own material into the therapeutic arena. The ongoing therapeutic relationship is a very important source of information for both sides. This becomes critical for effective psychotherapy as the therapist monitors and analyzes his or her resonance with the patient's expressed and hidden feelings. The resonance includes the therapist's spontaneous emotions in the here and now, activated by the patient's psychopathology (diagnostic countertransference) not merely the nonconscious emotions toward his or her (the therapist's) objects of the past (countertransference proper or personal countertransference). Affective resonance as a *diagnostic tool* helps the therapist identify the patterns of the patient's earlier object relationships and the ensuing feeling, behaviors, and meanings that the patient attaches to him or herself and others in the present interpersonal relationships. Simply put, the therapist uses his or her own emotions as data in the here and now. Once the therapist clears his or her emotional blind spots (supervision is recommended), he or she should be able to distinguish between his or her own feelings and those stirred up by the patient (Yalom, 2011). Affective resonance is also used as a *treatment tool*: communicating feelings is a powerful method for confrontation and clarification. Paradoxically, such confrontation can be introduced earlier and more directly in therapy of individuals with personality disorder, who respond to it by a tendency to integrate, than it can with persons functioning at a higher level of organization, who respond to confrontation with increased anxiety. Being aware of the feelings the patient engenders in the therapist and other people helps the patient develop mentalization, learn social skills, and discover empathy, particularly as a lack of these led to the disturbed interpersonal relationships in the first place. RIT encourages the patient to inquire about the therapist's feelings or thoughts. Such questions are answered openly and honestly, but tactfully and with full consideration for the patient's feelings. After a good rapport has been established, interchanges of this kind become an amazing catalyst that takes therapy to the level of realistic rather than fantasized understanding of the patient's own interpersonal contacts.

Countertransference and/or reactive emotions: when uneasiness becomes a useful tool. Countertransference and real reactive feelings are common in a therapeutic relationship with individuals with personality disorder. Continuous focus on the intrapersonal and the interpersonal enables the therapist to monitor his or her countertransference and natural reactions to the patient's psychopathology as well as the patient's reactions and transference (optimally, countertransference is analyzed in supervision, but this could be done by self-analysis as well). Working with "fragmented" patients stirs up a panoply of feelings in the therapist, accompanied by a sense of unease in the background at all times. The patients' primitive defenses, especially splitting and projective identification, generate complex and chaotic transferences in the therapeutic situation. Inordinately intense affect states expressed by the patient make the therapist feel like he or she is always dealing with a life-and-death struggle (Kernberg et al., 1989), something everyone working with these patients has at some point experienced. The therapist frequently has the impression that he or she is walking on eggshells because these patients are extremely sensitive to one's choice of words and even the smallest nonverbal signs of disinterest or inattention (rejection sensitivity). These, as it were, "continual-crisis" patients may inspire a strong drive in the therapist to "do something" or "speed things up," which increases the danger of overstepping professional boundaries. The feelings commonly aroused in the therapist include *guilt* (the patients accuse the therapist of not taking proper care of them, not liking them, being unprofessional, or being responsible for the deterioration in their condition, etc.); *rescuing fantasies and behaviors* (perceiving the patient as really helpless, allowing the sessions to last longer, disclosing personal problems, failing to bill the patient, meeting in inadequate settings, attempting to cure through unconditional acceptance and love etc.); *anger and hatred* (these patients project their negative raw affects onto therapist who may identify with such affects); sense of *helplessness, confusion, and worthlessness* (the patient devalues the therapist's efforts; the therapist feels that he or she indeed may indeed lack the requisite skills or is incompetent, and consequently withdraws or becomes defensive); *anxiety and dread* (the therapist always expects that he or she will say something wrong and thereby provoke an angry outburst or a sarcastic comment; Kernberg et al., 1989).

The therapist frequently continues to think about the "difficult" patient or to experience strong good or bad emotions long after the session, thus may feel burdened in his or her (the therapist's) free time. Incidentally, these emotions are more frequently negative, especially hostility and boredom. They fluctuate, much like the patient's affects, and can become extreme: for example, the patient may initially delight the therapist with an insight only to later disappoint with regression. In summary, the therapist uses countertransference both as a diagnostic sign indicative of fragmented personality and as a therapeutic tool, which is useful for the patient's insight as to how he or she affects people in general.

Professional boundaries have to be redefined in work with these patients, who need not only to be confronted but to be comforted as well. One of the ways in which the therapist can retain control of boundaries and still not become overcautious and guarded is to determine what it is that needs to be done in therapy that the parent of the patient did not do. This includes meeting the patient's unmet needs to be safe, to be close, to understand, and to be understood and accepted. As noted, supervision is recommended, not just to recognize the countertransference feelings but to use them as a tool in psychotherapy: projective identification becomes more than just a defense mechanism- it becomes a therapeutic tool through the analysis of countertransference.

In the here and now: removing the posters of primary objects from the actual faces. It is important to allow transference to develop, which helps the patient to separate the past from the present. The contents from the past are revived in RIT and treated as if happening in the here and now. They are then processed until a corrective experience is reached. To this end, the "empty chair technique" is commonly used (developed by Fritz Pearls in Gestalt therapy). Here the patient expresses different attitudes—rational, emotional, critical, and so on—toward the imagined person sitting in the chair (either the parent or someone else). Similarly, the "parent interview" technique enables the therapist to talk to the patient's introjected projections of the parent and to reveal the hidden motives (of which the patient, as a child, was not aware) of the real parent in the past. The patient can then accept his or her parents and their motives in a new way, or, if the patient cannot do this, the therapist may help "vanquish the powerful enemy" in the chair. This opens possibilities for correcting earlier biased decisions about oneself and others as well as expands options in experiences and behavior. It should be noted that this powerful technique for work with transference is applied cautiously and only in later stages of therapy, after some progress in overcoming splitting has occurred (as it might otherwise deepen the splitting).

Corrective emotional experience as a "way out" of the fragmented world. In the course of RIT, corrective emotional experience arises from the experience of object constancy (this time with the therapist) and the internalization of clinician's permissions to exist, feel, and think. The permissions are gradually "granted" by the therapist throughout the course of therapy. They are antithetical to the prohibitions the patient received in the formative period, which were later transformed into biased and typically flawed conclusions about self and others and even about life in general. The experience of object constancy is achieved in the relationship with the therapist which is maintained despite the patient's extreme behaviors and negative feelings during therapy. Rejection by the therapist does not happen even though the patient is constantly attempting to provoke it by playing psychological games (the "kick me game"; Berne, 1972). Extreme behaviors are confronted and controlled by protective contracts, but warnings of rejection are never made as these would only reinforce the early conclusion that "others can't be trusted" or that "one should never show one's true feelings." Of special importance is to contain the patient's sadistic feelings and fantasies. A supportive therapeutic setting in which permissions are granted instead of prohibitions enacted enables the patient to repair developmental defects and to mature and experience freedom to be who he or she really is. Within the context of object constancy, this helps patients develop whole, realistic representations of themselves and the therapist, which is subsequently generalized to other people as well.

In the early stages of therapy the therapist contains the patient's suppressed anger, sadism, fear, and emotional pain and facilitates both the expression and processing of contents associated with these feelings. It is precisely at this point that the therapist has to demonstrate patience and courage in order to contain and "survive" the assault of extreme affects. Such empathic persistence sends a powerful message to the patient that a relationship is still possible despite the destructive affects, that is, that the latter will not destroy the interlocutor. The work on developing trust is critical in advanced stages of therapy. The corrective relationship almost never requires less than a year just for the traces of trust to appear. If the therapist can manage through this relatively difficult phase, which is fraught with negative transference and complicated countertransference, he or she can expect to begin to see the early signs of trust. It could take years before the patient becomes stably confident that if he or she shows what he or she feels, there will be people around who will endure all the attacks of panic, anger, or sorrow. This is the period when the patient usually begins to develop attachment to the therapist (reflecting the reparenting process) as the therapist does not abandon the patient nor is he or she "destroyed" by the patient. This is key to establishing adequate relationships, both in and out of therapy. Within this framework, the therapeutic process can continue, gradually leading toward a reconstruction of personality.

The need for reparenting. Most authors agree that the psychopathology of personality disorder is rooted in the sensitive rapprochement subphase of the separation-individuation process (15–24 months of age per Mahler et al., 1975). In some cases, the mother, whether because of her own immaturity or mental disorder, would not allow the child to strive for autonomy without projecting anxiety, emotional blackmail, rejection, and so on. It has been both observed and hypothesized that children of these "not-good-enough mothers" were inadequately loved, as their mothers either "clung" to them and were preoccupied with them (overprotection), were uncaring (neglect), were aggressively dismissive (rejection), exhibited cold affectionless control, or some combination thereof. All of this took place during the period when the child needs unconditional support in order to feel safe to explore the world and develop self-confidence and mentalization. These observations are supported by research showing that mothers of children who later developed personality disorder were frequently emotionally unstable, or latently, transitorily or openly psychotic or borderline/cycloid, had an affective disorder, or were depressed (Maffei, 1993). Children raised by such mothers either never develop whole object relations or regress to partial object relations during the separation-individuation phase (the regression can be both mental and neural, as prefrontal networks can be fractured under stress, as discussed). Emotionally insensitive, troubled, or unstable mothers have a tendency to convey messages with "double meaning" (e.g., "Go away but don't leave me"), which generates confusion, deep uncertainty, or disappointment in the child. For example, a child may experience a sudden rejection from an otherwise overly devoted but stressed-out mother. Confused and uncertain, he or she has to accept the new reality immediately so as not to further complicate the relationship on which he or she (the child) realistically depends. The child of course at this stage is unable to cognitively analyze the confusion but rather sacrifices real experiences, gives up on exploration, and resorts to rescuing fantasies. The latter may lead to sadism, mistrust, and/or dependency as the main characteristics of the child's self-image and his or her later relationships with objects. As adults, these individuals do not move forward out of fear that in so doing they may lose the people upon whom they depend. Yet, they also do not develop closeness with the same people out of fear of becoming overpowered ("swallowed") in the relationship (this in part because these patients have difficulty understanding other people's real intentions and motivations). Since these experiences are something which patients cannot overcome or resolve, they behave impulsively with intense primitive affects. This is why the interpersonal relationships of persons with fragmented personality are plagued by misunderstandings. Corrective emotional experience through reparenting (Schiff et al., 1975) develops knowledge and establishes trust in one's own self and interpersonal relationships.

The psychotherapeutic practice of reparenting. Reparenting through psychotherapy is a long-term process which requires persistence on the part of the patient and a great deal of patience on the part of the therapist, not unlike the work of the parent bringing up a child in real life. This is why the therapist is sometimes described as a "third parent" (Berger, 1980). It is not possible to overstate both the degree of responsibility implicit in this third-parent position as well as the high level of integrity and professional competency it requires from the therapist.

In contrast to therapeutic work with neurotic patients where symbiosis is not advised, in persons with personality disorder symbiotic dependence may be a necessary first step in therapy, much like the mother-child relationship. After progress has been achieved in therapy, the work subsequently focuses on overcoming (abandoning) this symbiosis as the patient learns how to separate without guilt or fear. It can be fascinating to observe how the therapist's unconditional strokes with respect to the patient's inherent uniqueness can have a healing effect particularly as the patient might be hearing such praise for the first time. In order to be effective, of course, these positive remarks have to be genuine.

Reframing into positive connotation: the royal road in psychotherapy. As Milton Erikson famously said, "people come into therapy with problems they cannot solve, and we (therapists) give them those they can." Early in psychotherapy, as new light is shed on the patient's life story, his or her past attempts to solve problems are validated as understandable and creative, perhaps even lifesaving given the circumstances. This process of positive connotation assigns meanings and reasons to past experiences and behaviors. Placing old contents into a new frame allows the patient to accept him or herself even before making the desired changes. In fact, the humanistic approach postulates that the therapeutic change is most likely to stem from patients' acceptance of themselves the way they are, before they even begin to change. By attaching new meanings to the existing contents, patients become motivated to appreciate, rather than dismiss, alternative options and begin to develop confidence in their own ability to choose. Positive connotation of old decisions and solutions frees the patient from feeling helpless and inadequate and takes away the false superiority of the therapist's position. Only after experiencing acceptance, do these patients begin to embrace responsibility and grow up.

However, the surge of unconditional self-love in postmodern society threatened to bring the humanistic idea of self-acceptance to absurdity. If used uncritically, positive connotation can cause the patient to stagnate, if not get worse in therapy, while both the patient and the therapist operate under the mutual illusion that the therapy is facilitating some sort of progress. It is important that individuals with personality disorder develop the capacity to relate with positive connotation towards other people. Simply put, these individuals need to realize that positive connotation applies to other people as well, not only to them (the seeds of empathy), while neurotic patients need to learn that positive connotation applies to them, not only to others (the seeds of freedom from guilt).

PRACTICAL TIPS FOR PSYCHOTHERAPY OF PERSONALITY DISORDER

How to love what you don't like? It is not easy, but it is important to love your patient the psychotherapeutic way. The challenge is to find soothing yet effective ways to handle crises in a relationship imbued with aggression. How does one maintain a "good place" within oneself, amidst the patient's relentless attacks and accusations? Although expected, crises in the therapeutic relationship may still surprise the therapist, and supervision may not be immediately available to formulate the solution. At the same time, patients often, directly or indirectly, desire to know whether the therapist loves or at least likes them, and wish for an affirmative answer, although, if they receive it, they for long do not really believe it. The answer therefore must be authentic, not comforting. As most therapists really do care about their patients, this becomes their common answer. The way we accept the patient and nurture our positive emotional attitudes despite these challenges is an important aspect of the therapeutic relationship, particularly as it adds an enormous amount of stability to it. We find it useful to ideate the wounded child inside the patient who is in fact doing the attacking: he or she is doing so in order to cover his or her fear of abandonment and therefore checks the stability of the therapist`s "love." In such challenging situations we are guided by the thought that psychotherapeutic love is "when you love even what you don't like."

Psychotherapeutic love is similar to parental love. It does not mean unconditional approval of everything the patient does or says. Rather, it denotes the therapist's unconditional and emotional *presence* in the process. A genuine acceptance of the patient the way he or she is comes before the expectation for him or her to change. In therapy, the natural (real) relationship has a healing power equal to that of the transference relationship. In fact, the real relationship can be and often is more important than interpretations, especially at the later stages. The change and insights come after rather than during transference, amidst the torment of intense transference feelings. Years after the completion of therapy, these patients do not remember interpretations or insights but they will remember support they received from the therapist. A patient of ours (MDJ), suffering from panic attacks generated by her fragmented personality, years later confided to us that the therapist's supporting SMS messages at the moments of crisis "meant the most" to her and that she even saved them to look occasionally at.

The following point cannot be overemphasized: *We understand the patient through transference and countertransference but heal him or her trough the relationship.* The latter is characterized by constancy, presence, predictability, and authentic motivation. The patient and the therapist are close but not intimate. It is important to keep support, love, and confrontation balanced and spontaneous. The therapist should be spontaneous in the relationship but thoughtful and measured in the therapeutic process. Such "good-enough" environment has to be enduring and constant in order to assist the integration of the underlying fragmented personality.

Is psychotherapy of fragmented individuals difficult? There is a widespread view among clinicians that psychotherapy of persons with personality disorder is extremely difficult and demanding. Indeed, the treatment of these individuals does not only involve psychotherapy proper but also an overall strategy in the therapist-patient relationship, which may be particularly effective with advanced communication technologies. We use the term "strategy" because the treatment goes beyond the framework of traditional practices and formal sessions. There are simply no rules or precedents for many of the situations in which a therapist may find him or herself when working with these patients. In fact, strictly relying only on rules usually fails to deliver progress. Creativity, flexibility, readiness to step away from the rules, and individualized interventions are constantly needed in response to shifts between primitive defenses predominantly used by these patients. They are quick to devalue everything, including interventions and the therapist. Much like industrial molds that are more expensive if made for a small series, the therapy of persons with fragmented personality can be similarly viewed as an expensive small series. It is not difficult once an effective mold for a given patient has been established. It challenges the therapist's creativity, and, paradoxically, offers more freedom than the work with some other patients who are traditionally regarded as less difficult, for example, neurotic individuals.

There can be no doubt that psychotherapy of individuals with personality disorder is challenging. Primitive defense mechanisms elicit intensely unpleasant or professionally problematic countertransference reactions and spontaneous feelings. Still, the therapy can be gratifying to a composed and patient therapist, even when it appears that there is nothing more that can be done. The therapist has to avoid feeling guilty about lack of progress but rather accept it as part of the therapeutic process. Many patients are capable of surprising their therapist by making substantial progress out of seemingly dead-end situations.

In contrast to psychotic and neurotic persons with acute symptoms, therapy is not obligatory for persons with personality disorder—only desirable. These patients enter therapy convinced that things are wrong with the world, and not with them. Many of them engage not to correct their own behaviors or feelings but endeavor instead to test their own perception of the world (to tell their story) in order to get someone to finally take their side. In contrast to some neurotic or psychotic patients, who seek therapy because they feel guilty or scared (wanting to "get rid" of some parts of themselves), persons with personality disorder are looking for approval (wanting to "unite" with parts of themselves). These individuals understand guilt and responsibility diametrically differently than the way in which neurotic patients understand them: in the beginning of the therapeutic process they project guilt onto others, while the end of therapy is, symbolically, the moment at which they introject guilt.

Will they stay in therapy? Confrontation and humor can help. We sincerely admire people who engage in therapy. By that act they show exceptional courage to embark on an uncertain journey. It is up to us as therapists to remove the obstacles along their path (Yalom, 2009). Despite our best efforts, individuals with personality disorder may suddenly decide to terminate therapy, rationalizing the decision by exclaiming: "I am not learning anything new" or "I know more than my therapist," and the like. Direct confrontation is indicated here. Paradoxically, confronting patients with their responsibility for what is happening to them usually re-energizes their interest. As they are battling for control, they try to prove us wrong. Here, it is important to direct the patient's attention to his or her own role in the repetitive events which form the subject of their complaints: "Isn't it awful," "Look what they are doing to me," and the like. Such shifting of responsibility should be confronted as self-deception but in a nonthreatening manner and backed with plans for alternative actions or interpretations. In contrast to neurotic and psychotic patients, individuals with personality disorder react well to both confrontations and interpretations even early in therapy. Their interest is aroused by the challenge of confrontation, which galvanizes their battle for control with the prospect of being able to respond/return what they perceive as "aggression." This increases chances of continued engagement in therapy.

Individuals with personality disorder also react very well to humor, one of their favorite mechanisms to discount the significance of their problems or even that they experience (have) problems. Their humor is either an expression of passive aggressive mechanisms (laughing at others) or unhealthy laughing at their own failures and fiascos ("gallows humor"). Using healthy humor (laughing together) early on in therapy is a good way to establish positive rapport and buy additional time for more serious interventions. Alluding to the fact that a significant therapeutic change requires the energy of the inner child within us, Mary Goulding, a famous TA therapist, said that some of the most profound therapeutic changes in her practice happened amidst of salvoes of laughter (McClure Goulding & Goulding, 1979). An unusually frank, humorous, or plain spoken comment or confrontation may motivate the patient to stay in the conversation with someone who is perceived as nonstereotypical.

In working with these patients, it is important to consistently confront their tendencies to negate, discount, or minimize their own problems. One should not forget that the same discounting was once a functional defense against the sense of feeling inadequate, threatened, or rejected. Once patients are drawn into talking about early difficulties and traumas, we realize how their suffering was indeed great. Freely expressed and genuine empathy are a natural response during these periods, allowing the therapist to give positive connotation to all of the patient's earlier solutions, including the maladaptive ones. The patient will, in turn, have an authentic experience of being understood without being judged, the feeling of strength and resiliency despite suffering, and this facilitates their psychological growth.

How relevant is intelligence for the outcome? We bring this topic out in the open because it is an important topic in supervision. Our intention is to clarify the problem as this can help a realistic assessment of treatment planning. Some therapists struggle with certain patients, who keep regressing to the previous stages of work despite a full range of interventions. The therapist usually understands this in terms of resistance. The last thing to come to mind is that the patient may simply not have the cognitive capacities that would enable him or her to make progress in therapy. By "intelligent' we mean a relatively specific set of abilities that are not necessarily included in the traditional concept of IQ but are essential determinants of therapy outcome; namely, the ability to attach importance to thinking and decision-making, the ability of introspection, psychological mindedness, and determination (will) and perseverance in implementing new decisions, among others. Individuals with personality disorder struggle with social intelligence, owing to problems with mentalization. In our experience, outcomes may be decided by the aforementioned specific cognitive abilities. Specifically, the outcome is better with patients whose cognitive abilities were originally high or those who were able to develop or enhance such abilities during therapy.

Are moral values an issue in psychotherapy of personality disorder? The answer is affirmative: these patients characteristically have permissive (opportunistic) and nonprincipled (personal, non-abstracted) morality, particularly when it comes to external social norms (biological roots of morality are underdeveloped and dormant, as discussed). While respecting personal rights, the therapist raises the issue of the morality of behavior as needed. The therapist represents the broader social community, advocates desirable outcomes, and comments on his or her own value system with the expectation that the patient will realize the importance of these questions and dilemmas. For example, a therapeutic intervention as a patient was discussing suicide as the "best solution" for her during an agitated depressive phase was the statement (by the therapist) that self-aggression is not a solution, is absolutely unacceptable, is really not a way out but a way toward "nothing," is a misconception and a permanent "exit" from a temporary problem. The therapist (MDJ) here insisted on her own values and successfully conveyed to the patient who eventually gave up the ideation. Of course, a strong therapeutic alliance had previously been established, making this intervention effective in formulating the antisuicide contract.

In periods of acute crisis, the psychotherapeutic approach can be quite directive but should never come from a position of power. A clear and open message is that the patient has the freedom to make his or her own decisions, as well as to accept the responsibility for these decisions. Direct positive messages can influence the patient's views and values in a powerful manner. With patients struggling with severe identity problems, the therapist is advised to suggest more functional solutions for certain life situations. This part of therapy may take the form of reparenting, but here it works in terms of completing the hitherto incomplete system of rules for adequate functioning in the world as it is. Figuratively, this involves parenting a mis-parented child. Directive statements have drawn criticism as "imposing," but therapists working with personality disorder know very well that this is a necessary risk, which is small in comparison to the benefits of such directions.

How to handle therapy of fragmented couples: mediation from distance.

Psychotherapy of persons with personality disorder frequently combines different formats in order to meet the unique dynamics of the patient. The formats are individual, group, family, or partner therapy, which are sometimes combined after careful consideration. Family members, such as a parent, spouse, or significant partner may join therapy at the later stages. Partner therapy with personality disorder initially involves mediation rather than therapy proper. The therapist frequently engages in representing (interpreting) the patient's feelings to his or her partner or vice versa, whether relevant to their relationship or in general. Only after this new "introduction" to each other takes place can the partner therapy proper really begin because the root problem was bidirectional misunderstanding of emotions and motives.

In cases where just one partner has a personality disorder (the one not in therapy), that person often refuses to get involved even after being told that the participation would be useful in improving the outcome of his or her partner's therapy. In the context of such noncooperation, partner therapy is designed as "therapy from a distance": the therapist tries to influence the patient-partner system through the improved communication patterns of the patient. The person seeking help (for any reason but personality disorder) is not only the identified patient but may become an instrument of change in his or her partner with personality disorder. The strategy is surprisingly effective in practice given all the things that could go wrong during such meandering, indirect approach. In the significant majority of cases, the correction of the patient's behavior indirectly achieves a positive change in both partners. A plausible explanation of the efficacy is that in patients with personality disorder the main channel of communication is nonverbal–behavioral, which is exactly what the noncooperative partner is facing with the changed behavior of his or her partner (the patient).

When both partners have a personality disorder, and both are in partner therapy with the same therapist, their relationship can be disrupted to the point of no possibility of dialogue, which requires the therapist to first engage in mediation, rather than proper partner therapy. The need for preparatory, pre-therapy mediation is especially common with the "dramatic" variants of personality disorder (narcissistic, antisocial, histrionic), as these represent a mutually attractive nonconscious choice. Mediation in this case is a method of choice, since regular sessions are quickly and easily disrupted. Transformative mediation is a process focused on understanding the needs and feelings of partners with the aim of improving communication. With the consent of both sides, the therapist serves as an explorer and interpreter of the feelings underlying their behavior. Joint sessions, at which plans and tasks for both sides are defined, can be combined in a balanced manner with individual sessions. Contrary to the "rules" (and many times one has to break the rules when working with these patients!), it may be better if the same therapist does individual sessions with both partners despite the fact that this requires additional effort on the part of the therapist to not be seen as the culprit and/or arbiter. When the partners are involved in individual therapy with two different therapists, because of intensified splitting, they are more likely to grow apart and break-up their relationship without any improvement in mutual understanding.

In some cases the partners combine a "fearful" and an "eccentric" variant of personality disorder (anankastic or negativistic-dependent with paranoid or schizoid), also a frequent mutually attractive nonconscious choice. Here, they may develop an intensely symbiotic relationship, which excludes others from the system. This makes therapy a great deal more difficult, with strong resistance and ambivalence encountered from both sides. The patients frequently view the therapist as the arbiter who is expected to choose sides or else risk being devalued along with the therapy. The therapist needs to balance interventions carefully to make sure he or she comes across as the interpreter. To this end, again, the therapist's seeking to reveal authentic feelings behind certain behaviors is very useful. For example, a submissive passive-aggressive partner realizes that behind a paranoid attack by his wife lies her feeling of intense fear of abandonment, not anger, which the submissive partner fears. After this type of interventions, partners frequently manage to overcome splitting and resistance and stay in therapy as well as in the relationship.

Does psychotherapy of personality disorder ever end? The answer is it does not, but this requires elaboration. Individuals with personality disorder rarely enter therapy ready for change, and in fact do everything they can to avoid feelings because they often seem insuperable. They enter therapy to tell their side of the "story," to experience being cared for, or to vent anger or all of the above. They constantly escalate the position of the "righteous victim," which may urge the therapist to rescue or prosecute them. This trap can be avoided from the neutral position, which involves asking relevant questions to explore the patient's understanding of the world. The therapist must have patience and must be willing to give up control from time to time. It is essential to let the patient, rather than the therapist, have the initiative early in therapy.

These patients react very well to the permission to "control" the therapeutic process as well as to the idea that things can move forward even without their formal "work." Both help them overcome not only the fear of change but also the fear of taking responsibility for the change. For the same reason (the need to be in control), these patients do not take interpretations of resistance well in the early stages of therapy. They need freedom to resist and the freedom to leave therapy when "bored" (as both express control). Even when the latter is an expression of resistance, it should be respected, with a clearly conveyed understanding that the patient is welcome to return anytime. We suspect that this is quite similar to what Yalom (2009) meant when he said that "we should meet the patient at a place where he/she is instead of trying to bring him/her to the place where we are."

The psychotherapy of fragmented personality is frequently intermittent, progresses unevenly, and involves handling different stages of therapy at the same time. The impression that "nothing is happening in therapy" (the patient) or that it is "boring" (the therapist) may lead to breaks and cancellations. Both sides feel surprisingly bad about sudden breaks even though it seemed to both parties that the therapy was really going nowhere in the first place. Patients come and leave the therapeutic process following their subjective rhythms, and it is up to the therapist to review each break and develop a plan for future work. It should be made explicit upfront that the door to the therapy room always remains open for the patient. This way, therapy may span a number of years of which only a portion is spent doing the actual therapeutic work. Sometimes a break is followed by a surprising but frequently crucial change for the better. Of course, change is never as sudden as it appears, and this is the time for the patient to realize that he or she was engaged in the therapeutic process even when he or she was not coming to sessions. It is advisable to use one such return to therapy to set the boundary that there will be no more interruptions until everything that is important in therapy is accomplished. In conclusion, the therapy of persons with personality disorder may or may not take a long time; it usually is spread out over time in a discontinuous manner. It is essential that the therapist has the patience to wait for the patient; otherwise the patient wins the battle for control which, as a rule, is his or her "area of expertise". The phrase "once a therapist, always a therapist" especially applies to work with individuals with personality disorder many of whom, for many years after the therapy is formally finished, occasionally reappear to get support and "recharge batteries" .

Is it difficult to become an expert therapist of personality disorder? It takes serious training and a natural aptitude to become a competent therapist. Although the prerequisite for "natural aptitude" may sound discouraging, here it means no more than the capacity for empathy and psychological mindedness (aka "capacity for mentalization"), which most trainees considering this career path will likely already have. Other personal features, such as patience, ability to contain, and a belief that a person can indeed change, are learned in training and advanced through supervision and practical work. Training in psychotherapy takes between two and four years (depending on the modality) but can be completed in parallel with residency (psychiatry) or postgraduate studies (clinical psychology). It is indeed possible to be a physician and an expert therapist (e.g., Kernberg). Once the formal training is completed, it is the continuous supervision and analyses of sessions that hone the therapeutic skills. The benefits for the therapist are both personal, in terms of lifelong contact with his or her own personality and behavior (a sort of self-analysis through work), and professional, in terms of developing a deep understanding of the human mind which work in this field provides.

FINAL COMMENTS ON PSYCHOTHERAPY

A casual look at Table 4.1 titled "Evolution of Psychotherapy and Coping" and covering several centuries may leave the impression that psychotherapy is coming full circle. It started out with common sense and counseling and now has returned to using some of these same directive interventions.

We believe that psychotherapy, quite similar to people, evolves along an upward spiral with a progressively expanding radius, which keeps adding not only new perspectives and understandings but also new problems and adaptive tasks, as well as maintains its openness to use old (new) tools for new (old) tasks. Contemporary psychotherapy is entering a neoclassical period, returning to some of the classical methods, not just the revitalized psychodynamic approach but also that of common sense, counseling, conversation, and narrative therapy. As we see it, the reintroduction of direction and common sense reflects a natural need today to sort out the multiplicity of lifestyle and psychological alternatives in the present nondirective society, to arrive at an optimal personal choice. This is a new adaptive task in front of an unprecedented volume of information (dubbed "infomania") creating "new" naiveté ("ignorance in abundance"), with little ability to separate the wheat from the chaff that requires directive guidance and common sense. Direction is of course canonically combined with other paradigms, as discussed earlier and shown in Table 4.1. In our opinion, by integrating different paradigms into a unified transtheoretical model, psychotherapy shall remain one of the leading professions in our cyber-liquid future, as it contains healing powers of traditional interpersonal

Table 4.1 EVOLUTION OF PSYCHOTHERAPY AND COPING

Period	Generation	Problem	Need (Adaptive Strategy)	Therapy and Coping
<u>**Pre-psychotherapy era**</u>				
CLASSICAL Greco-Roman, late antiquity	**Unnamed**	**Ignorance, naivete & fear about nature**	**Future telling** (belief systems)	**Prophecies** **Religion/God**
POSTCLASSICAL and PREMODERN ERA ended c. 1880	**Lost generation** Born 1880s–1900 Fought WWI	**Lost ideals**	**Advise seeking** (story sharing)	**Common sense** (by common people)
<u>**Psychotherapy era**</u>				
MODERNISM Late 19th century–1950s	**GI Generation** Born 1901–1924 Fought WWII	**Anxiety, guilt,** suppressed urges	**How to fit?** (over-adaptation, disguise of needs)	**Psychoanalysis and psychodynamic therapies**
	Silent Generation born 1925–1945 Fought WWII, Korean War, Vietnam War	**Lost motivation**	**Disengagement** (indifference, absurdism)	**Group psychotherapy** ("golden age") Chemical stimulation (tobacco epidemics) Chemical coping (alcohol, cannabis epidemics)
POSTMODERNISM 1960s–2000s	**Baby Boomers** born 1940s–1960	**Self-actualization and individuation**	**How to self-actualize?** (capitalistic entrepreneurship)	**Humanistic therapies** Chemical exploration (hallucinogens)
	Generation X born 1960s–1980s	**Search for meaning**	**What to think?** (mental correctness)	**Constructivism** **Systemic therapies**
	Generation Y (millennials) born 1980s–late 1990s	**Search for new social models-relationships**	**What is right?** (political correctness)	**Cyber socialization**
LIQUID MODERNITY (Neoclassical?) 2000–present	**Generation Z** iGeneration, born late 1990s–mid-2000s	**Infomania** (new ignorance) **Search for choice and fear of passing up**	**What to choose?** (cyber advise sharing [internet forums])	**Integrative psychotherapy; Narrative therapy; Cyber identity updates; Common sense**

relationships, i.e., enables he mind to heal within the same framework it has been pathologized.

One may ask whether the powerful discourse of relativism in modern psychology might interfere with the healing effect of psychotherapy. It is true that the wisdom of the client possessing as he or she does a firsthand experience of the pathological is powerful, perhaps rivaling that of the wisdom of the therapist who has the knowledge. Yet a therapist's knowledge is critical in order to actually help by means of substantive change, rather than simply just understand and accept, which may have only a limited impact. The therapist is required to know *why* is he or she doing something in psychotherapy and *when* and *what* is he or she doing. The therapist first has to gain knowledge so that he or she can move forward and beyond knowledge (must "forget" that knowledge) in order to apply it authentically through his or her own behavior in the healing relationship with the patient. The increasing flexibility of the psychotherapeutic process merely reflects the evolving intersubjectivity and interpersonal culture in which it takes place, as well as the awareness of the crucial role of the corrective emotional experience as the main healing mechanism of psychotherapy. It is hard to predict the goals and methods of psychotherapy in the future, given the monumental impact of new technologies on our mental life and needs.

EMPIRICAL STUDIES: IS THERE EVIDENCE THAT PSYCHOTHERAPY OF PERSONALITY DISORDER WORKS?

An increasing number of methodologically sophisticated studies are addressing both the efficacy and the effectiveness[9] of various psychotherapy modalities in personality disorder. A consensual understanding is that personality disorder (fragmented personality) is very much treatable (amenable to integration) provided that the (i) *relevant processes of change are activated within the patient* during treatment and (ii) the *specific therapeutic techniques that bring about such changes are used.*

Short-term psychodynamic psychotherapy in personality disorder. A recent review (Town et al., 2011) of eight published randomized controlled trials (RCTs) reports that this modality may be considered

9. Efficacy of a treatment (internal validity) is established by highly controlled studies that test whether a proposed intervention would have the desired effects under ideal circumstances. Effectiveness (external validity) establishes whether the proposed intervention achieves the desired effect in less controlled and more real-life situations. Efficiency (cost vs benefit) depends on whether the intervention is worth its cost to individuals or society.

an effective treatment option for personality disorder, with significant medium- to long-term improvements for a large percentage of patients. The reviewed studies employed extended follow-up periods, on average 18 months. The use of manualized approaches, adherence ratings, and expert supervision ensured that treatment fidelity was maintained within the trials. A recent meta-analysis (Abbass et al., 2014) included 33 RCTs of 2,173 patients with common mental disorders[10] including personality disorder who received short-term (40 or fewer hours) psychodynamic therapy (controls were wait-list, minimal treatment, or treatment as usual). The analysis found modest to large treatment effect sizes that increased in long-term follow-up (effect sizes of 0.42, 0.50, 0.51, for interpersonal problems, depression, and social adjustments, respectively; all secondary outcomes). The trend toward larger effect sizes at follow-up suggests that psychodynamic therapy sets in motion psychological processes that spur further progress, even after therapy has ended. The authors advise cautious interpretation of the results as not all outcome measures improved at follow-up.

Long-term psychodynamic psychotherapy in personality disorder. Leichsenring and Rabung (2008) report a meta-analysis of 11 RCTs and 12 observational studies employing long-term psychodynamic psychotherapy lasting for at least a year, or 50 sessions, and a total of 1,053 patients with complex mental disorders (personality disorder, chronic mental disorders, multiple mental disorders, complex depressive and anxiety disorders associated with chronic course). No difference in effect size was found for RCTs (efficacy) and observational studies (effectiveness). Long-term psychodynamic therapy showed significantly better outcomes in target problems and personality functioning than shorter forms of therapy (CBT, DBT, cognitive analytic, supportive therapy, family therapy, treatment as usual). After long-term psychodynamic treatment, patients with complex mental disorders on average were better off than 96% of the comparison groups (effect size 1.8). Specifically for personality disorder, five studies (134 patients) of long-term psychodynamic therapy alone yielded significant effect sizes (all more than 0.80) for overall outcome, target problems, general psychiatric symptoms, and social functioning at posttest time points. Of note, due to the atypical methodology employed, the reported effect sizes have been questioned (Thombs et al., 2009), however a valid elaboration was provided (Leichsenring and Rabung, 2009). Long-term psychodynamic therapies are in general more effective than

10. Nonpsychotic symptom and behavior disorders commonly seen in primary care and psychiatric services (e.g., nonbipolar depressive disorders, anxiety disorders, somatoform disorders).

short-term and psychodynamic-based support (see review in Leichsenring and Leibing, 2007).

DBT in personality disorder. DBT is widely considered the gold standard for individuals with severe personality pathology. At least 10 independent RCTs assess DBT in personality disorder (reviewed in Robins et al., 2010). The data support the efficacy of DBT for women with borderline personality. The treatment meets the American Psychological Association criteria for "empirically supported." In four RCTs, DBT was superior to control treatments in women with borderline personality, chronic suicidality, and self-injurious behavior. DBT effectively reduced the frequency and medical severity of suicide attempts, self-injurious behavior, the patients' anger, and the frequency and total day duration of psychiatric hospitalizations. The improvements appeared to remain over at least one year at follow-up. In one study, the comparison group to DBT was treatment by clinicians nominated by their peers as experts in the treatment of borderline personality disorder, adding further weight to the findings regarding DBT effectiveness (Robins et al., 2010).

With respect to *conventional CBT*, a meta-analysis examined the effectiveness of psychodynamic psychotherapy (14 studies) and CBT (11 studies; Leichsenring and Leibing, 2003). The analysis assessed the effect size of the pretreatment–posttreatment difference for the reported follow-up period and the recovery rate from personality disorder (no longer meeting index criteria). For psychodynamic therapy, the average length and follow-up time was 37 weeks and 1.5 years, respectively. The pre–post treatment effect size was 1.46 (very large) and the recovery rate was 59% (three studies). For CBT, the average length of treatment and follow-up were 16 and 13 weeks, respectively, with an effect size of 1.0 (large) and a mean recovery rate of 47% (one study). The analysis provided evidence that both psychodynamic therapy and CBT are effective treatments for personality disorder.

Psychodynamic therapies designed for personality disorder: MBT, TFP, SFT. A number of studies find MBT effective in borderline patients. Bateman and Fonagy (1999) report that MBT-treated patients in a psychoanalytically oriented day program objectively showed a significant decrease in the frequency of suicide attempts, inpatient admissions, and use of psychotropic medication relative to controls. The patients subjectively reported significantly improved symptoms, interpersonal functioning, and social adjustment. Better functioning and improvement on social and interpersonal variables continued through 18-month of follow-up in comparison to the treatment as usual controls (Bateman and Fonagy, 2001). A more recent report (Bateman and Fonagy, 2008) compared the effect of

18 months of MBT by partial hospitalization plus 18 months of mentalizing group therapy as maintenance versus treatment as usual for borderline personality disorder eight years after entry into a RCT and five years after all MBT was complete. The MBT group continued to show clinical and statistical superiority versus treatment as usual on suicidality (23% vs. 74%), diagnostic status (13% vs. 87%), service use (2 years vs. 3.5 years of psychiatric outpatient treatment), use of medication (0.02 vs. 1.90 years taking three or more medications), global function above 60 (45% vs. 10%), and vocational status (employed or in education 3.2 years vs. 1.2 years). The general social adaptation of patients in the MBT group based on the Global Assessment of Functioning Scale remained impaired, however, with about half of the patients showing mild and another half moderate difficulties in social, occupational, or academic functioning.

TFP was tested in a prospective RCT (Clarkin et al., 2007) that compared three outpatient treatments for borderline personality disorder: DBT, TFP, and a dynamic supportive treatment. Ninety severe borderline patients were randomly assigned to one of the treatments and received medication when indicated over one year of outpatient treatment. Before the trial, as well as in four-month intervals, blinded raters assessed primary outcome variables (suicidality, aggression, impulsivity) and secondary outcome variables (anxiety, depression, social adjustment) in a multiwave study design for longitudinal continuous outcome measures (individual growth curve analysis was used to measure change in the dimensions of symptoms and functioning over time). The major finding was that TFP, DBT, and dynamic supportive treatment showed a significant relation to positive change in borderline personality disorder across multiple domains (suicidality, impulsivity, aggression, depression, anxiety, and social adjustment). As for the differences, for the primary outcome variables (suicidality, aggression, and impulsivity), TFP and DBT were associated with significant improvements in suicidality, whereas TFP and dynamic supportive therapy were associated with improvement in anger. Only TFP was significantly predictive of improvement in aggression (impulsivity, irritability, verbal assault, and direct assault), one of the deeply rooted distal mechanisms perpetuating personality disorder. Regarding secondary outcome variables, each of the treatments was predictive of the rate of change in a positive direction for depression, anxiety, global functioning, and social adjustment. TFP was predictive of significant improvement in 10 of the 12 variables across the six domains, DBT in 5 of 12, and dynamic supportive treatment in 6 of 12. The general equivalence in these broad positive changes suggests that the three modalities might be influencing symptoms through different routes, for example, learned skills in regulating emotions in DBT versus developing greater self-control through the integration of mental representations of self and other as they are activated in the relationship with the therapists (TFP) (Clarkin et al., 2007).

SFT was tested versus TFP head to head (the former more cognitive-experiential, but both psychodynamically oriented) in a sample of 88 patients with severe borderline personality disorder using a multicenter, randomized, two-group design. Patients in the study received two sessions per week of SFT or TFP for three years. SFT involved a range of behavioral, cognitive, and experiential techniques that focused on the therapeutic relationship, daily life outside therapy (also including homework assignments), and past (traumatic) experiences. Recovery was achieved whenever dysfunctional schemas no longer ruled the patient's life. TFP involved a negotiated treatment contract between the patient and therapist as the treatment frame, and the approach included analysis and interpretation of transference focusing on the here-and-now context. The main techniques were exploration, confrontation, and interpretation. Recovery in TFP was reached when good and bad representations of self (and of others) were integrated and when fixed primitive internalized object relations were resolved (Giesen-Bloo et al., 2006). After three years, full recovery was achieved in 45% of the patients in the SFT condition and in 24% of those receiving TFP. One year later, the percentage of fully recovered increased to 52% in the SFT group and 29% in the TFP group, indicating continuing improvement in subsequent years, as with other psychodynamically oriented treatments. Both SFT and TFP had positive long-term effects, with SFT found to be more successful. The Society of Clinical Psychology (a division of the American Psychological Association) classifies SFT as "probably efficacious" and modestly supported by research (one or more methodologically sound studies).

ARE SOME PSYCHOTHERAPIES BETTER THAN OTHERS?

Virtually any professionally administered psychotherapy is likely to have some benefit for individuals with personality disorder—and for that matter patients with any other mental problem. Such global, albeit modest positive impact must reflect a nonspecific factor, such as the quality of the working alliance (agreed-upon tasks, goals to achieve, patient-therapist bond based on trust) or simply the value of the patient setting aside time to tell his or her story to a supportive listener and hear him or herself talking about issues which are usually not shared with others. The latter may help some internal integration of blatant discrepancies. Working alliance is a reliable predictor of positive, albeit modest clinical outcome independent of the psychotherapy approach and outcome measures. A meta-analysis found it to have an overall effect size of 0.26, or about 9% of effectiveness of any psychotherapy (Horvarth and Symonds, 1991). To illustrate the need for a more specific psychotherapy effect, we cite here the old adage that "psychotherapy begins where common sense ends."

When it comes to specific impact, psychodynamically oriented therapies, especially long term, appear to provide the best fit between the *healing ingredient* of therapy and the *postulated causes and maintenance* of severe personality pathology. Long-term psychodynamic therapies consistently yield better results on multiple outcome measures in personality disorder, at the level of both general functioning and at the level of individual symptoms. The psychodynamic prototype of treatment (reviewed in Shelder, 2010) (i) involves unstructured, open-ended dialogue (e.g., discussion of fantasies and dreams); (ii) identifies recurring themes and patterns in the individual history of the patient (thoughts, feelings, self-concept, relationships, life experiences, among others); (iii) links the patient's feelings and perception in the here and now with the corresponding feelings and perceptions in the there and then; (iv) draws attention to feelings regarded by the patient as unacceptable (e.g., anger, envy, sadism, shame); (v) points out defensive maneuvers; (vi) interprets warded-off or nonconscious contents; (vii) focuses on the therapy relationship (transference) as a topic of analysis; and (viii) draws connections between the therapy relationship and other relationships outside of therapy. Such an approach activates deep integrative processes, rendering the polarized object relations, as the substrate of the mind and its subsystems, more coherent. A number of independent reports have shown that the benefits of psychodynamic therapies not only continue but also tend to increase over time, after the therapy is completed. In contrast, the benefits of nonpsychodynamic but real-time effective approaches tend to dissipate over time (reviewed in Shedler, 2010). It appears as though psychodynamic therapies trigger fundamental changes in the patent that subsequently come to take on a life of their own and continue to "work" from the inside long after the treatment is over. This, we believe, reflects a successful creation of a *good internal object* in therapy, now providing internal support on its own, a replica of normal childhood experience. Incidentally, the concepts of "good internal object" and "whole objects relations" are equivalent in our opinion. Accumulated empirical data now place psychodynamic psychotherapy of personality disorder in the group of "evidence-based" treatments. Individual format is preferred over groups, the former facilitating the establishment of trust and intimacy, development of transference, and individualized attention, although the latter (the group format) makes use of support and advice, practicing of skills, and modeling with peers (Beutler and Clarkin, 1990). In contrast, the CBT prototype emphasizes dialogue with a more specific focus, as the therapist structures the interaction and introduces topics, functioning in a more didactic or teacher-like manner and offering explicit guidance or advice. CBT focuses on the patient's current life situation and cognitive themes, explains the rationale behind the treatment and techniques, and discusses tasks or activities ("homework") for the patient to attempt outside of therapy (Beutler and Clarkin, 1990). Incidentally, CBT also meets criteria for "evidence based."

In a commentary on the Clarkin et al. (2007) study, Levy et al. (2006) point out that it was only the psychodynamically based TFP, but not the DBT and dynamic support, that was associated with changes in attachment coherence and reflective function, both suggestive of enhanced personality integration. Mechanisms of change at the level of the patient may involve the integration of polarized representations of the self and others (Levy et al., 2006). Mechanisms of change at the level of the therapist's interventions might include the structured treatment approach and the use of clarification, confrontation, and transference interpretations in the here and now of the therapeutic relationship, all of which provide the opportunity to integrate cognitions, motivations, and emotions that were previously split and disorganized (Levy et al., 2006). Such fundamental integration of polarized elementary units of self- and object representations are likely to propagate, that is, to be higher order represented by the general network of cognition into more balanced mental faculties (conscious thought, emotion, motivation), as postulated by neuroscience (LeDoux and Brown, 2017). The integration of object relations and the related balancing of mental faculties could become the instrument of long-term change in the subsystems of the mind (which are configured from these same mental faculties), making the subsystems thus more effective as adaptive mediators to the internal and external environment. Supportive evidence for the hypothesized dynamics comes from a study by Bond and Perry (2004), which showed how immature defense mechanisms (by definition reflecting a low degree of integration of object relations) change to a higher level of defensive functioning, improved symptoms, and better general adaptation in general in long-term psychodynamic psychotherapy for personality disorder.[11] Such profound personality change appears to be mediated by the integration (depolarization) of object relations and the maturation of defense mechanisms, both distal processes in comparison

11. Also included were subjects with chronic and recurrent anxiety and depression.

to other measured clinical outcomes in the study (these were: better therapeutic alliance and global functioning, reduced distress and depression). MBT and SFT appear to be working long term as well (Bateman and Fonagy, 2008; Giesen-Bloo et al., 2006).

Reflecting their specific impact, psychodynamic psychotherapies can be discriminated with sufficient accuracy from other forms of psychotherapy by blinded raters assessing which interventions were actually applied (reviewed in Leichsenring and Leibing, 2007). The outcome of psychodynamic psychotherapy is significantly related to psychotherapeutic techniques and therapist skillfulness, competent delivery of interpretive techniques, and accuracy of the interpretation. Specific changes in transference patterns are also related to the outcome of psychodynamic psychotherapy. A working alliance is a significant but modest predictor of treatment outcome in psychodynamic psychotherapy, as is the case with other therapies as well (Leichsenring and Leibing, 2007). Psychodynamic therapies can be thought of as environmental intervention targeting the exact same issues previous environments were unable to address, either due to overpowering biogenetic biases or the suboptimal environment itself. Psychodynamic therapy thus promotes a specific corrective cognitive-emotional experience though a significant relationship with the therapist that generalizes to other relationships and continues after therapy is completed, much like the natural course of personality and psychosocial development.

Mechanisms of change embedded in the intervention do not have to reflect theoretical postulates of a psychotherapy. Contradicting CBT theory, cognitive changes during CBT for depression do not necessarily precede improvement in symptoms (Kazdin, 2008). In fact, nonpsychodynamic therapies may be effective in part because practitioners, knowingly or more likely intuitively, utilize techniques that are central to psychodynamic theory and practice (reviewed in Shedler, 2010). When transcripts and video recordings of session are analyzed, regardless of the therapy the therapist believed he or she was administering, the therapist's adherence to the psychodynamic prototype predicted successful outcome in both psychodynamic and CBT modalities (Shedler, 2010).

CHAPTER 5

Pharmacotherapy of Personality Disorder

Mechanism-Based and Symptom-Based Approach

A relatively large space in the book is allocated to a review of pharmacotherapy of personality disorder which may strike the reader as unusual given the historically psychological understanding of the syndrome. However, neuroscience has made significant inroads into the complex neurophysiological architecture of the mind, which has uncovered a host of new target processes for pharmacotherapy. Real time neuroimaging, such as functional magnetic resonance imaging (fMRI) and optogenetics, as well as computer science, particularly machine learning and pattern recognition, have been instrumental in delivering this progress. Substantial personality change, which of course is invariably needed for individuals with personality disorder, is a complex process that begins with control of disruptive affect states and behaviors (a short stabilization phase) and then goes on to involve reorganization of fundamental patterns of mental functioning (a much longer reconstruction phase) with integrative effects on the mind as a whole. Treatment of personality disorder relies on precise diagnosis (not only of clinical symptoms but also of the underlying organization of personality), individualized treatment planning (combining expert pharmacotherapy and in-depth psychotherapy), a patient determined to change (preferably one who appreciates psychological mechanisms to achieve change), and an expert-trained clinician genuinely interested in this type of psychopathology (preferably one with personal features of high integrity–low narcissism, high energy–low authority, and the creativity needed to find solutions to frequently "no way out" situations). Here we review relevant neuroscience and clinical nosology of traits and symptoms of personality disorder used to guide pharmacotherapy of specific trait vulnerabilities and symptom domains.

Pharmacotherapy of personality disorder is either

1. *Mechanism based*, aimed at correcting heritable neurobiological dispositions acting as "trait vulnerabilities" that not only increase the risk of personality disorder, but continue to perpetuate its core psychopathology, and/or to shape its clinical presentation or
2. *Symptom-domain based*, aimed at correcting clinical symptoms of personality disorder arranged into domains by co-occurrence.

MECHANISM-BASED PHARMACOTHERAPY OF PERSONALITY DISORDER: A PIONEERING CONCEPT

Mechanism-based pharmacotherapy draws from the modern psychobiology of excessive temperament, one of the major risk factors for personality disorder.[1] In prior work, we labeled the approach "causal" but here use a less ambitious term, since precise causes of any psychiatric illness are not fully understood.

The development of personality disorder can be thought of as a positive feedback mechanism by which biological vulnerabilities and psychological weaknesses reinforce each other. Diverse lines of evidence indicate that a child's heritable excess of temperament (fear, anger, detachment) and/or adverse early environment (neglect, abuse, psychological trauma) may set in motion aberrant, albeit reversible, brain and mind development, resulting in personality disorder. These pathogens, singly or in concert, interfere with early integrative processes of the mind rendering it polarized into contradictory units of memories and affects (the mental part) and hinder normal organization of brain networks, even fracturing the ones that have already formed (the neural part); in a vicious circle, the neural and mental aberrances perpetuate each other. With this in mind, pharmacotherapy of biological vulnerabilities, which perpetuate inner fragmentation, and psychotherapy of mind fragmentation, which perpetuates hypoactive brain networks, both qualify as mechanism based treatments, as discussed. Indeed, modern psychotherapy of personality disorder is in depth and reconstructive, while mechanism-based pharmacotherapy of

1. The other being inadequate early care or psychological trauma.

root vulnerabilities is introduced here. At one point in treatment, a positive feedback loop will be formed whereby improved neurobiology and psychology support each other, thereby reversing the vicious circle. At this point, the healing of the brain/mind is not limited to treatment sessions but continues through experiences in nonsupervised real-life situations.

Beyond "one transmitter—one disorder" concepts. To achieve a full neurobiological understanding of psychopathology, we first need to understand how individual neural activities and intercellular signals are organized into local and distributed networks and how these networks function individually and collectively as dynamic interacting systems. When damaged beyond homeostatic self-correction, any of these processes may turn into a neurobiological substrate of mental dysfunction, disturbing to a degree the function of the mind as a whole. Despite great progress in recent years, we still do not fully understand how the human brain, cobbled through evolution, integrates its modular components into a functioning mind.

Complex neurophysiological processes underlying mental faculties are not modulated by any particular neuroactive molecule but comodulated by most of them, directly or indirectly. Excitatory neurons (using glutamate as a neurotransmitter) are counterbalanced by inhibitory interneurons (using *gamma*-aminobutyric acid [GABA] as a neurotransmitter) and both systems are the major drivers of brain activity. Both types of these executive neurons express receptors for numerous neurotransmitters (mediating fast, point-to-point effects) and neuromodulators (mediating slower, spatially distributed effects, affecting groups of neurons with appropriate receptors, aka "volume transmission"). Both types are thus open to regulation by numerous neuroactive molecules, resulting in complex and coregulated suppressing, facilitating, or preparatory influences. Subcortical limbic regions and midbrain nuclei coparticipate in cognitive processes but are themselves regulated by cortical top-down feedback control. With the above in mind, the time has come to move beyond simplistic hypotheses that any particular neuroactive molecule can be the sole neuropathological substrate of any particular mental disorder. The rapidly advancing fields of network genetics and clinical neuroscience continue to inform molecular neuropharmacology to identify all the relevant neural players in the pathogenesis of mental syndromes as targets for psychoactive medications. For example, responding to the influx of data about complex psychobiology of depression, pharmacotherapy is diversifying its targets aiming to include all the relevant neural players in the pathogenesis of the syndrome, proximal and distal alike. Accordingly, current pharmacological approaches to depression include multimodal drugs (targeting monoaminergic receptors and transporters, such as vortioxetine and vilazodone), drugs targeting multiple monoamines (e.g., serotonin [5-HT]-norepinephrine [NE] reuptake inhibitors—aka "serotonin norepinephrine reuptake inhibitors" [SNRIs] and dopamine [DA]-NE reuptake inhibitors, e.g., bupropion), drugs targeting dopaminergic and reward circuitry (aripiprazole), drugs targeting glutamate and impaired neuroplasticity (e.g., ketamine), among many other targets. In fact, complex action antidepressants which target multiple neuromodulatory circuits (e.g., SNRIs) are modestly more effective than single-system antidepressants (e.g., selective serotonin reuptake inhibitors [SSRIs]). Meta-analyses consistently suggest that venlafaxine (an SNRI) may have greater efficacy than the SSRIs as a class. The magnitude of the advantage is modest, with differences in remission rates of 5% to 10%, and no advantage has been demonstrated versus escitalopram, perhaps the best SSRI (Thase, 2008). However, as Thase (2008) points out, even such modest differences in antidepressant efficacy, if sustained, may have important public health implications given how common and disabling depression can be.

Can homeostasis be harnessed to deliver treatments? One of the brain's main functions is to maintain homeostasis in the organism's internal environment (e.g., electrolyte balance, glucose levels), including its own neurochemical environment. The following few examples indicate that the brain's homeostatic functions can be harnessed to deliver treatments. Electroconvulsive therapy (ECT), introduced in the 1930s, is still one of the most effective treatments for major depression and a number of other syndromes. One established predictor of ECT efficacy is the brain's ability to robustly terminate the ongoing epileptic seizure. Although the precise mechanism of action of ECT is not known, the leading candidate is homeostasis. The latter, presumably activated by electricity-induced generalized seizure, helps to reorganize the pre-existing neuropathological balance of depression into a new and healthier equilibrium via multidirectional co-regulatory optimization processes. The class of SSRIs provides a pharmacological example of such on-demand homeostasis. The antidepressant and/or anxiolytic effects of SSRIs can be summarized as "disturb and wait" for homeostasis to heal (discussed later in the chapter). The process is reminiscent, in terms of nonlinear system dynamics, of the simulated annealing method for solving unconstrained and bound-constrained optimization problems in physics: a system stuck in a less than optimal minimum, which is externally and suddenly excited from its nonoptimal stable configuration into a disorder, is expected to subsequently settle into a more stable state which is closer to global stability. About 10 years ago, one of our colleagues said: "If I give Prozac to all my clinic patients, regardless of their presenting problems, 80% are going to improve." Taking into account selection bias (most outpatients seek help for anxiety and depression), the powerful placebo effect, and the nonspecific healing of the therapeutic alliance, there was indeed some truth to this observation. We believe that our colleague, a great clinician, was describing the widespread homeostatic perturbations caused by acutely increased extracellular 5-HT in the brain (a Prozac effect), which subsequently goes on to recruit homeostatic corrections towards a lower serotonergic equilibrium and stabilize depression and a number of other mental phenomena, such as aggression or anxiety, for example (a homeostatic effect).

Temperament: a clean target for mechanism-based pharmacotherapy. Temperament traits are rooted in subcortical and midbrain circuits involved in a variety of affect states (fear, anger), their respective behaviors (submission/escape, aggression) and a number of other instinctive social and sexual behaviors (aka "subcortical social behavior network"; Newman 1999). In humans, these circuits usually work in conjunction with cortical networks but can also function independently. Given its functional independence from the neocortex and the well-defined subcortical circuitry, temperament may be viewed as a relatively clean pharmacological target. Excessive temperament traits arise from a pathological equilibrium among involved neurophysiological processes occurring within the respective subcortical circuits, resulting in either hypo- or hyperreactivity. Disturbance of any natural equilibrium, whether normal or pathological, triggers homeostatic optimization affecting all components, modulating in the process the equilibrium in question. This dynamics of homeostatic optimization is the conceptual basis of the mechanism-based pharmacotherapy of personality disorder. Although still in its infancy, a rather detailed review of the approach may both inform the reader and inspire research interest. At the moment, symptom-domain pharmacotherapy is the standard of care for these individuals. To discuss neurobiology of temperament, we borrow from our prior work (Cloninger and Svrakic, 2017) and cite other work as indicated.

Cloninger (1987) pioneered a model of temperament traits rooted in discernible neurophysiological systems of learning and memory, each mediated in turn by a specific mix of neurotransmitters and neuromodulators and each underlying a specific motivational bias (inhibition, initiation, maintenance, and persistence) of behavior. Excessive temperament traits may turn into a trait vulnerability for personality disorder by restricting mind development to suboptimal (immature) outcomes, both in terms of poor personality integration (low self-directedness) and secondarily its maladaptive interpersonal features (low cooperativeness; Svrakic et al., 1996). With this in mind, pharmacological modulation of temperament qualifies as a bona fide mechanism-based approach. Such pharmacotherapy does not directly affect the fragmented personality core, only its root and/or perpetuating mechanisms. It is thus most effective if combined with expert psychotherapy, where the two engage in a significant

Table 5.1 FOUR DISSOCIABLE BRAIN SYSTEMS INFLUENCING STIMULUS-RESPONSE PATTERNS UNDERLYING TEMPERAMENT[a]

Brain System (Related Temperament Dimension)	Principal Neuromodulators	Relevant Stimuli	Behavioral Response
Behavioral Inhibition (Harm Avoidance)	**GABA** **Serotonin** (dorsal raphe)	Aversive conditioning (pairing CS and UCS)	Passive avoidance Extinction
Behavioral Activation (Novelty Seeking)	**Dopamine**	Novelty CS of reward CS or UCS punishment	Exploratory pursuit Active avoidance/escape
Social Behavior Activation (Social Reward Dependence)	**Norepinephrine** **Serotonin** (median raphe) **Oxytocin** **Dopamine** **Endogenous opiates**	Social reward (UCS)	Attachment
Partial Reinforcement (Persistence)	**Glutamate** **Serotonin** (dorsal raphe)	Intermittent (partial) reinforcement	Resistance to extinction

UCS = unconditioned stimulus; CS = conditioned stimulus; GABA = gamma aminobutyric acid.
[a] Modified from Cloninger (1987) (used with permission from the Anthropedia Foundation).

positive feedback, as discussed. Table 5.1 presents a simplified summary of complex, functionally coregulated and anatomically overlapping neurophysiological systems involved in temperament traits (modified from Cloninger and Svrakic, 2017).

The big four: evidence supports four main biogenetic trait vulnerabilities. Human behavior traits vary quantitatively along a continuum with no natural breaks that separate trait normalcy from trait pathology. Personality disorder therefore cannot be validly conceptualized by extreme traits alone but requires a measure of impairment that would be more indicative of personality disorder. This central impairment is fragmented personality in our model. Notwithstanding, a valid trait construct of personality disorder provides important insights into the psychobiology of the syndrome and ultimately its specific treatment.

One of the hardest problems in personality theory is the identification of higher order dimensions (natural "building blocks") that underlie and quantify individual differences in personality and behavior. The dimensions have to be both fundamental (i.e., reflect truly essential behavior tendencies) and sufficiently broad to capture an umbrella trait rather than isolated behavior acts. Solid evidence exists that the clinical construct of personality disorder arises from four underlying latent dimensions (a) emotional dysregulation, (b) antisocial and impulsive, (c) inhibition with emotional disinterest, and (d) compulsivity (Livesley et al., 1998). Importantly, the phenotypic structure of personality disorder traits was also found to closely reflect the underlying genetic architecture (Livesley et al., 1998). Note that the four latent dimensions identified by Livesley et al. correspond to the outlying (extreme) ends of normal temperament, notably high harm avoidance (HA), high novelty seeking (NS), low reward dependence (RD), and high persistence (PE), respectively. These temperament dimensions appear to be the general determinants of fundamental but distinct phenomenological and behavior patterns that vary quantitatively, are heritable (up to 60%), and stable over time and across situations and various cultures. The big four appear to be the natural building blocks that "carve nature at its joints" as a true neurobiological organization of personality (or more precisely temperament) and personality disorder (excessive temperament traits as trait vulnerabilities).

To summarize, neurobiological, psychometric, quantitative genetic, normative, and clinical studies of personality disorder at various levels of inquiry yield a consistent association among the four biogenetic vulnerabilities (excessive temperament traits), latent genotypic-phenotypic dimensional organization of the clinical construct, and chronic symptoms organized into four symptom domains (Table 5.2). As such, the big four are useful to assess individual differences in temperament and to design a mechanism-based treatment plan of trait vulnerabilities more so than to conceptualize personality disorder.

With the above in mind (Table 5.2), one may postulate a rather straightforward functional connection between heritable neurobiology of excessive temperament, latent biological and genetic organization of personality disorder, and manifest behavior symptoms arranged in four domains. A notable exception to such a direct relationship are symptoms of cognitive distortions which tend to load within the emotional dysregulation dimension (Table 5.2), perhaps reflecting the dominating influence of dysregulated mood and anxiety on cognitive processes, common in personality disorder. Furthermore, symptoms of cognitive distortions include the primary process or magical thinking, prevalent with obsessive-compulsive disorder (OCD) and anankastic personalities, which may explain the correspondence with the temperament trait of PE (Cloninger), particularly the facets of perfectionism and industriousness as well as with the Livesley's latent dimension of compulsivity with similar facets (Table 5.2).

Table 5.2 CORRESPONDENCE AMONG NEUROBIOLOGICAL TEMPERAMENT TRAITS, GENOTYPIC-PHENOTYPIC DIMENSIONAL CONSTRUCT OF PERSONALITY DISORDER, AND SYMPTOM DOMAINS OF CLINICAL MANIFESTATIONS

Neurobiological Trait Vulnerability[a]	Latent Dimensional Genotypic-Phenotypic Architecture[b]	Symptom Domains (Chronic symptoms of personality disorder)
Harm Avoidance	**Emotional Dysregulation**	**Mood and Anxiety Dysregulation**
Worry and pessimism	Anxiousness	Mood instability
Fear of uncertainty	Submissiveness	Core dysphoria ("default mood")
Shyness	Identity problems	Depression
Fatigability	Social avoidance	atypical
	Insecure attachment	typical
	Cognitive dysregulation	Trait anxieties
	Affective lability	Neurobiological (constitutional)
	Oppositionality	Fragmentation anxiety ("core" anxiety)
	Suspiciousness	Disintegration anxiety
		Existential anxiety
		Somatic (hypochondriasis)
Novelty Seeking	**Dissocial**	**Behavior Dysregulation**
Exploratory excitability	Stimulus seeking (impulsivity, recklessness, sensation seeking)	Impulsive-affective aggression (hostile, non-gain-oriented outbursts)
Impulsiveness	Callousness	Controlled aggression (planned, gain-oriented predation)
Extravagance	Interpersonal rejection (hostile, judgmental)	Propensity to interpersonal conflicts
Disorderliness	Conduct problems	
Reward Dependence (Low)	**Inhibition**	**Emotional Detachment**
Practical (non-sentimental)	Intimacy problems	Lack of empathy
Aloof	Restricted expression (restricted affects, difficulty sharing)	Social detachment/ isolation
Cold		Restricted expression of emotion
Independent		Intimacy problems
Persistence	**Compulsivity**	**Cognitive Distortions and Psychotic Symptoms**
Industriousness	Self-discipline	Brief reactive psychosis
Determination	Dutifulness	Sub-psychotic cognitive distortions
Ambitiousness	Ambition	Loose mental functioning: magical thinking (primary process)
Perfectionism	Lack of spontaneity	Biased mental functioning: egocentric perception of reality

[a] Cloninger et al. (1993). [b] Livesley et al. (1998).

Next we review mechanism-based pharmacotherapy for excessive HA, NS, low RD, and high PE. There are no big surprises to report in this approach, perhaps with the exception of oxytocin and buprenorphine, but we discuss the existing medications through its prism. Pharmacotherapy of adult aggression is discussed in this section as well. Anger and aggression, be it passive or active, fantasized or executed, perpetuate the psychopathology of personality disorder and are thus included with mechanism based treatments.

MECHANISM-BASED PHARMACOTHERAPY OF TRAIT VULNERABILITY ASSOCIATED WITH HIGH HA

The temperament trait of HA and its facets are described in Chapter 1. Under normal circumstances, HA mediates motivation to avoid threat or danger, perhaps the highest survival priority of all. As a trait vulnerability, excessive HA increases the risk for the majority of personality disorder variants (four out of seven: narcissistic, anankastic, passive- dependent, paranoid). The psychobiology of HA is believed to be rooted in overactive subcortical circuits involving the amygdala and the bed nucleus of the stria terminalis (BNST) as the main players. The BNST may respond to more generalized stimuli to trigger projections to the hypothalamus in anxiety-related conditions in comparison to the central nucleus of the amygdala which responds to more explicit fear-related conditions (Nestler et al., 2015). Synaptic plasticity has been documented for the extended amygdala (includes BNST) which in fact can learn fearful responses; the strong connections to the hippocampus (responsible for declarative memory and processing of novelty and context) are believed to underlie the generalization of anxiety on all stimuli that are similar to the original one (Zorumski and Rubin, 2011). The BNST is also connected with the brainstem nuclei, thalamus, hypothalamus, VTA, PAG, and the neocortex, which explains a spectrum of neuroendocrine, autonomic, and cognitive facets of anxiety. A relatively weak connection to the dorsolateral PFCx may explain why amygdala can function independently from and even suppress rational thinking[2] (Zorumski and Rubin, 2011). A heritable overactivity in these subcortical circuits is believed to modulate preconceptual sensory processing of fearful stimuli, leading to associative conditioning of excessive HA, notably worry and pessimism, fear of uncertainty, shyness, and fatigability. The overactivity is maintained by a hypofunctional PFCx, caused by the heightened vulnerability to stress in the first place, now with a compromised ability to exercise top-down cognitive control, thereby forming a perpetuating loop. Cautioning against simplification, an *overactive 5-HT modulatory system* and/or *underactive GABA-ergic*

2. The opposite is also true, as conscious thought may override the amygdala, an important mechanism in CBT

inhibitory neurotransmission are thought to mediate individual differences in HA. Mechanism-based pharmacotherapy targets either or both systems.

The serotonergic system: jack of all trades but master of none. The evolutionarily ancient serotonergic system originates in a small number of midline serotonergic cells (nuclei) in the pons and medulla. Projections from the pontine raphe nuclei, median (MRN) and dorsal (DRN), are numerous and diffuse, with overlapping terminal fields (reviewed in Jacobs and Azmitia, 1992). These projections contact almost every neuron in the brain, suggestive of their modulatory roles in many functions rather than precise information transfer. 5-HT is involved both in basic brain functions (sleep-wake cycle, hunger and feeding, processing of sensory information, energy balance) and more evolved functions (attention, cognition, novel stimuli recognition, mood regulation, fear/aggression, impulse control). 5-HT participates in these functions by modulating the activity of multiple types of neurons (most neurons express 5-HT receptors, even if they do not synapse directly with serotonergic neurons) and by varying the release of other neurotransmitters, such as glutamate, GABA, acetylcholine, and DA. In return, multiple brain areas, cortical and subcortical, provide inputs to pontine MRN and DRN. The inputs (glutamatergic, cholinergic, GABAergic, histaminergic, dopaminergic, adrenergic, neuropeptidergic, among others) mediate activation and deactivation of midbrain serotonergic nuclei in response to diverse stimuli and demands. With respect to attention, there is often an inverse relationship between the activity of serotonergic neurons and strong attentional shifts (Jacobs and Fornal, 1999) as sensory information processing of novel or imperative stimuli is suppressed during the act of motor behavior and vice versa. The serotonergic system can be thought of as a switch that redirects the organism from the "act of doing" to the "act of assessing" and vice versa (Jacobs and Fornal, 1999), a function also supported by the brain's noradrenergic modulation of attention. The 5-HT system is distal in anxiety and depression syndromes, as both also involve cortical networks and other neurotransmitters, such as glutamate and GABA. Pharmacological manipulation of the serotonergic system is certain to affect numerous other brain functions, neurobiological and mental alike.

Overactive serotonergic system at the core of excessive HA. Amounting evidence points to an overactive serotonergic system at the core of diverse anxiety syndromes, most with a common feature of passive avoidance of conditioned fear-provoking stimuli. High expression of the tryptophan hydroxylase-2[3] gene and high amygdala 5-HT levels are found in anxious, avoiding animals (Naslund et al., 2015). In shy, socially inhibited humans, an overactive serotonergic system has been identified both presynaptically (e.g.,

3. Tryptophan hydroxylase is the main enzyme catalyzing 5-HT synthesis from tryptophan.

increased 5-HT synthesis and transporter availability) and postsynaptically (e.g., downregulation of 5-HT1A inhibitory autoreceptors) in the amygdala, raphe nuclei, caudate, thalamus, putamen, hippocampus, and anterior cingulate cortex (ACCx) (reviewed in Frick et al., 2015). Serotonergic cells of the DRN project to the dopaminergic substantia nigra pars compacta and the VTA (regions involved in movement and reward) which (the DRN projections) appear to be essential for conditioned inhibition of behavior by signals of punishment and frustrative non-reward. The anterior serotonergic cells in the DRN intermingle with dopaminergic cells of the VTA, and both groups innervate the same structures (basal ganglia, accumbens [NAc], amygdala) providing opposing dopaminergic-serotonergic influences in the modulation of approach and avoidance behavior (reviewed in Cloninger and Svrakic, 2017).

Serotonergic medications modulate HA by means of homeostasis. SSRIs are the standard of care in both anxiety and depressive syndromes, with somewhat greater effectiveness deomonstrated for anxiety. The precise anxiolytic and antidepressant mechanisms of long-term SSRI administration are not fully understood. SSRIs acutely, within hours, increase extracellular 5-HT by blocking its removal from the synaptic cleft ("reuptake inhibition"). Despite this acute effect, SSRIs take weeks to impact the symptoms ("therapeutic delay"). In fact, SSRIs can worsen anxiety and depression in the first week of treatment, as would be expected in the context of an already overactive serotonergic system in both syndromes. One explanation of the therapeutic delay involves the process of homeostasis: the acute increase ("disturbance") in extracellular 5-HT leads to neuroadaptive desensitization and/or downregulation (decreased number) of 5-HT2A receptors and tonic activation of 5-HT1A/B somatodendritic autoreceptors on DRN and postsynaptic inhibitory hetero-receptors in many brain regions ("homeostatic optimization reaction"). The net effects are *inhibition of 5-HT synthesis, decreased intra- and extracellular 5-HT, and "clamped" transmission* (reviewed in Andrews et al., 2015). These adaptive responses coincide with adaptations in other circuits, for example, mesolimbic dopaminergic (involved in anhedonia), glutamatergic (involved in ruminative cognition), and neuroendocrine/metabolic (cortisol), among others (Andrews et al., 2015). In the end, the brain's homeostatic adaptive response to the acute increase in extracellular 5-HT and the subsequent attenuated pre-existing pathological equilibrium among the coregulated components may underlie improvement in depression and anxiety, rather than the direct chemical effects of the antidepressants. Alternative explanations for the delayed response to SSRIs include neuroplastic and structural changes in neurons as well as neurogenesis in the dentate gyrus of the hippocampus[4] that are found to occur with

4. SSRIs increase the expression of glucocorticoid receptor, a transcription factor

most effective antidepressants. An interesting recent hypothesis points to energy homeostasis as the engine behind the neuroadaptive changes which are stirred by SSRIs, improving in the process high-energy states of depression and anxiety (Andrews et al., 2015).

Sertraline and escitalopram show linear pharmacokinetics and appear to be more effective and better tolerated than other SSRIs. Notwithstanding, the choice of SSRI is customized based on the side effect profile, drug interactions, and/or patient treatment history and preference. Recent antidepressants, such as vilazodone, combine inhibition of 5-HT reuptake with partial agonism at 5-HT1A inhibitory autoreceptors and thus maximize the downregulation of the overactive serotonergic neurotransmission. The same effect can be achieved by combining an SSRI with 5-HT1A partial agonists, such as pindolol (a beta blocker) or buspirone (a partial or full 5-HT1A agonist and 5-HT2A inverse agonist). Even newer antidepressants, such as vortioxetine, combine 5-HT reuptake inhibition and partial 5-HT1A agonism with antagonism at 5-HT3 receptors (the sole ligand-gated ion channels among G-protein coupled 5-HT receptors), the last of which is thought to lead to decreased anxiety, reduced seizure propensity, and reduced neuronal excitation. Although not yet sufficiently studied, based on its profile of action, vortioxetine may be a promising modulator of high HA.

Medications that activate 5-HT1A autoreceptors expressed on DRN cell bodies inhibit this main source of 5-HT, leading to other homeostatic and epigenetic adaptations beneficial for individuals with high HA. Buspirone monotherapy (six weeks at 15–45 mg per day) is modestly effective in treating generalized anxiety disorder (GAD), the clinical "face" of heritably high HA.

The GABA inhibitory system of the brain. GABA, a small amino acid not incorporated into proteins, is the primary inhibitory neurotransmitter in the brain (operates in about 30% of all brain synapses). Similar to glutamate, GABA neurons, mainly interneurons, are modulated by the midbrain monoamines (histamine, 5-HT, DA, DA, and NE, among others) and a number of other neuromodulators (e.g., neuropeptides such as neuropeptide Y, oxytocin/vasopressin, orexin, or opioid peptides, among others). The variable binding affinity of different subunit configurations of GABA receptors coupled with their variable expression in the brain account for functional and regional specificity of GABA modulatory effects on memory, anxiety, arousal, and excitability. GABA receptors are expressed throughout the cortical, subcortical-limbic, and midbrain regions.

GABA's effects are mediated through fast (GABA A) and slow (GABA B) receptors, and both types are expressed on neurons throughout the brain. Slow GABA B receptors are G-protein coupled and upon activation open K+ channels, decrease Ca++ conductance, and inhibit adenylyl cyclase. Fast GABA A transmembrane receptors are ligand-gated ion channels composed of five glycoprotein subunits, usually expressing α, β, and γ or Δ subunits, but others have also been recognized. The subunits are arranged to form a central pore, a Cl^- ion channel. Upon activation, GABA A receptors undergo a conformational change and allow Cl^- ions to enter the neuron, typically resulting in hyperpolarization and decreased excitability. GABA A receptors are heterogeneous with respect to subunit composition, and this influences their affinity not only for GABA, but also for neurosteroids, and GABAergic drugs. The main targets for antianxiety medications are GABA A receptors, although GABA B agonists are being investigated for this and other indications (e.g., in depression and as cognition enhancers).

Underactive GABA underlies excessive HA. High HA and underactive GABA are related at several levels. First, GABA receptors are densely expressed on DRN serotonergic cells. An underactive GABA system may leave the DRN cells without sufficient inhibitory balance, thereby engendering overactive serotonergic neurotransmission, a proposed contributor to high HA. Second, GABA receptors are densely expressed in key way-stations in the network of anxiety signaling, including the amygdala, hippocampus, and PFCx (Roy Byrne, 2005). In the amygdala, GABA modulates excitatory circuits that use glutamate and corticotropin-releasing factor (CRF) (Roy Byrne, 2005). Individuals with high HA (clinically showing as GAD, as discussed) have a downregulated GABA activity in these brain regions (reviewed in Lydiard, 2003) and lower levels of plasma GABA than healthy controls, although the latter finding is inconsistently observed (Roy Byrne, 2005). Finally, GABA drugs also modulate proximal cortical mechanisms (e.g., glutamatergic activity), and rather directly dampen the ruminative thinking of high HA individuals.

GABAergic medications modulate HA in a mechanism-based manner. GABAergic drugs have a trifold effect on anxiety: (i) suppress DRN serotonergic overactivity, (ii) inhibit excitatory subcortical (amygdala) circuits, and (iii) modulate PFCx circuits. All three mechanisms are important in the neurophysiology of high HA. The term "GABAergic" refers to two types of medications: (i) positive allosteric modulators of GABA receptors (PAMs) and (ii) drugs that increase extracellular GABA. In the presence of GABA, PAMs allosterically modulate Cl^- channel subunits, promoting more frequent or longer duration openings of the channels. PAMs include benzodiazepines, barbiturates, etomidate, propofol, certain neuroactive steroids, non-benzodiazepine "Z" hypnotics, and alcohol, among others. PAMs are rarely used to modulate HA as they are to potentially lethal in overdose (barbiturates, many anesthetics) and carry abuse/ addiction risks. More frequently used are GABAergic drugs which increase the availability of GABA, either by blocking its reuptake (tiagabine) or by inhibiting its degradation by GABA transaminase (vigabatrin) or through multiple or different mechanisms (valproate, pregabalin, gabapentin). Structural derivatives of GABA, gabapentin and pregabalin, have multiple mechanisms, one of which is to block voltage-activated Ca^{++} channels and reduce the release of glutamate from presynaptic terminals, the latter is one of the proximal mechanisms in chronic anxiety (pregabalin has been approved in Europe for GAD and it appears to be as effective benzodiazepines (meta-analysis by Generoso et al., 2017). Both drugs also enhance GABA transmission either via increasing its synthesis from glutamate (gabapentin) or via enhancing its functional transport (pregabalin). In summary, low to moderate doses of GABAergic drugs effectively disinhibit passive avoidance, reduce apprehension, and improve other facets of high HA, and in so doing affect direct (amygdala, BNST), distal (serotonergic), and proximal (glutamatergic) mechanisms.

MECHANISM-BASED PHARMACOTHERAPY OF TRAIT VULNERABILITY ASSOCIATED WITH HIGH NS

The temperament trait of NS and its facets (exploratory excitability, impulsivity, extravagance, disorderliness) are described in Chapter 1. We add here that human motivation is associated not only with reward (physical or intellectual) and expectations (defined by personality) but also with seeking novelty (with or without reward) and includes exploration of the environment as one of the independent behavior motivators. In fact, both NS and RD (another primary behavior motivator) are related although not identical components of the motivational system of humans. Both NS and RD are in some part modulated by the brain's mesocorticolimbic DA system, although with some important differences as discussed later.

As main trait vulnerability, excessive NS increases the risk for antisocial and histrionic variants (Table 2.1). The complex psychobiology of NS is postulated to arise from a heritably strong disposition to an appetitive approach which is conditioned during the first year of life into propensity for *behavior initiation*, a biased response to novelty, signals of reward, active avoidance of conditioned signals of punishment, and escape from unconditioned punishment (all of which Cloninger hypothesizes to covary as part of one heritable system of learning). At the risk of oversimplifying, it may be said that NS is primarily modulated by *mesolimbic DA pathways* originating in the VTA. Important VTA projections involve the amygdala, hippocampus, the cingulate, and PFCx. Practically all of these VTA projections are reciprocal feedback connections, suggesting that DA has a role in modulating higher order cognitive functions of the neocortex, as well as the subcortical limbic areas involved in novelty and reward-based learning, to name but a few functions.

Exploratory approach and stimulus hunger in novelty seekers. The VTA, with substantia nigra the main source of the brain's DA neurons, projects widely to the PFCx, including its limbic parts (ventromedial, orbitofrontal, anterior cingulate), paralimbic insular cortex, as well as the subcortical structures (e.g., hypothalamus, NAc, amygdala, and the septal area, among other regions). Originating in the VTA and acting in diverse terminal fields, dopaminergic neurotransmission confers motivational (incentive) salience ("wanting") of the reward itself or associated cues (NAc shell region), updates the value placed on different goals in light of this new experience (orbital PFCx, a component of the ventromedial PFCx), helps consolidate multiple forms of memory such as location and cues of reward (amygdala and hippocampus), and encodes new motor programs that will facilitate obtaining this reward in the future (NAc core region and dorsal striatum; Nestler et al., 2015). VTA dopaminergic neurons fire prior to behavior activity elicited by cues predictive of reward. To coordinate responses to such cues, the VTA receives inputs from diverse brain regions involved in coming up with a valuation of the reward (e.g., glutamatergic inputs from orbitofrontal cortex, among others) and systems involved in arousal, attention, and memory, such as orexinergic inputs from hypothalamus, noradrenergic inputs from the locus coeruleus (LC), serotonergic inputs from the DRN, and GABAergic inputs from the NAc and ventral pallidum (Nestler et al., 2015). DA itself is not a reward signal, but rather an error-detection signal that communicates whether a perception meets expectations. In a "better than expected" scenario, the VTA neurons fire at increased rates resulting in more DA in other components of the reward-network, including the PFCx, and this determines the "salience" of the activity in question. The opposite holds true for the "worse than expected" scenario. As Zorumski and Rubin (2011) note, DA signaling mediates error prediction in the posterior medial PFCx, including the rostral cingulate and the supplemental motor area, while focusing attention and working memory are mediated by the dorsolateral PFCx. Hence, DA can be thought as "volume control" that sets neurons to only respond to strong (salient) stimuli, rewarding and aversive, and reduces the noise of the less salient ones (Zorumski and Rubin, 2011). The described processes are pivotal in reward-based learning. Incidentally, pleasure ("liking") is part of all intrinsic (primary) rewards, but not of all rewards (i.e., those learned by association, like money). Pleasure "hubs" in the reward system are functionally co-recruited (parallel activity) and appear to include NAc shell, ventral pallidum, parabrachial nucleus, and orbitofrontal and insular cortex; the activation is mediated by endogenous opioids, orexin, endocannabinoids, and benzodiazepine receptor agonists (the role of DA at least in some aspects of pleasure is also postulated).

The most distinctive behavior of NS is termed the exploratory approach. Functional MRI (fMRI) studies show increased striatal activity of (presumably) dopaminergic neurons triggered by novel stimuli regardless of whether they predict reward or not (Krebs et al., 2009), suggestive of the independent motivational value of novelty. The effect was anticorrelated with striatal dopaminergic activity triggered by novel cues that predicted reward, indicating that differential midbrain DA responses to novelty and reward may reflect individual differences in temperament traits of NS and RD (Krebs et al., 2009). Krebs et al. showed that the proportion of the midbrain pool of dopaminergic neurons recruited into stimulus-specific burst firing (novelty vs. reward anticipation) might help determine whether an individual is biased toward seeking novelty or reward or whether, in simpler terms, the personality traits RD or NS are predominantly modulating dopaminergic neuronal activation elicited by reward-predicting versus novel non-reward-associated stimuli in the substantia nigra/ventral tegmental area. As Heinz et al. (2009) postulate, stored hippocampal information on reward- or novelty-related features of sensory input and its (hippocampal) control of the striatum and ventral pallidum may modify the state and the population of midbrain dopaminergic neurons activated by the appropriately novel or rewarding stimuli, thereby explaining their relevance to both NS and RD (noradrenergic mechanisms, among others, are additionally involved in social RD).

High scores on NS are associated with reduced D2/D3 autoreceptor control of the midbrain dopaminergic nuclei (Zald et al., 2008), leading to accentuated dopaminergic responses to novelty and other conditions that induce DA release. The increased striatal DA release in response to novel stimuli occurs in tandem with higher density of DA-reuptake transporters in the region and increased reuptake of DA at presynaptic terminals, requiring frequent and novel sensorimotor stimulation to maintain optimal levels of postsynaptic stimulation by DA ("stimulus hunger") (reviewed in Cloninger and Svrakic, 2017).

Dopaminergic drugs modulate high NS. At present, the first-line medications to modulate excessive NS are partial D2/D3 receptor agonists, due to their unique ability to target the postulated DA overactivity without much disturbance of the DA-driven reward system. D2 and D3 autoreceptors are preferred targets, because of the abundance of these receptors in the striatum and midbrain. The candidate medications are aripiprazole, brexpiprazole, and cariprazine. Aripiprazole has been referred to as a "biased ligand" and "smart drug" to illustrate its unique DA action profile: it can act as a full antagonist, partial antagonist, and partial agonist at D2/D3 receptors, determined by the local DA levels, cell type, and functional and signaling status of the target system. In the abundant presence of DA (a full agonist), aripiprazole acts as a partial or full *antagonist*, reducing high NS in a mechanism-based manner. Aripiprazole was found effective in children with disruptive behaviors, aggression, and impulsivity associated with a number of syndromes, including conduct disorder and attention deficit hyperactivity disorder (ADHD) perhaps in ADHD acting as a partial dopamine agonist in the context of dopamine deficiency (reviewed in Greenaway and Elbe, 2009). The D4 receptor, abundant in the midbrain, hippocampus, and probably PFCx, may also be a promising target for pharmacological correction of high NS. In a meta-analysis, *lower* scores on approach-related traits (NS, sensation seeking, impulsivity) are weakly correlated with the D4 receptor promoter 521 T allele, which is associated with a 40% decrease in expression of the D4 receptor and *lower* DA activity. Inversely, *high* scores on NS are expected to have the C allele instead, translating into an *increased* central DA activity (Munafo et al., 2008). Flibanserin, a weak partial agonist at the D4 receptor (also a full agonist at 5-HT1A receptors and antagonist at 5-HT2A receptors) has been approved for the treatment of hypoactive sexual desire disorder, but to our knowledge it has not been tested for any personality disorder-related indications.

Although the D4 receptor was also implicated in ADHD, which created a mis-impression about its shared genetics with high NS, it is the D4 exon III 7-repeat polymorphism acting to dull the response of dopaminergic cells to DA, making ADHD a low DA condition (Faraone et al., 2005; Todd et al., 2007). Also, tandem polymorphisms, the 7-repeat exon III and the 521 T allele, might coparticipate in the deficient dopaminergic neurotransmission in ADHD (McCracken et al., 2000).

High NS and ADHD: similar presentation, different neuropathology and treatments. As discussed, high NS is postulated to involve heritably increased DA activity in the mesocorticolimbic DA circuits. We hypothesize that such DA overactivity not only makes people hungry for novelty (the limbic part) but also affects their cognitive functioning, which is thought to make them impulsive and inattentive (the cortical part). The postulated effect on cognition is based on the inverse U-shape pattern of optimal levels of cortical DA and NE, whereby small changes (up or down) can produce large effects (Arnsten and Rubia, 2012). Simply put, high DA-high NS individuals may manifest ADHD-like features but do not have ADHD. Rather, individuals with ADHD have a *deficient* cortical DA and NE activity, thinner PFCx, decreased volumes of subcortical structures, and impaired interregional structural and functional connectivity in the PFCx circuits involved in mediating attention and inhibitory control (reviewed in Arnsten and Rubia, 2012). Many consider ADHD to be a disorder of executive function because of reduced PFCx ability to exert and maintain cognitive top-down control over decision-making, attention, and "hyper-emotional" behavior (aka "supervisory attentional system") (Nestler et al., 2015). The mesocortical DA system) is pivotal for executive function, but other circuits, neurotransmitters, and neuropeptides have significant modulatory roles as well. Optimal D1-receptor stimulation in the PFCx suppresses neuronal processing of irrelevant information (i.e., reduces "noise"), rendering the PFCx firing rate more selective. High levels of D1 stimulation in PFCx impair working memory (reviewed in Arnsten, 2006). Similarly, optimal NE levels improve PFCx function through actions at the postsynaptic alpha-2A-receptors, which increases the "signal strength." Monoaminergic (5-HT, NE, DA) modulatory effects on PFCx anatomically overlap and are frequently complementary (Goldman Rakic et al., 1990).

Clinical similarity between children high in NS (a variant of normal temperament) and those with ADHD (a structural and functional brain disorder) can be remarkable. Both are characterized by inattentiveness, distractibility, impulsivity, and hyperactivity, but for diametrically different reasons. Such clinical similarity could lead to misdiagnosing and treating a high NS child as having ADHD. Psychostimulants are effective in bona fide ADHD but may worsen impulsivity and/or distractibility of children high in NS (and high central DA activity), perhaps accounting for about 25% of ADHD-like children nonresponders. Nonpharmacological modification of behavior may be sufficient to channel high-NS children into functional adaptation. In contrast, ADHD children may learn to compensate but rarely completely outgrow structural and functional deficits on tasks of inhibitory control, attention, and timing (Langley et al., 2010), and pharmacotherapy is usually long term.

MECHANISM-BASED PHARMACOTHERAPY OF TRAIT VULNERABILITY ASSOCIATED WITH HIGH PE

The temperament trait of PE and its facets (industriousness, determination, ambition, perfectionism) are described in Chapter 1. High PE does not appear as major trait vulnerability for personality disorder. It is not associated with heightened negative affects and rarely by itself is it able to cause a disturbance in early relationships with caregivers. It acts as a powerful modifying trait, in fact decisive for the perpetuation of the anankastic variant of personality disorder (which is why we discuss it among other mechanism-based treatments) and also contributes to chronic symptoms of the paranoid variant (both variants, have high HA as the main trait vulnerability).

The complex psychobiology of PE. PE is defined as a conditioned bias in the *maintenance of behavior* despite failure, frustration, fatigue, and inconsistent reinforcement. In a complex functional interaction with other temperament traits, high PE is facilitated by low HA (high energy, optimism), high NS (exploratory excitability), and high RD (reward-seeking). The dynamics are supported by genetic studies: high PE is associated with *interacting* polymorphisms between the DA-reuptake gene (*DAT1*) and the serotonergic *5-HT2A* receptor gene (Schosser et al., 2010) associated with NS and HA, respectively. All this points to PE as a resulting vector outcome of search for reward and novelty competing with avoidance of frustration. The trait of PE can also be thought of as effortful control of temperament traits with heightened affects (high HA and fearful avoidance, high NS and impulsivity) that interfere with task completion and undermine fitness. Hence, the distinct circuitry involved in PE (Gusnard et al., 2003) might also be involved in top-down regulation of subcortical areas involved in heightened affect reactivity as hypothesized by Posner and Rothbart (2006). High PE also involves greater arousal and focused attention, both of which are functions of the brain's noradrenergic mechanisms, as measured by salivary alpha-amylase activity (Monasterio et al., 2016). The above regulatory effects of PE on affects and cognition are protective against personality disorder.

The trait of PE can be measured by the partial reinforcement extinction effect (PREE), a phenomenon in which partially reinforced operant responses persist longer in extinction than those acquired under continuous reinforcement. The integrity of the PREE depends on glutamatergic projections from the hippocampal subiculum to the NAc. This projection may be figuratively described as a short circuit (a "switch") from the behavioral inhibition system to the behavioral activation system, which converts a conditioned signal of punishment into a conditioned signal of anticipated reward. High PE individuals manifest a positive bias in reward perception, as neutral stimuli are perceived as more intrinsically motivating (Gusnard et al., 2003). PE is alternatively defined as the ability to maintain motivation internally in the absence of immediate external reward. Accordingly, high-PE individuals show greater activation of reward-related ventral striatum and medial and lateral PFCx (Gusnard et al., 2003) in the context of intermittent reinforcement, thus giving rise to the PREE.

Anankastic personality: when compulsive perfectionism organizes internal fragmentation. High HA is the primary trait vulnerability for the anankastic variant of personality disorder. Singly or in concert with environmental pathogens, excessive early fearfulness leads to insecure attachment, inadequate emotional development, and low empathy, all present in anankastic personality disorder (reviewed in Diedrich and Voderholzer, 2015) and suggestive of inner fragmentation. Excessive PE, a modifying trait for the anankastic variant, completes the clinical picture with perfectionism, preoccupation with rules and order, rigid morality, and excessive devotion to work. Ordinarily, anxiety interferes with persistence in behavior; with anankastic personality, however, it appears that excessive worries of high HA are somehow calmed by high PE. The dynamics is unique, as HA and PE are always inversely correlated except in the anankastic and paranoid variants. In the former, compulsive perfectionism, ordinarily a maladaptive trait, appears to help the mind to consolidate internal fragmentation by means of rigid external structure.

Modulation of trait vulnerability associated with high PE: ketamine and lamotrigine. The literature on this subject is scarce. Antiglutamatergic medications (lamotrigine, riluzole, memantine, ketamine) may help disrupt the mentioned glutamatergic switch which is involved in turning signals of punishment into anticipations of reward. This would be a mechanism-based approach, albeit with no empirical evidence to support it. Of interest are lamotrigine and ketamine, with some evidence for OCD proper, as discussed next.

Augmentation of an ongoing SSRI treatment of resistant OCD patients with lamotrigine was found effective in several randomized controlled trials. The main mechanism of lamotrigine's action is thought to occur via inhibition of voltage-sensitive Na+ channels with stabilization of neuronal membranes. By also blocking Ca++ channels, lamotrigine may diminish presynaptic excitatory transmitter release (glutamate, aspartate), which becomes most evident during high-firing neuronal activities (reviewed in Hahn et al., 2004). In addition to direct effects of Na+ and Ca++ channels, other mechanisms may contribute to the mood stabilizing, antimanic, antiaggressive, antiobsessive, or antidepressive effects of lamotrigine. Some of these mechanisms may be downstream consequences of the ion channel effects; for example, neuroprotective effects are postulated to reflect an inhibitory influence on glutamate release. Other lamotrigine's mechanisms include 5-HT-reuptake inhibition, and 5-HT3 receptor antagonism, perhaps explaining its anxiolytic and antidepressant properties (reviewed in Hahn et al., 2004). Lamotrigine's impact on GABA function is actively debated, but seems likely.

Ketamine has not been studied in anankastic personality but has shown some effects in OCD. Ketamine is a direct antagonist at the *N*-methyl-D-aspartate (NMDA) glutamate receptor, but its effects also include dopaminergic, opiodergic, cholinergic, serotonergic, and adrenergic mechanisms. A single intravenous subanesthetic dose of ketamine (up to 1 mg/kg) relieves depressive symptoms within hours. Powerful antianxiety effects are also reported by patients, including a reduction in obsessive ruminations, which in many cases are reported to occur before the improvement in depression takes place (L. Giuffra, personal communication). Therapeutic effects tend to disappear when ketamine is stopped, hence most responders need repeated administrations every one to four weeks. Maintenance doses of ketamine in rapid succession after the first administration over 10 to 14 days may prolong the duration of remission, but this has not been adequately studied; potential adverse effects of longer term ketamine administration in psychiatry have also not been studied (Zorumski and Conway, 2017). Intramuscular administration is a reasonable alternative to intravenous ketamine, but again this approach has not received adequate systematic study. Intranasal S-ketamine appears to be headed for Food and Drug Administration (FDA) approval. Precise mechanisms of ketamine's effects on depression and anxiety are unknown. Although a NMDA antagonist, ketamine paradoxically leads to increased release of glutamate, enhancement of fast-acting α-amino-3-hydroxy-5-methyl-4-isoxazolepropionic acid (AMPA) glutamate receptors, and a cascade of postsynaptic events, notably the activation of brain-derived neurotrophic factor (BDNF) and mammalian target of rapamycin (mTOR), a protein kinase involved in a number of vital cellular functions. Interestingly, low BDNF and low expression of mTOR have also been implicated in depression. Synaptogenesis in response to mTOR activation is hypothesized to contribute to ketamine's acute and sustained antidepressant effects (review in aan het Rot et al., 2012).

In what represents an indirect tactic, high PE could be approached through mechanism-based pharmacological modulation of high HA, which is, as we have noted, the main trait vulnerability in the anankastic variant. Correcting high HA may help reduce the mind's need for its functional coalition with high PE, whereby the latter tends to attenuate the former.

MECHANISM-BASED PHARMACOTHERAPY OF TRAIT VULNERABILITY ASSOCIATED WITH LOW RD

The temperament trait of RD and its facets (attachment, sociability, sentimentality, dependence on others) are described in Chapter 1. The trait is defined as a heritable bias in the *maintenance* of behavior in response to cues of *social* reward and is thus more accurately labeled "social RD," although it may facilitate other types of reward conditioning, including addictions. Low RD is the main trait vulnerability for the schizoid variant of personality disorder, and a modifying trait for the paranoid and antisocial variants. In contrast, high RD is protective against personality disorder (sociable children are biased toward positive social emotions), but appears as a modifying trait in narcissistic, histrionic, and particularly dependent variants.

Social motivation for acceptance or approval by the group has played a major role in the evolutionary success of many species, most impressively in humans. The link with survival puts social reward in the class of unlearned primary positive reinforcers,[5] together with food, mating, and water. Propensity for social interaction is observable early in development, even in newborns (reviewed in Bicks et al., 2015). Importantly, for most pharmacological treatments of low social RD, whether mechanism-based or symptomatic, at least some interest in genuine social exchange with others increases the chance of success. These first prosocial steps are usually achieved in psychotherapy which, here, sets the stage for pharmacotherapy and they continue together (and not the other way around as is generally the strategy in treating personality disorder).

The complex psychobiology of social RD. In higher animals, social signals and cues are processed by two main subcortical networks: (i) the social behavior network (Newman, 1999), composed of limbic structures involved in primordial social behaviors evolutionarily conserved across mammalian species, and (ii) the mesolimbic dopaminergic reward pathway, adding the incentive and perhaps some hedonic aspect to social communication. In humans, information processed by the networks is represented in the PFCx as well as other components of the general network of cognition. Representational knowledge about social signals within working memory (a function of the general network of cognition) provides motivational valuation of instinctive social behaviors. Cortical mechanisms send feedback to conceptualize and contextualize subcortical processing of social information, together called "social cognition."

Human social life: not so human after all. Cooperation *and* competition are integral to social interactions in most animals. Dominance relationships effectively organize intraspecific interactions and are important in the formation of social bonds (Caldwell and Albers, 2016). The subcortical social behavior network (Newman, 1999) refers to an interconnected network of limbic areas which are gonadal-steroid hormone sensitive and rich in oxytocin and vasopressin receptors (both peptides are synthetized in the hypothalamus). These networks include a number of nodes, for example, the medial extended amygdala (the medial amygdaloid nucleus and BNST), lateral septum, periaqueductal gray (PAG), and hypothalamus (Newman, 1999). The areas are reciprocally connected, and each is an important site of regulation or activation in more than one primordial social behavior which are closely related, such as male mating behavior, female sexual behavior, parenting behavior, social recognition memory, communication of social hierarchy, and offensive and defensive aggression (Newman, 1999). These complex behaviors emerge from a temporal pattern of activity across the network, rather than being a product of any particular node.

5. Primary reinforcers motivate and strengthen behavior per se.

Subcortical oxytocin and dopamine in human social behaviors. Being produced already in utero, hypothalamic neuropeptides and hormones oxytocin and vasopressin are activated early postnatally, through skin-to-skin contact, breastfeeding, and face recognition. Quantitative levels of oxytocin and vasopressin are heritable, which likely accounts for individual variability in social information processing and affinity for bonding, both pivotal for social RD. Both peptides are regulated by multiple inputs, e.g., gonadal and steroid hormones, social engagement with parents, and growing cognitive-emotional prosocial capacities. Early activation of the oxytocin-vasopressin system modulates the development of brain networks underlying adult social behaviors, including not only cooperation and bonding but also aggression and competition. The organization of these brain networks is mediated epigenetically through social experiences and circulating levels of modulating hormones and neuropeptides. The networks are open to lifelong plasticity based on social experience.

Instinctive social behaviors regulated by the social behavior network include (i) approach and avoidance motivation toward positive (rewarding) and away from negative (threatening) stimuli, (ii) incentive salience ("wanting"), (iii) consummatory pleasure ("liking"), and (iv) reward-related learning of motor function ("approach"). The mesolimbic dopaminergic reward pathway mediates the incentive salience (wanting) of social behavior and might co-participate in its pleasurable aspects (liking), the latter together with endogenous opiates and orexin. fMRI studies show that social rewards (e.g., positive feedback, a beautiful face, or a good reputation) are processed by the same mesolimbic reward network as nonsocial reward and addictions. Oxytocin, vasopressin, and their receptors are abundant in the reward network as well, perhaps providing the connection between the specific elements that are processed by each. Oxytocin augments the NAc response to viewing the faces of romantic partners and to reciprocated cooperation from human partners (reviewed in Caldwell and Albers, 2016). These authors cogently propose that the lateral septum and the medial extended amygdala, including BNST, functionally connect the social behavioral network with motivational information, which leads to an appropriate behavioral response (Caldwell and Albers, 2016).

Oxytocin: the prosocial molecule for those who are sociable. There is accumulated data to suggest that in healthy individuals, intranasal oxytocin mediates prosocial behaviors and attenuates negative social effects: specifically, it reduces amygdala reactivity to negative emotional and social stimuli, reduces neuroendocrine reactivity to stress and anxiety in social challenges, is released in response to positive social interactions with stress-protective effects in these interactions, reduces uncertainty and increases trust about the predictive value of a social stimulus, inhibits social defensiveness and promotes social cognition, and facilitates approach in social interactions (reviewed in Heinrichs and Domes, 2008). These numerous prosocial effects vary depending on gender, context (familiar vs. unfamiliar people), perceived threat, childhood experiences, and personality features, the most notable of which is quality of attachment. For example, intranasal oxytocin increases bonding and cooperation within one's own group but triggers competition and envy with nonfamiliar people. It can even increase aggression when the partner is perceived as untrustworthy. Instead of being the universal "love" molecule, intranasal oxytocin may simply increase the salience of perceived social cues and is thus likely to be prosocial only in individuals who already possess the tendency to trust others while it may rather increase antisocial behavior among those who distrust others.

People high in social RD show greater discrimination of facial emotions and social cues, presumably mediated by larger oxytocinergic regions in the hypothalamus. RD scores are positively correlated (r = 0.425) and explain about 17% of the variance in plasma oxytocin levels, making this neuropeptide the most powerful predictor of the trait (Bell et al., 2006) and a key player in human prosocial behaviors. In summary, oxytocin might be a fundamental factor for the development of the personality dimension of social RD and perhaps a specific medication for individuals with low RD. Psychiatric uses of oxytocin to improve sociability are discussed next, vasopressin is mainly used in internal medicine.

Low oxytocin in social detachment (low RD) and social distrust (personality disorder). With respect to temperament and low RD, low plasma oxytocin was found in callous–unemotional postpubescent boys, both key features of low social RD. Low oxytocin was associated either with an epigenetically silenced (hypermethylated) promoter for the oxytocin receptor gene (*OXTR;* Dadds et al., 2014a) or with *OXTR* mutation (Dadds et al., 2014b). These findings implicate the oxytocin receptor, either epigenetically silenced or mutant, in a host of structural and functional aberrances relevant to sociability, from differential amygdala reactivity (Dadds et al., 2014b) to aberrant brain networks of social cognition (Hammock, 2015), the last of which becomes especially compromised in ambiguous situations per some reports.

With respect to personality disorder, oxytocin has been studied mostly in borderline personality, which is characterized by rejection sensitivity and negative relationship representations. Overall, intranasal oxytocin tends to hinder trust and cooperation in these individuals (Bartz et al., 2011a). The effect is postulated to reflect childhood adversity and a deeply rooted bias toward negative interpretation of social cues (reviewed in Bakermans-Kranenburg and van IJzendoorn, 2013). Such negative bias tends to undermine the sociability effects of oxytocin, as discussed. Women with borderline personality have low baseline oxytocin levels, which tend to correlate with the experience of trauma in childhood (Bertsch et al., 2013). Epigenetic silencing (methylation) of the oxytocin receptor gene in the context of early adversity is believed to be maintained by low-circulating oxytocin and chronic interpersonal insecurities via negative feedback. Thus early dysregulation of the oxytocin-vasopressin system could be instrumental in connecting childhood adversity and/or innate excessive affects, under-development of neural networks involved in social cognition and empathy, disorganized-ambivalent attachment, amygdala hyperreactivity with bottom-up negative emotion domination, social distrust and hypersensitivity toward negative emotions, impaired social cognition, and poor top-down cortical control of emotional behavior, all of which perpetuate each other in a vicious circle in personality disorder.

Noradrenergic mechanisms in social reward. The dorsal ascending noradrenergic system originates in the locus coeruleus (LC-NA) and widely innervates the spinal cord, VTA and the midbrain reward system, dorsal striatum, basal ganglia, limbic system (amygdala, hippocampus), hypothalamus, thalamic relay nuclei, and neocortex. It is the second most widely projecting modulating system, next to serotonin. The inputs to LC are numerous, including the orexin sleep-arousal system, hypothalamus, amygdala, and several cortical regions, among others. Inputs from the ventromedial PFCx are most relevant here, because this is where the reward value, the expected value, and the hedonic experience of reward are represented. Through widespread pre- and postsynaptic receptors, the LC-NA system modulates neural processes involved in sensory signal detection, alertness, and arousal and comodulates various aspects of cognition (attention, working memory, learning, long-term memory), behavior flexibility, and emotion, especially anxiety. Tonic (basal) firing of the LC-NA neurons occurs during the waking state, decreases during sleep, and bursts en masse during sensory stimulation. Stimuli that portend threat and activate defensive/aggressive instincts seem to generate the highest rate of firing of the LC-NA neurons which mediates attention shifting and focus on the threatening stimulus.

Noradrenergic exploration, exploitation, and disengagement, but not the pleasure of reward. The LC-NA system appears to play a role in processing information concerning attentional orientation toward and incentive value of conditioned rewarding stimulus but not reward itself (Bouret and Sara, 2004). LC-NA activation occurs at the moment of attentional shifts toward anticipated reward and interrupts other behaviors, right up to the reward-directed behavioral response, before it begins to subside during the delivery of reward. LC-NA firing inhibits medial PFCx prelimbic regions during the increased attention phase and the presentation of clues of reward, thereby "allowing" more cognitive cortical regions to dominate when a task demands a high level of attention (Bouret and Sara, 2004). During the anticipation phase, the LC-NA neurons are less active, while prelimbic medial PFCx and VTA neurons are activated, as discussed. Experiencing of a reward also involves the medial caudate nucleus, putamen, dorsal caudate and supplemental motor cortex (Zorumski and Rubin, 2011). Pursuit of signals of reward is an integral part of NS, illustrating the close functional relatedness between the two temperament traits.

LC-NA activity regulates bottom-up, affect-generated attention motivated by long-term subjective goals of increasing pleasure and avoiding pain. The LC-NA activity interacts with cortical and subcortical hubs of the emotional salience network that facilitates learning and survival by enabling organisms to focus on the most pertinent subset of the available sensory data. Moderate levels of NE influence the brain reward system by increasing the signal strength of sensory processing, which allows for more efficient formation of paired associations. In humans, short-term reduction of NE release by the alpha-2 presynaptic agonist clonidine selectively impairs paired-associate learning, particularly the acquisition of novel associations. During pair associate learning, LC-NA neurons acquire the association before it is behaviorally expressed, while the ventromedial cortical neurons activate only after the behavior is learned and during reward delivery (Bouret and Sara, 2004). LC-NA is located at the same posterior level of the brain stem as the serotonergic MRN, and both innervate structures important to attentive orientation towards a stimulus, a goal-purposeful behavior, or a formation of reward conditioning by paired associations, highlighting the interactive complexity of the brain's distal neuromodulating systems.

The strength of social RD is inversely related to NE levels as measured by urine metabolites (Garvey et al., 1996). It appears that a constitutionally high baseline NE tone leaves little room for phasic bursts in NE to accentuate salient stimuli including social rewards, and thus flattens the need for social approval, manifested as low social RD (detached introverts). Inversely, individuals high in social RD and presumably low baseline NE activity are more "reward vigilant," engaging in social reward (people-oriented extraverts) and other rewarding activities, including addictions (task- or object-oriented extroverts).

Modulation of trait vulnerability associated with low RD. The neuropathology of social detachment and disinterest involves dysfunctions in the social behavior network and reward system, specifically pursuit of signals of social reward and social anhedonia, as discussed. Modulations of oxytocinergic, noradrenergic, and dopaminergic components are all mechanism-based strategies for low social RD; however none has been studied systematically, hence our discussion is limited to theoretical possibilities and the author's (DMS) clinical experience. None of the below cited drugs have been approved for social detachment or distrust, but the clinician may use them off label at his or her discretion and based on risk/benefit analysis.

Intranasal oxytocin for sociability. At least some cases of schizoid personality disorder are characterized by low plasma oxytocin (Bell et al., 2006). These individuals manifest primary low social RD (social disinterest, defective emotion recognition and interpretation of social signals, low social proficiency) not necessarily associated with interpersonal distrust (in sharp contrast to all other variants). In this context, oxytocin may be beneficial even without preparation in psychotherapy (reviewed in Bakermans-Kranenburg and van IJzendoorn, 2013). Noradrenergic and dopaminergic drugs, combined or not with oxytocin, may be helpful as well. For other variants of personality disorder, the previously cited negative trials question the benefits of oxytocin in the context of high distrust but high need for social relations. Here, prosocial effects of oxytocin may be facilitated by trust-building psychotherapy. In summary, oxytocin is a promising "sociability" molecule in syndromes of social detachment and disinterest (schizoid personality disorder) and social distrust (other variants) but is bound to carry large individual differences in responses. The differences could reflect genetic and/or acquired variations in the oxytocin-vasopressin system, age, gender, context, pre-existing personality features, or specific environmental influences during sensitive periods in mental development. An interactionist approach in which stable individual differences and contextual factors are taken into account, could maximize the desired effects of exogenous oxytocin on social cognition and prosociality in healthy and clinical populations (Bartz et al., 2011b). There is insufficient knowledge of how oxytocin interacts with vasopressin, glucocorticoids, gonadal hormones, or dopaminergic, serotonergic, and noradrenergic drugs, which affect other key neurosystems in the experience of social reward. Any combination of medications, whether intuitively logical and/or likely to be of low risk, is nevertheless a march into unknown territory.

Noradrenergic drugs may focus attention to social signals. Noradrenergic mechanisms seem like a plausible target to strengthen the signal of social clues via distal mechanisms. Medications that enhance noradrenergic transmission include SNRIs (venlafaxine, desvenlafaxine, duloxetine, milnacipran, levo-milnacipran), norepinephrine reuptake inhibitors (NRIs; reboxetine, atomoxetine), and the unique bupropion (weak NE and DA reuptake inhibitor). Reboxetine was found to selectively enhance detection of emotionally arousing but not neutral stimuli, likely due to an increase in extracellular NE occurring as phasic bursts (De Martino et al., 2008). Such bursts result in both facilitating and impairing effects on attention: attentional gain in the PFCx but at the same time an increased refractory period after the burst at the level of LC-NA via alpha-2 autoreceptors. Only the boost in NE elicited by *emotionally salient stimuli* can have a positive net effect and selectively improve target detection of such stimuli (De Martino et al., 2008).[6] To our knowledge, noradrenergic medications have not been systematically studied in socially detached individuals, with the exception of individuals with autism. With mixed success, atomoxetine improved social withdrawal in developmentally disabled young individuals, including those with autism which is characterized by low social RD and social disinterest (Aman et al., 2014).

Dopaminergic drugs may improve social disinterest. As discussed, dopaminergic mechanisms appear to be involved in reward prediction in social interactions based on a summation of the past history of reward delivery.[7] History of pleasant social interactions incentivizes pursuit of new social interactions with the anticipation of rewarding and pleasurable experience. Rewarding novelty is valuated and pursued based on that history. Brain structures involved in reward-based learning are rich in DA receptors, which are crucial in reward receipt (e.g., the basal ganglia, supplemental motor cortex) and reward prediction error signals (i.e., to reflect whether an outcome is less than, equal to, or exceeds expectations, as discussed). Pleasure is a component of most rewards[8], including social reward. Pleasure hotspots in the reward system that mediate the hedonic or the "liking" aspect of activity are subcortical (NAc shell, ventral pallidum) and cortical (ventromedial PFCx, insular cortex) and in addition to DA also involve mediation by endogenous opioids and orexin (Berridge and Kringelbach, 2015).

A hypoactive mesocorticolimbic dopaminergic system, postulated to underlie low NS, may also contribute to reduced anticipation of reward in social contacts observed with low RD. Such social disinterest is typical of the schizoid variant of personality disorder and occasional with the

6. Reboxetine has no enhancing effect on detection of neutral stimuli which are unable to break the equilibrium between facilitation and impairment in attention; propranolol, a beta noradrenergic blocker, impairs attention regardless of stimulus salience (De Martino et al., 2008).

7. Anticipation of reward or reward prediction error (Schultz) based on summed history of reward delivery is mediated by the DA system.

8. Not all rewards are pleasurable (e.g., money).

paranoid and anankastic variants. There is some, albeit scarce, evidence that medications which enhance central DA activity may enhance the incentive salience of social interactions. Psychostimulants and bupropion are thought to increase extracellular DA and NE via reuptake inhibition and possibly also via presynaptic release (bupropion). In humans, amphetamines increase sociability both by diminishing responses to threatening stimuli (angry faces) and enhancing responses to rewarding social signals (happy faces). The effect is postulated to reflect decreased activation of the amygdala by the threatening stimuli in parallel with increased activation of the NAc by the rewarding stimuli (Bedi et al., 2009). Figuratively, drugs enhancing central DA and NE neurotransmission may increase sociability by decreasing the noise of social insecurities (a dopaminergic effect) and increasing the strength of social signals (a noradrenergic effect). Caution is advised with psychostimulants because of the risk of abuse and cognitive disorganization with high doses. Second-generation partial DA agonists (aripiprazole, brexpiprazole, cariprazine) may be of interest, especially the latter, which has a strong affinity for the D3 receptor, abundant in the NAc.

Opioids may increase hedonism and reduce anxieties of social contacts. The hedonic aspect of social reward appears to be in part mediated by the endogenous opiate system. In healthy individuals, high social RD, but not other temperament traits, was associated with increased density of opiate receptors in the NAc and ventral striatum (major hubs in the brain's reward system) (Schreckenberger et al., 2008), presumably mediating warm attachments to other people. Buprenorphine, a partial mu opiate receptor agonist with low risk of addiction, may benefit individuals with chronic social disinterest by activating the VTA-NAc pathway, although it has not been studied for this indication. Through its kappa receptor antagonism, buprenorphine may decrease dysphoria and improve frustration tolerance in social interactions.

PHARMACOTHERAPY OF ANGER-AGGRESSION, THE PERPETUATING AFFECT-BEHAVIOR STATE OF PERSONALITY DISORDER

The phenomenology and symptoms of trait-aggression in personality disorder are discussed in Chapter 2. In all animals, aggression is a complex adaptive behavior that can be motivated by a spectrum of affect states and vital sensations. It has evolved to deal with overlapping selection pressures for survival and reproduction, that is (i) a defense against threat to oneself or one's offspring (*defensive rage*, a rapid and sudden attack towards the threat which can be followed by fleeing); (ii) presence of a prey as food (interspecific[9] *predatory aggression* with disguising, stalking, planning, and surprising the prey); and (iii) intraspecific competition for resources, territory, and opportunity to mate (*offensive aggression*, a sequence of pursuits, threats, and bursts of attacks separated by pauses). Human adaptive aggression is a corticalized derivative of these animalistic antecedents: for instance, defensive aggression as a contextualized albeit still sometimes adrenalized response to a threat to ourselves, our kin, or our property. Offensive aggression has been transformed into assertiveness, competitiveness, and other socially acceptable strategies employed to earn, rather than seize, status, resources, or a mate. In contrast, pathological[10] aggression refers to aggressive behaviors that exceed species-typical levels of adaptive aggression. In humans, escalated aggression is facilitated by the influence of disinhibiting substances (most notably alcohol), or when aggressive responses are exaggerated in relation to the social provocation (very relevant in personality disorder) or as a premeditated violation of sociolegal norms for personal gain (as in adults with character disorder) to name just a few scenarios in which aggression can take place. The term "violence" refers to human aggression characterized by a threat or actual use of physical force, usually indicating the aggressor's intention to harm.

Most definitions of aggression emphasize the intent to harm. However, harm is not necessarily the intent of aggressive outbursts seen in personality disorder, as these individuals usually fight to change rather than to physically harm others, with the exception of what is occasionally seen in antisocial personalities.

Pharmacotherapy of impulsive aggression associated with excessive NS (trait vulnerability for histrionic and antisocial variants of personality disorder) directly qualifies as mechanism-based. Chronic interpersonal aggression and conflicts, not as a heritable drive but as a consequence of a perceived threat to self, further reinforce the fragmentation into "black-or-white" extremes of experience in all variants of personality disorder, as discussed. Such perpetuation of root psychopathology by what in essence is an epiphenomenon places pharmacotherapy aggression closer to mechanism-based than to symptom-based in our opinion.

On human aggression: the bimodal classification. The bimodal theory postulates two major types of escalated aggression in humans: *affective*

9. The terms "interspecific" and "intraspecific" (or conspecific) refer to between and within species, respectively.

10. Concepts of "nonadaptive," "escalated," and "pathological" aggression are equivalent.

(aka "reactive," "defensive," "impulsive") and *predatory* (aka "premeditated," "controlled," "gain-oriented"). The bimodal classification is a simplification because of the difficulty inherent in parsing human aggression into pure types. One can expect a certain degree of coexistence of these two subtypes in human naturalistic interactions (Vitiello and Stoff, 1997), as discussed later. Most legal systems appreciate the difference between premeditated and impulsive aggression, holding those who engage in the latter less criminally responsible.

Affect states of anger and fear, mediated by the fight-or-flight subcortical circuitry, intervene between threats and defensive/offensive behavior. Affective interpersonal aggression in personality disorder is explosive ("hot-blooded"), occurs in response to a perceived, usually misattributed threat to own idealized image and is frequently followed by paranoid fears. The "provocateur" is important for the psychological stability of the provoked, who thus cannot just avoid confrontation but instead feels compelled to re-establish the image through the conflict, as discussed throughout the book ("conflict as the only resort"). With respect to human-on-human predatory aggression, elements of classical predation[11] (disguised intention, premeditation and planning, mismatched attack on vulnerable targets) are combined with elements of offensive aggression (seizure of resources, sexual predation). Such combined aggression also includes a premeditated plan for cover-up to avoid punishment. Next we review the neuroanatomy and neurochemistry of aggression as the groundwork for pharmacotherapy, in which we mainly focus on impulsive-affective aggression. Our review of the literature turned into a humbling experience due to the complexity of the subject; we are going to be satisfied if we manage to inform rather than confuse the reader.

The neuroanatomy of human aggression: cortical and subcortical mechanisms. Two neuroanatomical networks, one primarily subcortical (instinctive) and the other primarily cortical, each having the amygdala as the key informant, are postulated to underlie the complex phenomenon of human aggression (Victoroff, 2017). The cortical network is involved in the conscious processing of stimuli to which an aggressive response might be appropriate. The subcortical network mediates nonconscious processing of affect states as well as behavioral and sexual instincts that may be associated with "reflexive" aggression (Victoroff, 2017). Such shared responsibility for aggression between rational analysis and affect

11. In humans, interspecific predatory attacks on prey as food within an ecosystem have become obsolete with agricultural revolution, except as hunting or fishing hobbies.

driven instincts perhaps reflects an adaptive process in group living animals, which culminated in human civilization. As discussed, in personality disorder, both of these loops contribute to trait aggression. First, the hypofunctional PFCx renders subeffective feedback regulation of affect-driven behaviors. Second, most variants of personality disorder have a heritably heightened fear and anger reactivity, both of which predispose them to aggression. Heritably decreased limbic volumes, increased amygdala reactivity to aversive memories, and increased arousal to threats have been demonstrated in aggression-prone individuals with personality disorder (in some cases, such limbic overactivity is associated with a mutation of a gene encoding for MAO A, in other cases with early trauma). The same MAO A mutation can be associated with a decreased prefrontal activity as well, thereby creating a vicious circle that perpetuates aggression through both cortical and subcortical loops. The neuroanatomy and neurophysiology of aggression are substantially more complex than the neuroanatomy and neurophysiology of temperament, making pharmacotherapy of aggression also substantially more complex than is the case with temperament traits. Escalated aggression is a global problem, both in clinical and general populations. For all these reasons we allocate significant space in the book to address aggression, both in terms classification and phenomenology and treatment. To discuss the neuroanatomy of aggression we borrow from Victoroff's (2017) excellent review. Other work is cited as indicated.

The amygdala: the brain's "watchdog." As summarized by Zorumski and Rubin (2011), the amygdala is a component of an extended system that interconnects the amygdala, the BNST (involved in associative learning and anxiety), the striatum (including the NAc, relevant to motivation and reward), the hypothalamus (regulates hormone output via the pituitary, particularly relevant is cortisol which mediates stress which is associated with impulsive aggression), and brain-stem nuclei (regulate dopamine, serotonin, and norepinephrine modulatory outputs). Most amygdala connections are bidirectional. Simplified, the basolateral amygdala (BLA) receives input from the sensory systems, whereas the central-medial amygdala are the main outputs for the BLA, which projects to numerous cortical, subcortical, and brainstem structures. The amygdala receives sensory input from the thalamus and sensory cortices, the hippocampus (works synergistically with the amygdala to form long-term emotion-regulated memory), the brainstem (taste, pain, viscera), and olfactory bulb, among others. The amygdala information is sent to the medial and ventral-orbital PFCx (involved in valuation of reward, decision-making, impulse control, emotional regulation, and associative learning), hypothalamus (regulating autonomic and neuroendocrine responses),[12] PAG (movement freezing), ventral striatum including NAc (important in stimulus-response associative learning, aka "instrumental actions"), and brain stem nuclei governing arousal and motivation (serotonin, dopamine, and norepinephrine). With this connectivity in mind, the amygdala is positioned to have a major role in regulating brain functions involved in emotion and motivation, including defensive-offensive affect states of fear or anger, which drive evolutionarily crucial behaviors. Hence the amygdala is sometimes called the brain's "watch-dog" that detects challenges (threat, danger).

In humans, the amygdala is critical for the formation and storage of memories associated with emotional events (aka "emotional learning"). It is bidirectionally connected with the hippocampus, believed to be a pointer to stored episodic and semantic memories, but also helps process novelty and context, adding complexity to emotional learning (Zorumski and Rubin, 2011). These two limbic structures are linked to two independent memory systems which, as Phelps (2004) described, work in concert when "emotions meet memory": the amygdala can modulate both the encoding and the storage of hippocampal-dependent memories. The hippocampus, by forming autobiographical memories of the emotional significance of events, can influence the amygdala response when emotional stimuli are encountered. The hemispheric specialization of amygdala functions and for that matter of aggression in general is beyond the scope of this book.

The subcortical aggression network: aggression as an instinct. As noted by Victoroff (2017), the subcortical loop of aggression involves the amygdala, the hypothalamus, the NAc/septal region, and the brain stem, most notably the superior and inferior colliculi, the dopaminergic VTA, the serotonergic raphe nuclei, and the dorsal PAG. Upon reaching the thalamic relay nuclei, the perception (any sense) of environmental threat is dispatched by these nuclei, the brain's "traffic controller" of information flow. In contrast to the thalamus-amygdala shortcut in lower animals, where aggression is executed without much deliberation, in mammals with large cortices, the main route from thalamic nuclei to the BLA is a slower indirect pathway by which information is first passed to primary and then to higher order, tertiary sensory association cortices (e.g., the inferior parietal lobule) (Victoroff, 2017) to reach both the BLA and the ventromedial PFCx, perhaps reaching the amygdala a split second earlier. As noted, the BLA is involved in the detection of potential threats

12. The amygdala is connected with the dorsal motor nucleus of the vagal nerve (fast regulation of parasympathetic responses) and the sympathetic system (via anterior cingulate).

or predatory opportunities; that is, the amygdala assesses whether this is an aggression-provocative stimulus, whether it is defensive or offensive, or whether it requires fleeing (the decision is made either unilaterally by the subcortex in emergencies or in collaboration with the neocortex as the most appropriate response, as discussed below). Behavior inhibition or "freezing" is mediated by PAG. Many of these "flight-or-fight" responses are learned by amygdala (which is capable of synaptic plasticity) and can be automatically activated. This allows amygdala to hijack physiological and behavioral responses via its own connections to the hypothalamus and brain stem as well as with the striatum and motor system before the neocortex gets involved (Zorumski and Rubin, 2011). However, cortical involvement and even control of these subcortical instincts is also available in humans, as discussed later. The subcortical paths of defensive and predatory aggression appear to separate and in fact inhibit each other at the level of the medial versus lateral hypothalamus and the dorsolateral versus ventral PAG, respectively. Predatory aggression includes little arousal, some sympathetic activation (e.g., focused attention), and cortical planning. Defensive rage is associated with high noradrenergic arousal and high autonomic activation.

The cortical aggression network: aggression as a decision. As noted, sensory signals about potentially aggression-provocative stimuli travel from higher order association regions to reach both the amygdala and the ventromedial PFCx (Victoroff, 2017). Although the amygdala is reached a split second earlier (leaving open the option of automatic subcortical reaction when needed), these regions rapidly interact to assess the threat, opportunity, social significance, and potential reward value of aggression (Victoroff, 2017). This is a partly conscious process capable of suppressing automatic amygdala reactions. The ventromedial PFCx *complex* (includes the orbitofrontal cortex, ventromedial PFCx, and ACCx) is believed to play a role in restraining reactive/impulsive aggression (Victoroff, 2017). Specifically, the centro-medial amygdala is connected via ventral amygdalofugal pathway to the medial orbitofrontal cortex, which is in turn connected with ACCx and dorsolateral PFCx—a circuit by which amygdalar nonconscious processing of threats is integrated with higher order assessment of social circumstances and appropriateness of aggression. The ACCx can be thought of as "error and conflict detector" which enables a person to deliberate before acting on impulsive, emotionally driven, socially inappropriate planning. The dorsolateral PFCx is involved in conscious working memory and reasoning as well as with motor planning necessary to execute behavior. At this level aggression becomes a decision. As summarized by Victoroff (2017), acting under the influence of ventromedial PFCx (involved in social cognition and empathy), the orbitofrontal cortex (social decision-making, valuation of different experiences), and the ACCx (error and conflict detection processes), the dorsolateral PFCx combines new sensory data within working memory alongside long-term memories in order to generate a plan, anticipate its consequences, and materialize the selected plan through the motoric action of behavior.

Next we review some selected functions of the hypothalamus and the "stress axis" relevant to aggression.

The hypothalamus: the home of the attack area. The hypothalamus, a part of the limbic system, can be thought of as the organism's homeostatic control center, or as Zorumski and Rubin (2011) call it a homeostatic "thermostat" which adjust bodily functions, whether basic or more complex, to meet demands (metabolism, heart rate, respiration, body fluids, hormone levels, circadian rhythm, fear and rage processing, sexual behavior, parenting and bonding, among many others). The hypothalamus controls the autonomic nervous system (as the head ganglion it projects neurons directly to the dorsal vagal nucleus and spinal intermediolateral sympathetic columns), the neuroendocrine system (via the pituitary gland and humoral pathways), and the limbic system (via dense bilateral neuronal connections). Most connections of the hypothalamus are bidirectional and subcortical. Cortical inputs from the temporal lobe and medial PFCx, whether direct or via basal ganglia, as well as the projections back to the cortex, whether direct or via the thalamus, are important for the execution of instinctive behaviors related to fluid intake and feeding, reproduction, and attack/defense. The relevance of the so called "hypothalamic attack area,"[13] from which attacks can be induced by electrical stimulation for human aggression is not clear. In fact, because serotonergic drugs that activate the 5-HT1 type receptors reduce hypothalamic impulsive aggression, the hypothalamus is one among several subcortical sites where 5-HT may act as an antiaggressant, the other sites are PAG, basal ganglia, hippocampus, lateral septum. In contrast, activation 5-HT2 type receptors in this region increases defensive rage (complex serotonergic influences on aggression are discussed later in more detail).

13. "Hypothalamic attack area" (HAA) includes ventral portions of the ventromedial (VM) and lateral nuclei of the hypothalamus.

The hypothalamus-pituitary-adrenal (HPA) axis: to fight or fight effectively. The subcortical circuits processing threatening stimuli almost simultaneously activate the HPA, which renders the organism ready to fight or flight effectively. The adrenal production of norepinephrine activates the sympathetic nervous system resulting in mobilization of energy stores and cardiovascular system readiness ("peripheral arousal"). Incidentally, descending fibers from the medial hypothalamus project, among other targets, to the LC-NA, which provides noradrenergic fibers back to the hypothalamus, the rest of the limbic system, and the forebrain (increasing vigilance, enhancing memories of similar experiences, etc); this is believed to be the noradrenergic feedback for *potentiation* of defensive and offensive aggression ("central arousal").

The neurochemistry of human aggression. Human aggression is mediated by numerous neurotransmitters and neuromodulators (e.g., serotonin, norepinephrine, dopamine, GABA, glutamate) and neuropeptides and hormones (testosterone, cortisol, vasopressin-oxytocin, CRF). These are discussed within relevant neurophysiological mechanisms of aggression and as potential pharmacological targets in treatment. Selected genetic factors that increase propensity to aggression are discussed with their respective neuroactive molecules.

Why some people can't control their temper? As summarized by Siever (2008), the most frequently cited mechanisms for propensity towards impulsive aggression are suboptimal "top-down" cortical modulation of aggressive responses to anger provoking stimuli, an imbalance between prefrontal regulatory influences and hyper-responsivity of the limbic regions involved in affective evaluation, insufficient serotonergic facilitation of "top-down" control (aka "serotonin deficiency"), excessive catecholaminergic stimulation, subcortical imbalances of glutamatergic/GABAergic systems, and pathology in neuropeptide systems involved in the regulation of affiliative behavior. Caution is advised when extrapolating results from animal research to human aggression, due to the corticalization and socialization of human behavior.

The role of PFCx. Functional and structural abnormalities of the network involving the orbital, medial, and dorsolateral PFCx, ACCx, and the amygdala have been postulated to underlie subeffective prefrontal (executive) regulation of aggression (Davidson et al., 2000). The midbrain monoaminergic systems, 5-HT in particular, are important modulators of both the limbic-amygdala reactivity and cortical network organization which take place during interactive processes of brain and mind development. In return, the medial PFCx sends glutamatergic feedback to the DRN nuclei to auto-regulate cortical 5-HT release. Complex serotonergic modulation of the PFCx is reviewed in Puig and Gulledge (2011). Activation of 5-HT1B receptors in subregions of PFCx potently inhibits escalated aggression (Miczek et al., 2007). If this effect can be attributed to actions on postsynaptic 5-HT1B receptors, then compromised medial PFCx glutamatergic feedback to the DRN may be the neurobiological substrate for the expression of escalated aggression versus adaptive aggression (Miczek et al., 2007). Namely, increased cortical glutamatergic activity during escalated aggression appears to result from serotonergic dysmodulation of the PFCx resulting in increased glutamatergic input to the DRN. This results in phasic spikes of 5-HT release to the projection areas in the medial PFCx (Takahashi et al., 2015) which is a documented mechanism contributing to the initiation and maintenance of aggressive outbursts in social conflicts.

5-HT deficiency in escalated affective aggression. 5-HT is the main inhibitory modulator of aggression, both at the cortical and the subcortical level. The transition from adaptive aggression to escalated aggression is postulated to involve regulation of the midbrain 5-HT nuclei via 5-HT1A and 5-HT1B autoreceptors, as well as GABAergic and glutamatergic regulatory inputs to the DRN (reviewed in Miczek et al., 2007) to name just a few among many aminergic and peptidergic influences (e.g., CRF, opioids, vasopressin, oxytocin). Deficient 5-HT synthesis, release, receptor activation, and metabolism (aka "serotonin deficiency hypothesis") makes up the classical neurobiological model of *escalated* affective aggression. Low tonic brain levels of 5-HT have been found to be related to escalated affective aggression, supporting the deficiency hypothesis (reviewed in Takahashi et al., 2011). Increased 5-HT2A receptor availability, presumably reflecting receptor upregulation in the context of 5-HT deficiency, has been demonstrated in physically aggressive patients with personality disorder (reviewed in Comai et al., 2012a). In contrast, episodes of *adaptive* aggression are positively related to the central and peripheral serotonergic function (de Boer and Koolhaas, 2005).

With this in mind, the brain's serotonergic activity certainly appears to have different roles in adaptive and escalated aggression, at least in animal models: 5-HT deficiency holds for escalated but not for adaptive aggression. Both forms of aggression are controlled by a rapid but short release of 5-HT during the aggressive act. In escalated aggression, the phasic spikes occur in the context of a low baseline serotonergic tone (5-HT deficiency). Such low basal 5-HT in escalated aggression could reflect an upregulation of pre- and/or postsynaptic inhibitory somatodendritic 5-HT1A as well as terminal 5-HT1B autoreceptors, perhaps as an adaptive compensation for the high reactive state (i.e., frequent 5-HT spikes before and during angry outbursts) of the brain's serotonergic system in habitually high aggressors (de Boer and Koolhaas, 2005). Such compensatory upregulation of 5-HT1 family of autoreceptors, and the respective hypofunction of serotonergic neurons, might turn into a neurobiological vulnerability for affective aggression as a trait (de Boer and Koolhaas, 2005). The 5-HT deficiency model has been expanded over recent decades to include a more detailed set of modulatory and regulatory mechanisms, proximal (cortico-limbic) as well as distal (midbrain; Miczek and de Almeida, 2012). Ascending mesocorticolimbic projections and descending cortical glutamatergic and GABAergic feedback, as well as peptidergic modulation of these circuits, have emerged as the substrate for different forms (offensive, defensive) and different phases (initiation, execution, termination) of aggressive behavior (Miczek and Fish, 2005).

The role of CRF, stress, and hyperarousal in affective aggression. Affective aggression involves activation of the HPA axis, increased circulating glucocorticoids, and autonomic hyperarousal. Stress-induced glucocorticoids facilitate aggressive outbursts demonstrating a positive feedback loop. The mechanisms may include a secondary increase in certain neurosteroids, which at lower concentrations would facilitate aggressive outbursts by disinhibition of cortical control mechanisms (higher concentrations induce sedation and suppress motor activity). In addition, hyperarousal aggression could be mediated by stress-induced hypothalamic hyperproduction of CRF, which may result in increased firing rates of DRN serotonergic neurons. CRF1 and CRF2 receptors modulate the DRN cell firing and 5-HT output to the projection areas. CRF1 receptor antagonists improve alcohol-heightened aggression via action on the serotonergic DRN–PFCx pathway (Quadros et al., 2014). Combined multiple single nucleotide polymoprhisms of the CRF gene were found to be associated with physically aggressive behavior toward others in a Han population of Chinese men, which points to the role of one's predisposition to stress as a biological initiator of aggression (Chen et al., 2014).

The role of reward-based learning in aggression. Once aggressive behavior is established in the repertoire of an individual, its likelihood becomes more predictable due to reinforcing effects. The experience of victories or defeats result in epigenetically altered neural activity in the DA cells of the mesocorticolimbic circuits as well as in altered tonic brain levels of serotonin (reviewed in Miczek et al., 2007), and several of these neuroadaptive changes appear to mediate the sensitized response to challenges: victorious aggressors become more aggressive, defeated aggressors more timid. The role of the mesocorticolimbic DA system in aggression has not been fully clarified. High DA levels in the PFCx and in the ventral striatum-NAc, are associated with visceral "fight-or-flight" responses and helping in learning of rewarding or aversive outcomes. The mesocorticolimbic DA system may be aggression permissive for both defensive rage and predation.

The mesocorticolimbic DA system, excepting the nigrostriatal arm, has been implicated in preparation for and initiation of victorious aggressive encounters (incentive value), but this is true of other motivated activities as well. Acting in concert, a serotonergic-dopaminergic dynamism has been described in aggression: increased prefrontal and accumbal[14] DA coupled with decreased prefrontal 5-HT may underlie the rewarding and thus the reinforcing aspects of aggression (Miczek et al., 2004). The incentive aspect ("wanting") of aggression is a possible DA effect (albeit other brain areas are also included), which may be related to seizing resources (aggression "pays"). Self-reinforcing effects of aggression are not necessarily implying pleasure ("liking") insofar as aggressive encounters usually mean stress, with a notable exception of "sadistic pleasure" hypothesized in human predatory aggression. To complicate things further, elevated DA in the corticolimbic areas is associated with both aggressive and submissive reactions to attacks (Miczek et al., 2004), which is not surprising given the role of DA not only in signaling reward but also in responding to aversive stimuli. In contrast to its permissive role in aggression, less support exists for the mesocorticolimbic dopaminergic system's role in direct modulation of affective aggression. The system's involvement in both aggression and submission indicate that DA antagonists might not be specific antiaggressants, and would perhaps be considered only to mitigate the permissive effect of dopamine on aggression. As a clinical observation, DA antagonists (typical antipsychotics) reduce motivation in general ("haloperidol apathy"), and perhaps may also decrease the incentive value ("wanting") of aggression.

Neurobiology of impulsive affective aggression: summary. To summarize a bit more simply, overactive serotonergic activity in individuals prone to escalated aggression leads to low basal serotonergic neurotransmission (a neuroadaptive response, as discussed) which in turn compromises cortical glutamatergic feedback to the limbic system and midbrain DRN, VTA, and LC-NA, resulting in, respectively: (i) phasic bursts in serotonin release

14. But not striatal dopamine involved in the execution of aggression.

to the medial PFCx (necessary for the initiation of aggression); (ii) dopaminergic permission and reinforcing of victorious aggressive encounters; and (iii) noradrenergic potentiation of aggression at the level of the limbic system and forebrain. With this in mind, glutamate may function to exaggerate the excitability of the neural players involved in aggressive behavior, particularly when aggression is intense; that is, glutamate may sensitize an individual to become more aggressive (Miczek and Fish, 2005). GABA, by contrast, generally inhibits aggression, as do opioids and serotonin.

The neurobiology of predatory aggression: rationally controlled versus cold-blooded. Predatory aggression is not modulated by the serotonergic system to the same degree as impulsive-affective aggression. The sympathetic nervous system is integral not only in defensive rage but also in predatory attacks, here mediated by hypothalamic projections to the LC-NA and downstream projections to the spinal intermediolateral column (Siegel et al., 1999). These hypothalamic projections increase readiness and focus via the sympathetic system without necessarily activating a full-scale HPA arousal (the latter of which could interfere with the effectiveness of predation). Human career predation also involves a better cortical control of emotions, but not a complete absence of heightened emotions (at the minimum it usually includes fear of consequences). However, the emotions are kept under control by an effective executive function. A subgroup of predators have low basal glucocorticoid levels, reduced adrenaline stress reactions, reduced autonomic, cardiovascular, and skin conductance in response to stress, and impaired fear conditioning ("hypoarousal predation"). Such hypoarousal aggression is reviewed in Haller et al. (2005a; 2005b). Here, low glucocorticoids and the absence of emotional associative ability (aka "cold-blooded" people) can be biogenetic ("natural-born predators") or epigenetic, molded by environmental influences within a subculture of crime ("homegrown predators"). As mentioned, predatory aggression is not frequent in personality disorder, thus a detailed review is not our priority here.

MECHANISM-BASED PHARMACOTHERAPY OF AFFECTIVE AGGRESSION

Here we focus on drugs targeting the circuitry involved in the neurophysiology of impulsive-affective aggression, much less on the treatment of predatory aggression. To strengthen cortical-cognitive control of aggression, pharmacotherapy of aggressive individuals *without* personality disorder is optimally combined with cognitive-behavioral therapy (CBT; aka "anger management"). For aggression-prone individuals *with* personality disorder, the in-depth corrective emotional experience is required to integrate personality and eliminate the root source of trait-aggression (combined with pharmacotherapy).

Serotonergic drugs (SSRIs) are first line for affective aggression. As a reminder, baseline 5-HT deficiency is and has been the leading model of escalated affective aggression. Long-term SSRIs ultimately reduce 5-HT synthesis and neurotransmission. Still, SSRIs are first line for this type of aggression (reviewed in Takahashi et al., 2011). The seeming paradox is related to the fact that long-term SSRIs cause a downregulation and/or desensitization of 5-HT2A receptors as well as upregulation of inhibitory 5-HT1A/B receptors, both as a result of homeostatic neuroadaptations in response to the acutely increased extracellular 5-HT. These neuroplastic adaptations make the postsynaptic neurons less responsive to the phasic spikes in 5-HT activity which are necessary for the initiation and maintenance of affective aggression. Other unknown pre- and postsynaptic mechanisms and neuroplastic changes may underlie the long-term antiaggressive benefits of SSRIs (reviewed in Takahashi et al., 2011). Also, SSRIs (fluoxetine in particular) may reduce impulsive aggression by modulating limbic effects of vasopressin, suggestive of interactions between the arginine-vasopressin and the serotonergic system (Victorof, 2017).

Chronic administration of SSRIs tends to *increase* aggression in placid, nonaggressive rats, but it *reduces* aggression in already aggressive animals. In nonaggressive animals, long-term SSRIs eventually lower 5-HT in the context of normal baseline serotonergic activity (creating 5-HT deficiency which facilitates aggression), while in aggressive animals the same mechanism (5-HT decrease and receptor downregulation) may curb the phasic spikes in 5-HT release and reduce aggression. Recently, 5-HT3 antagonists have been shown to have antiaggressive properties. In addition to mirtazapine, vortioxetine is promising given its combined 5-HT reuptake inhibition, 5-HT3 antagonism, and partial 5-HT1B and full 5-HT1A agonism, thereby affecting a number of steps in the development and execution of impulsive aggression.

Polymorphic genes relevant to the serotonergic circuitry, such as *5-HTT*, *MAO A*, tryptophan hydroxylase 2 [*TPH2*]), either singly or via epistasis, increase the risk of habitual affective aggression especially when coupled with early adversity and stress. The genetic effect disappears in environments with low stress, pointing to the importance of gene × environment interactions.

Taken together, the above observations may help in part to explain the variable responses to SSRIs among individuals with affective aggression and may also help clinicians to develop personalized treatment plans. We emphasize again that the majority of individuals with affective aggression improve on SSRIs. This makes drugs with modulatory influences on the midbrain DRN cells acting on their respective expressed receptors (e.g., GABA, glutamate, CRF, and opioid peptide receptors) relevant to modulating escalated aggressive behavior. Some are discussed next.

Can antidopaminergic drugs reduce the incentive salience of and/or revoke mental permission for aggression? Increased prefrontal glutamatergic output, a regular finding in the pathophysiology of aggression, activates the VTA dopaminergic cells, among other already mentioned effects. The resulting increase in accumbal and cortical DA, may play a role in the incentive salience but not in the significant modulation of offensive aggression as noted. The activated VTA also projects to the medial hypothalamus and other limbic structures, which also may facilitate both offensive and defensive rage. These observations are suggestive of some, albeit limited, antiaggression benefits of DA antagonists, although with no evidence that these drugs mediate the extinction of aggression via blocking reinforcement. Rather, typical and potent D2 antagonists decrease aggression via non-specific sedating and locomotor effects, hence the term "chemical restraints," as it is today known in shorthand, which comprise the last-resort intervention on inpatients units and in emergency rooms.

Second generation psychotropics (SGPs),[15] have been shown to have modest antiaggression effects, which is perhaps more reflective of their 5-HT2A antagonism and 5-HT1A partial agonism (both may render the cortex less sensitive to phasic spikes in 5-HT activity), than of their DA antagonism. Most SGPs also have anticholinergic and antihistaminic properties, adding non-specific sedating and locomotor effects. Studies of antiaggressive efficacy of SGPs (risperidone is studied most frequently) are limited to autism, youth with subaverage IQ, and individuals with Alzheimer's disease.

GABA and aggression: predictable and unpredictable GABA effects. As a general rule, direct activation of GABA receptors or higher plasma levels of GABA correlate with suppressing effects on aggression, perhaps by (i) stabilizing cortical glutamatergic pyramidal neurons and (ii) via subcortical inhibitory effects on the amygdala and hypothalamus. GABA A receptors in the medial and lateral hypothalamus suppress defensive rage and predatory attacks, respectively. GABA A receptors in the PAG also suppress defensive rage when activated by GABA neurons, the origin of which has yet

15. We prefer the term "psychotropics" over "antipsychotics" for these medications, as they are commonly used in nonpsychotic behavior syndromes, anxiety, and affective disorders.

to be identified (Siegel and Victoroff, 2009). Through distal afferents and interneurons, GABA inhibits serotonergic cell firings in the DRN cells, curbing in the process phasic 5-HT spikes in cortical, limbic, and striatal regions. As the reader will remember, these spikes are necessary for the initiation and maintenance of social conflicts (Takahashi et al., 2015). Antiaggressive effects of GABA are modestly specific, as they also reflect dose-dependent sedation and general brain slowing. PAMs of GABA A receptors (benzodiazepines, barbiturates, and alcohol, among others) impact impulsive aggression in a *dose dependent* pattern (some call it a bitonic pattern): at higher doses PAMs reduce while at lower doses they increase impulsive aggression; the latter effect is thought to be facilitated by the history of aggression (reviewed in Miczek et al., 2002), the former effect by non-specific sedation. Allosteric GABA A receptor facilitation in cortical and limbic regions is postulated to underlie this dose dependent pattern. As these GABA A receptors are modulated by the prevailing 5-HT tone, PAMs amplify aggression in habitually aggressive individuals with a pre-existing dysfunctional 5-HT flow to these areas (Miczek et al., 2004). Additionally, GABA inhibition of DRN cells alters the serotonergic impulse flow to the VTA dopaminergic cells, resulting in increased cortical and subcortical DA known to be associated with escalated aggression (Miczek and Fish, 2005). Interestingly, in animals with a history of social defeat, diazepam exaggerated the defensive flight response, providing further evidence that the aggression-heightening and -suppressing effects of PAMs are modified by previous social experience (Hebert et al., 1996). Hence, the type and history of aggression must be taken into account before GABA medications are prescribed.

In the context of unreliable effects of PAMs, a more predictable way to manage affective aggression would work via increased GABA availability, using GABAergic drugs. These drugs deliver antiaggressive effects via increased GABA synthesis, GABA reuptake transport blocking, or decreased GABA metabolism. Relevant drugs include valproate (multiple mechanisms), lamotrigine (multiple mechanisms), vigabatrin (blocks GABA metabolic degradation by GABA transaminase), tiagabine (blocks GABA reuptake), and pregabalin (increases GABA synthesis by L-glutamic acid decarboxylase-GAD1). In rodents, chronic administration of valproates correlates with increased brain levels of NE, DA, and 5-HT in some areas and decreased levels in other areas (Johannessen and Johannessen, 2003), which suggests that GABAergic drugs may treat impulsive aggression via multiple mechanisms.

Noradrenergic blockers may suppress potentiation of aggression. The brain's noradrenergic system may have a potentiating role in aggressive behavior, facilitating fight over flight in response to a challenge, perhaps at the level of the hypothalamus (reviewed in Siegel and Victoroff, 2009). The system is activated whenever an environmental signal conveys the possible need to become aggressive, during both offensive and defensive aggression. Increased cortical glutamatergic activity during aggression activates the LC-NA cells and NE projections to the medial hypothalamus which facilitates both defensive and offensive aggression. Disruption of the gene encoding for the NE transporter increases NE levels and defensive aggression (Miczek and Fish, 2005). Humans with point mutation of the *MAO* gene tend to be more aggressive, although the polymorphism recruits not only NE but 5-HT and DA mechanisms as well (Miczek and Fish, 2005). Beta adrenergic blockers have been used to control aggression in clinical work, although mostly in organic aggression with central nervous system lesions, rarely in personality disorder. Pindolol, a beta blocker and a weak partial agonist of 5-HT1A receptors, has been shown to decrease aggression when administered to augment antipsychotic treatment in Schizophrenic inpatients, perhaps by multiple mechanisms. However, a confounding factor is that beta blockers such as propranolol also act on the 5-HT1B receptor as agonists. Pre- and postsynaptic alpha-2 receptors may have different roles in aggressive behavior. Translating from animal research, the alpha-2 receptor agonist clonidine has been extensively used in the treatment of agitated and aggressive patients (review in Comai et al., 2012a), mostly hyperactive children and aggressive individuals with autism. In healthy humans, clonidine increases irritability, perhaps indicating that striking a balance between $\alpha2$ and β activity may be needed for healthy and socially appropriate aggressive responses (Victoroff, 2017).

Alternative pharmacotherapies of aggression: when nothing else works.

Can antiglutamatergic drugs suppress aggression? Glutamate has been implicated in aggression via multiple mechanisms. Glutamatergic projections from medial hypothalamus and basal amygdala to the PAG, acting through NMDA receptors, have been implicated in the facilitation of subcortically mediated defensive rage. As noted, increased cortical glutamate may exaggerate the excitability of all neural players involved in aggression. Still, less glutamate does not necessarily mean less aggression. The effect of NMDA antagonists depends on the animal's prior history and baseline levels of aggression (Miczek and Fish, 2005). PCP (a strong NMDA receptor antagonist) increases aggression in mice with little history of fighting but decreases aggression in habitually aggressive mice (Miczek and Fish, 2005). Low-affinity NMDA receptor antagonists, such as memantine, may modify escalated, rather than basal levels of excitation, which becomes particularly important in the treatment of aggressive symptoms associated with opiate and alcohol withdrawal (Miczek and Fish, 2005). Other medications that suppress glutamatergic neurotransmission, such as lamotrigine, are only modestly effective in reducing affective aggression. Lamotrigine's multiple other mechanisms, particularly those involving the 5-HT system, may in part explain its efficacy in several clinical trials of aggressive behaviors, two of which involve the *Diagnostic and Statistical Manual of Mental Disorders* (DSM) borderline personality disorder (reviewed in Comai et al., 2012b). Some antiglutamatergic effects on aggression may occur via the NMDA receptor on DA neurons in the VTA, via gating DA transmission (reviewed in Miczek and Fish, 2005).

Any antiaggressant benefits of monoamine oxidase inhibitors (MAOIs)? An interesting result illustrates the complex coregulation that takes place in aggression. Polymorphisms of the *MAO A* gene in humans and animals have been associated with a lifelong propensity to escalated affective aggression, especially in high-provoking situations. Aside from the increase in central DA and NE (both contribute to increased aggression), *MAO A* deficiency causes significant imbalances in synaptic expression of NMDA receptor subunits in the PFCx in escalated aggression (Bortolato et al., 2012). In other words, *MAO A* appears to facilitate affective aggression by modulating the structure and function of synaptic NMDA receptors in the PFCx, ultimately affecting cortical control of aggression. Clinically, MAOIs can be useful in the pharmacological management of affective aggression triggered by provocation in personality disorder.

Opioids have a serenic effect. Suppression of defensive rage can be mediated via μ-opioid receptors in the PAG. These receptors are activated by enkephalinergic neurons arising in the central nucleus of amygdala (reviewed in Siegel and Victoroff, 2009). This mechanism opens the door, at least theoretically, for partial μ-receptor agonists, like buprenorphine, to be tried in human affective aggression. Heroin addicts, many with personality disorder, typically report a significant serenic effect of buprenorphine treatment, although the experience might be partly related to the buprenorphine's blocking of kappa opiate receptors with antidysphoric effects.

How close are we to a specific treatment of aggression? Recent research points to the 5-HT1 family of serotonergic receptors as prime pharmacological candidates for selective antiaggressants. 5-HT1A and 5-HT1B receptors are underexpressed in aggression-prone individuals. 5-HT1A and especially 5-HT1B agonists potently and specifically reduce aggressive behavior, and some do so without causing significant motor slowing and sedation (reviewed in de Boer and Koolhaas, 2005).

5-HT1A receptors are somatodendritic inhibitory autoreceptors on serotonergic cell bodies in the raphe nuclei and postsynaptic heteroreceptors in other areas. 5-HT1B receptors are inhibitory autoreceptors on presynaptic axon terminals and postsynaptic inhibitory heteroreceptors[16] found in the serotonin system's terminal fields within several corticolimbic regions which mediate aggression. 5-HT1A and 5-HT1B agonists, systematically administered at relatively high doses, robustly decrease brain 5-HT release as a result of their inhibitory actions at both midbrain and cortical target neurons, respectively. Much like SSRIs and SGPs, the main antiaggressive effects of 5-HT1A/B agonists can be explained as suppression of the phasic bursts in midbrain 5-HT activity that are needed to initiate and execute aggressive conflicts. As an additional benefit, activated 5-HT1B inhibits the release of DA in the PFCx, a mechanism thought to be important in curbing aggression. In humans referred to treatment for aggression and violence (i.e., without high levels of anxiety), buspirone, a partial 5-HT1A agonist, has been shown to reduce impulsive aggression at higher doses (60–90 mg daily), albeit with some motoric side effects (Neppe, 1999). Lower dose buspirone (10–25 mg per day) has been found the reduce symptoms within days in patients with high levels of frustration and / or high levels of stress who have significant chronic irritability and impulsive verbal and physical aggression (Neppe, 1999). Unfortunately, these impressive pilot results have not been followed by larger studies of buspirone in habitually aggressive adults with or without personality disorder. Compounds with selective action at 5-HT1B receptors are more aggression specific, particularly when aggression is facilitated by previous moderate consumption of alcohol or triggered by social instigation (Miczek et al., 2002); these drugs are not available to use in human medicine at the present time. To complicate things further, 5-HT1A and 5-HT1B agonists in the medial PFCx or septal area can increase aggressive behavior under specific conditions in animals, pointing to the importance of regional specificity of action and context.

Mechanism-based pharmacotherapy targeting trait vulnerabilities of personality disorder is summarized in Table 5.3.

16. Heteroreceptors respond to multiple neuroactive molecules.

Table 5.3 MECHANISM-BASED PHARMACOTHERAPY OF TRAIT VULNERABILITIES AND AGGRESSION

Trait Vulnerability	Neurophysiological Mechanism	Mechanism-based Treatment
High Harm Avoidance	1. Overactive serotonergic system	SSRIs, Vilazodone, Vortioxetine, Buspirone
	2. Underactive GABA modulation of subcortical and midbrain anxiety signaling	GABA enhancers: Tiagabine, Vigabatrine, Valpraote, Pregabalin, Gabapentin
High Novelty Seeking	1. Overactive mesolimbic dopaminergic pathways	Partial D2/D3 agonists: Aripiprazole, Brexpiprazole, Cariprazine Partial D4 agonist (flibanserin?)
Low Reward Dependence	1. Hypoactive oxytocinergic system	Oxytocin (intranasal)
	2. Hypoactive noradrenergic system	SNRIs NRIs MAOIs Bupropion (DA and NE) Psychostimulants (DA and NE)
	3. Hypoactive dopaminergic system	Ligand biased D2/D3 partial agonists: aripiprazole
	4. Hypoactive endogenous opiate system	Buprenorphine
High Persistence	1. Overactive glutamatergic "switch" from inhibition to activation of behavior (positive bias in reward perception)	Riluzole, Memantine, Lamotrigine, Ketamine Mechanism-based treatment of HA[a]
Trait Aggression (impulsive-affective)	1. Phasic spikes in midbrain serotonin release (initiation of aggression)	SSRIs SGPs Buspirone (other 5-HT1 A/B agonists)
	2. Noradrenergic potentiation	Beta blockers
	3. GABAergic deficit	GABA enhancers
	4. Dopaminergic reinforcing (incentive salience)	SGPs

SGPs = second-generation psychotropics; SSRIs = selective serotonin reuptake inhibitors; MAOIs = monoamine oxidase inhibitors; GABA = gamma amino butyric acid; DA = dopamine; NE = norepinephrine; HA = harm avoidance; SNRIs = serotonin norepinephrine reuptake inhibitors; NRIs = norepinephrine reuptake inhibitors.
[a] Indirect approach.

SYMPTOM-DOMAIN PHARMACOTHERAPY OF PERSONALITY DISORDER

In addition to managing acute crises, most clinicians engage in pharmacological treatment of chronic symptoms of personality disorder, for example, dysphoria, mood swings, anger, impulsivity, interpersonal aggression, and cognitive distortions. The majority of these symptoms arise more or less directly as a result of a neurally and mentally subeffective personality, particularly the fragmentation of its substrate; thus integrative psychotherapy targets the core problem. Accordingly, systematic reviews of drug trials of borderline (fragmented) personality indicate that medications may be effective in treating turbulent affects and behaviors but not the overall severity of the disorder (Lieb et al., 2010). Importantly, medication-improved symptoms are not to be interpreted as reflecting personality improvement. Nonetheless, such symptomatic control facilitates corrective emotional processes in psychotherapy and better self-regulation of affects in real life. Despite methodological problems, including small samples and short trials, we agree with Blais et al. (2016) that modest empirical evidence and considerable clinical benefits continue to support the use of medications in the overall treatment of personality disorder.

In symptom domain–based approach, the symptoms are targeted outside of their larger mental or neurobiological context: dysphoria with antidepressants, unstable mood with mood stabilizers, and so on. The goal is to reduce symptoms as effectively as possible and at the same time avoid undesirable side effects, the priority is clinical benefit rather than theoretical purity. The rationale for drug choice is analogy with treatments proven effective for "major" affective, anxiety, and psychotic disorders, rather than a theory driven approach specific to personality disorder. Simply put, while similar clinical symptoms are not created equal, they all must materialize within a similar neural substrate (e.g., all conscious moods arise from their respective circuitry, combining subcortical and proximal-cognitive processes). In most cases, symptomatic pharmacotherapy of personality disorder merely "quiets down" the subjective experience of a symptom ("chemical suppression"), in few cases it is more specific (e.g., anxiety symptoms, brief reactive psychoses), and in yet fewer cases borrows from mechanism-based pharmacotherapy (e.g., social amotivation, restricted emotions). This lack of specific hypothesis to guide treatment is the fundamental difference between mechanism-based and symptom-based pharmacotherapy of personality disorder. The most frequently studied drugs are mood stabilizers (lithium and anticonvulsants), all classes of antidepressants, and SGPs.

The majority of symptoms, including mood disorder (e.g., dysphoria, unstable mood), fragmentation anxieties, biased cognition, and interpersonal aggression are not specific to any particular variant of personality disorder but appear to a variable degree in all of them, albeit with some predilection for certain variants (e.g., impulsivity is most impressive in histrionic, antisocial, and narcissistic variants). For this reason, symptomatic pharmacotherapy cannot be usefully organized either at the symptom level or at the level of individual variants of personality disorder but rather around four empirically derived domains of symptoms, shared by all variants to a variable degree. In other words, these domains are also dimensions, but phenotypic dimensions, comprised of manifest symptoms but with no expectation of shared neuropathology among the symptoms within a domain. The four symptom domains are:

1. Mood dysregulation (chronically unstable mood, core dysphoria, recurrent atypical depression, typical depression, trait anxieties);
2. Behavior dysregulation (affective and controlled aggression, poor impulse control, proneness to conflicts);
3. Emotional detachment (social disinterest, low intimacy, lack of empathy, restricted expression of emotion); and
4. Cognitive dysregulation (distorted, loose and biased cognition, transient psychoses).

Pharmacotherapy effects on these four domains are nonspecific, as medications simultaneously affect multiple domains. For example, SGPs are used for all four symptom domains (e.g., mood and anxiety dysregulation, behavior dysregulation [aggression], emotional disinterest, and cognitive symptoms of psychosis). Similarly, serotonergic antidepressants are the treatment of choice for mood, anxiety, and aggression. Such nonselectivity may reflect a number of factors, the most likely being that the four domains, while appearing as distinct at the phenotypic level, are not distinct at the deeper level of neuropathology, i.e., they are coregulated by anatomically overlapping, neuronally interconnected, and functionally interrelated brain networks involved in mood, motivation, cognition, and cognitive control of behavior. A change in one network reverberates through other networks and coaffects other system domains. With this in mind, recommendations for pharmacotherapy targeting symptom domains are summarized in Table 5.4.

The recommendations listed in Table 5.4 are made based on the available, albeit rather limited literature, as well as on one of the authors' (DMS) clinical experience. The evidence for the recommendations is generally weak, this reflecting the lack of good clinical studies rather than negative findings. Table 5.4 is self-explanatory; hence we have chosen to address a

Table 5.4 PHARMACOTHERAPY OF TARGET SYMPTOM DOMAINS OF PERSONALITY DISORDER

Target Symptom Domain	Drug of Choice	Comments
I MOOD DYSREGULATION (UNSTABLE MOOD, DYSPHORIA, DEPRESSION, TRAIT ANXIETY)		
Mood instability/ emotional lability	LITHIUM, VALPROATE, LAMOTRIGINE Low- to moderate-dose SGPs (aripiprazole, quetiapine) "chemical suppression"	PSYCHOTHERAPY (root treatment) "mind stabilization"
Core dysphoria (default mood)	No effective pharmacotherapy	PSYCHOTHERAPY (corrective emotional experience)
Atypical depression (frequent)	MAOIs (phenelzine) SGPs (aripiprazole, lurasidone, low-dose clozapine)	TCAs not indicated: catecholamine stress
Typical depression (rare)	SSRIs, SNRIs, TCAs Augmentation with SGPs and/or lamotrigine	
Psychobiological trait anxiety (excessive HA)	SSRIs, GABAergic DRUGS (PREGABALIN) Lamotrigine, mild NMDA antagonists (ketamine) Azapirones (buspirone)	
Fragmentation anxiety ("core" anxiety) (disintegration, existential)]	"comfort pharmacotherapy": SGPs, pregabalin	Tx of choice for functional anxieties: RECONSTRUCTIVE PSYCHOTHERAPY
Somatic anxiety		
Hypochondriasis	TCAs, SNRIs (milnacipran, duloxetine)	
II BEHAVIOR DYSCONTROL (IMPULSIVITY, AGGRESSION, VIOLENCE)		
Impulsive aggression (default affect state) (affective, unplanned, non-gain oriented)	LITHIUM, SSRIs, SGPs, GABA ENHANCERS Beta blockers (propranolol, pindolol), MAOIs, buprenorphine	
Controlled aggression (premediated, gain-oriented)	NO EFFECTIVE PHARMACOTHERAPY SGPs (dopamine blockade of reward) Beta blockers, Naltrexone	Limited effects of psychotherapy
"career predators" by character	Behavior correction by confinement	

Table 5.4 CONTINUED

Target Symptom Domain	Drug of Choice	Comments
III SOCIAL DETACHMENT, LOW INTIMACY. RESTRICTED EMOTIONAL EXPRESSION		
Social amotivation ("asociality")	Buprenorphine, SGPs (aripiprazole) Tx of choice: MECHANISM-BASED modulation of low RD	Pharmacotherapy largely ineffective Low motivation to change PSYCHOTHERAPY (metacognitive, mentalization)
IV COGNITIVE PERCEPTUAL DISTORTIONS and PSYCHOTIC SYMPTOMS		
Brief reactive psychotic episodes	SGPs (risperidone) STRESS SUPPRESSION (chemical) (mood stabilizers, antidepressants, anxiolytics) STRESS MANAGEMENT (coping) (exercise, meditation)	
Sub-psychotic chronic cognitive distortions ("loose" and/or "biased" mental functioning)	SGPs (risperidone, aripiprazole)	Tx of choice: RECONSTRUCTIVE PSYCHOTHERAPY

CAPITAL LETTERS = first line and major indication; lowercase letters = second line; SGPs = second-generation psychotropics; BNZD = benzodiazepines; SSRIs = selective serotonin reuptake inhibitors; SNRIs = serotonin norepinephrine reuptake inhibitors; NRIs = norepinephrine reuptake inhibitors; MAOIs = monoamine oxidase inhibitors; Tx = treatment; RD = reward dependence.

selected number of topics, some controversial, that might be of interest to the reader.

SYMPTOM DOMAIN I: MOOD DYSREGULATION AND ANXIETY SYNDROMES

As described in Chapter 2, this symptom domain includes mood fluctuations, core dysphoria, recurrent atypical depressions, episodes of major depression, and a spectrum of trait anxieties. Based on Livesley et al. (1998), we include anxiety syndromes in the mood dysregulation domain.

Stable mood instability is one of the hallmarks of personality disorder. Although nonbipolar in nature, it is treated by traditional mood stabilizers, lithium and lamotrigine in particular. As a second-line treatment, low to moderate doses of atypical SGPs stabilize mood by unknown but likely diverse mechanisms; all have been approved by FDA for bipolar disorder and show some efficacy in personality disorder as well. Normally, people can keep their everyday mood fluctuations private (subclinical) by leveraging cognitive self-regulation. With personality disorder, negative and positive stimuli easily activate polarized moods and the related self- and object images (be they positive or negative), while hypofunctional PFCx fails to deliver cognitive feedback control. Mood stabilizers are modestly and nonspecifically effective in subduing mood instability fueled by the specific dynamisms of personality disorder. As hinted earlier, all different moods, whether biological, self-generated, or reactive, ultimately operate within their specific neurobiological substrate and appear in consciousness by the work of the same general network of cognition. Reconstructive psychotherapy is more specific for mood instability of personality disorder and is thus the treatment of choice.

Not all mood swings are created equal: misdiagnosing personality as bipolar disorder. Individuals with fragmented personality may and frequently do present with bipolar-like symptoms (unstable mood, promiscuity, overspending, turbulent interpersonal relationships, inflated self-image, anger), which may be mistaken for bipolar II disorder and vice versa. Personality disorder should be diagnosed only when all domains of psychopathology are present: affective, impulsive, interpersonal, and psychodynamic. In everyday practice, one of the short defense mechanism questionnaires (Inventory of Mechanisms of Defense) and identity surveys (Identity Disturbance Questionnaire) can provide a quick but informative assessment of defense operations and overall maturity of personality to help differentiate fragmented personality from affective disorders, as the respective treatments greatly differ.

Different management for different negative moods of personality disorder. *Core dysphoria* is the default mood state of fragmented personality, and is notoriously refractory to pharmacotherapy. Some options are presented in Table 5.4. Corrective emotional experience in expert psychotherapy helps both the dysphoric mood and the co-occurring personality features indicative of fragmentation (Beatson and Rao, 2012).

Any form of *episodic depression*, typical or atypical, which is comorbid with personality disorder, is more resistant to antidepressants, including ECT, than the same type of depression in individuals with no personality disorder. The first hint that *atypical depression* could be biologically distinct from major depression was the inferior response to standard antidepressants (tricyclic antidepressants [TCAs] and ECT) and superior response to phenelzine, an MAOI. Reports of SSRIs being as effective as phenelzine in the treatment of atypical depression remain isolated. For phenelzine nonresponders, instead of switching to a non-MAOI antidepressant, augmentation with or switching to one of the SGPs may be more effective, although this has not been studied.

TCAs are not recommended for *typical melancholic depression* in cases when it *complicates* personality disorder. TCAs are otherwise superbly effective for melancholic depression in individuals with no personality disorder. TCAs may exacerbate the impulsivity and anger of personality disorder; the effect is believed to reflect cognitive-behavioral disorganization caused by a dramatic increase in catecholamine levels during TCA treatment ("catecholamine stress"). Given its frequent comorbidity with major depression, there have been proposals that borderline personality is merely an unusual manifestation of unipolar depression. As noted earlier, the most compelling evidence against such spectrum relationship is that treatment of depression does not improve core borderline symptoms, while psychotherapy of borderline personality tends to improve both personality and chronic depression (reviewed in Beatson and Rao, 2012).

Prozac "poop out": Is it time to use pulse treatments for the phasic illness of depression? In the early 1990s, only about 10% to 15% of patients with major depression were treatment-resistant. Nowadays the estimates are about 30%, often after a good initial response. The increase coincides with the expanding use of SSRIs. This pattern is dubbed "antidepressant treatment tachyphylaxis" (colloquially "Prozac poop-out"), a debatable term. "Tachy" actually means "rapid," which makes the term something of a misnomer, as this change is not fast; it is rather a more insidious development of treatment failure. Dual reuptake inhibitors, TCAs and SNRIs, appear to have lower rates of progressive decrease in response (Posternak and Zimmerman, 2005). Tachyphylaxis is hypothesized to reflect pharmacodynamic tolerance (desensitized receptors) and/or pharmacokinetic tolerance (decreased quantity of the substance reaching the target site), both documented with SSRIs.

Criteria for discontinuation of antidepressant drug treatments are soft and vague. Clinicians are reluctant to discontinue antidepressants to avoid relapse, a real risk for many patients. However, a significant number of patients taking antidepressants relapse anyway, so the rates cannot be much worse with discontinuation. A few logical strategies to reduce the incidence of refractory depression listed next have not been supported by systematic research. One possibility is to treat depression as *a phasic illness in a phasic manner* (aka "pulse treatment") with SSRIs. Drawing from our concept of harnessing homeostasis for healing, drug holidays from SSRIs during remissions may help preserve the brain's ability to activate its homeostatic response in case SSRIs are needed again, although there are no systematic studies to support such pulse treatment. Another benefit of intermittent treatment perhaps could be a reduction in the number of individuals who go on to develop SSRI-induced apathy. Mood stabilizers (lamotrigine in particular) may reduce the risk of relapse during the holidays. Another strategy is to alternate between SSRIs, NRIs, and SGPs at regular intervals, which would mean even switching patients who are doing well on a certain drug.

Comfort pharmacotherapy for trait anxieties. An unparalleled variety of *trait anxieties* observed with personality disorder are presented in Chapter 2. Treatment of choice is reconstructive psychotherapy. Pharmacological numbing of trait anxieties ("chemical coping"), whether separation, disintegration, or existential anxiety, does not address the root problem, and in fact may mask important cues in psychotherapy. Medication is thus not used beyond the minimum amount and time necessary to ensure some comfort ("comfort pharmacotherapy"). For *hypochondriasis,* reconstructive integrative psychotherapy is the treatment of choice, while relaxation techniques and CBT may be helpful. Antidepressants are not very effective, but TCAs may perhaps be more effective than SSRIs, although the latter have not been studied as frequently.

Revisiting GAD: excessive HA without personality disorder? Heritably high HA increases the risk of not only personality disorder but also of depression, dysthymia, alcoholism, sedative use, GAD, and various phobias, among others. Empirical studies show that individuals with GAD manifest substantially increased scores on the HA dimension, but not on other temperament traits (Starcevic et al., 1996). Excessive HA, notably worry and pessimism, fear of uncertainty, fatigability, and shyness, is indistinguishable from GAD, both phenomenologically and symptomatically: GAD is defined as excessive, uncontrollable worry about everyday events or activities, occurring for at least six months (DSM-5). Individuals with GAD also exhibit chronic fatigue, avoidant behaviors, and a variety of somatic symptoms. Median age of GAD onset is spread over a broad range, including childhood, here called "anxious temperament" which is strongly suggestive of heritably high HA. Rates of remission are low. It appears that, depending on risk and protective factors, heritably excessive HA may lead to personality fragmentation and personality disorder[17] or to GAD or major depression, the last two with a relatively integrated personality in the background. For example, some protective factors, whether biogenetic

17. Baseline HA scores in individuals with "depressive" personality disorder tend to be higher than in major depression or dysthymia.

(perhaps a co-existing high RD) or environmental (good parenting, functional families) can help ameliorate the impact of excessive HA on early integrations and prevent personality disorder. Here, excessive HA may continue to express itself as lifelong GAD in these mature individuals.

SYMPTOM DOMAIN II: DYSREGULATION OF BEHAVIOR (AGGRESSION, IMPULSIVITY, VIOLENCE)

Symptom-based treatment of affective aggression includes a series of behavioral, cognitive, and pharmacological approaches with mixed success. No medication listed in Table 5.4 has been approved by the FDA specifically for aggression control. A few psychotherapies specifically tailored toward aggression are discussed.

Lithium to the symptomatic rescue of aggression. Multiple double-blind trials have shown the efficacy of *lithium salts* in the treatment of affective aggression at therapeutic levels for mania. Similar efficacy has been reported for combinations of lithium either with SGPs or with many anticonvulsants (reviewed in Comai et al., 2012b). The exact nature of lithium's antiaggression effectiveness has not been clarified. It is likely multifaceted (reviewed in Beaulieu and Caron, 2008; Pasquali et al., 2010). Lithium's cellular effects on second-messenger pathways that modulate neuronal excitability, a possible antimanic mechanism, may also stabilize affective aggressive outbursts. There is some evidence that, in a chronic treatment paradigm, lithium upregulates glutamate reuptake and decreases glutamate release, another possible antimanic mechanism (reviewed in Hahn et al., 2004) which perhaps also reduces the propensity toward aggression.

Specific psychotherapy for affective aggression. Given the importance of cortical cognitive control of impulsive aggression, it comes as no surprise that CBT has proven beneficial for this indication, provided the patient is motivated. CBT trains patients to manage aversive stimuli in the day-to-day environment and thus may prevent aggressive impulses. Most "anger management" interventions for patients with impulsive aggression make use of CBT. High levels of arousal impair cognitive feedback control of affective aggression. CBT combined with relaxation techniques aims to improve cognitive functioning and cortical control of the subcortex while pharmacotherapy aims to prevent, decrease, or counteract the peripheral effects of sympathetic arousal (e.g., with beta blockers). They often work well together in impulsively aggressive youth (Vitiello and Stoff, 1997). Another approach to psychotherapy of affective aggression is suppression of negative affect in response to a stimulus that previously aroused such emotion. The method has been called *reversal learning*.

Any pharmacotherapy for predatory aggression? Low basal serotonergic activity is believed to underlie the propensity toward affective but not predatory aggression. There is no effective pharmacotherapy for premeditated predation. These individuals are usually not compliant, prediction of future violence is unreliable, and managing risk is thus made difficult. In theory, opioid antagonists (e.g., naltrexone) may reduce the hedonic aspects of sadistic predation (if it does really exist), and DA antagonists the incentive salience (the wanting) of predatory aggression, albeit neither with empirical support for the indication. Vitiello and Soloff (1997) report that children with the predatory-violent subtype of aggression (e.g., bullying) may respond to behavior therapy. Career nonviolent predation (fraud, Ponzi schemes) are addressed by the legal system.

SYMPTOM DOMAIN III: SOCIAL DISINTEREST, LOW INTIMACY, RESTRICTED EMOTIONAL EXPRESSION

The controversy surrounding schizoid personality disorder, its nosology and phenomenology, was discussed in Chapter 2. The variant is unique in that these individuals neither desire nor seek social contacts, as they appear to have withdrawn from the bilateral social world into the unilateral world of fantasy and daydreaming, in which they have full control over events. No data exist for pharmacotherapy of the globally hypoactive temperament of schizoid personalities. Clozapine has been shown to improve apathy, amotivation, avolition, social disinterest, lack of sexual interest, and other "negative" symptoms in patients with the negative subtype of Schizophrenia. Here, social withdrawal reflects "primary asociality" with specific neural correlates (Kaiser et al., 2016). It is not clear whether clozapine, or any other drug, may affect the secondary asociality of schizoid personality, a compensatory adaptive style. Aripiprazole, brexpiprazole, and cariprazine, all partial D2 and D3 agonists with documented benefits for schizotypal symptoms but no studies in schizoid personality disorder to our knowledge, are certainly attractive candidates to try. In summary, given the limitations of symptom based pharmacotherapy, perhaps excepting clozapine, mechanism-based pharmacotherapy described for low social RD preferably combined with metacognitive psychotherapy is the best available option for individuals with schizoid personality disorder.

SYMPTOM DOMAIN IV: COGNITIVE-PERCEPTUAL DISTORTION AND PSYCHOTIC SYMPTOMS

Brief reactive psychoses as well as loose and biased cognition observed with personality disorder are discussed in Chapter 2. Symptom-based medications are listed in Table 5.4; risperidone is the most frequently used agent. Stress reduction is an important indirect way to resolve brief reactive psychoses in the context of acute stress or personal crisis. For example, benzodiazepines (alprazolam) were shown to improve paranoia in borderline individuals, presumably due to anti-anxiety (anti-stress) effects. Short-term use of benzodiazepines for personality disorder increases the risk of behavior dyscontrol and aggression, while long-term use increases the risk of overuse. If prescribed, benzodiazepines should be monitored for abuse and used only until the reactive psychosis is resolved. Alternative approaches to reduce stress and emotional tensions include other GABAergic drugs, SSRIs, MAOIs, psychotherapy, relaxation techniques, and meditation.

THE ROLE OF ANTIPSYCHOTICS IN THE TREATMENT OF PERSONALITY DISORDER

Following the DA hypothesis of Schizophrenia (1960's), the group of antipsychotics evolved from low-potency, sedating compounds in the 1950s to potent D2 antagonists in the 1970s. These drugs are primarily used to treat the positive symptoms of psychosis, such as delusions and hallucinations. Administered to nonpsychotic individuals with personality or mood problems, typical antipsychotics have no desired specific effects[18] but a plethora of undesired effects, including major sedation and motoric incapacitation, and they may also cause irreversible tardive dyskinesia.

During the past three decades, a number of SGPs have been developed with multiple modes of pharmacodynamic actions, primarily targeting but not limited to DA and 5-HT neurotransmission. SGPs (aka "atypicals") cause less sedation and have a much more favorable side-effect profile in comparison with typical antipsychotics. In addition to antipsychotic effects, they also have impressive antidepressant, antimanic, mood-stabilizing, and anxiolytic effects, likely reflecting multiple modes of action and/or functional overlap among brain networks involved in mood and cognition.

18. Except perhaps for the incentive-blocking effect in predatory aggression, including sexual predation.

Clozapine and aripiprazole stand out in the group of atypicals. A unique place among the atypicals is reserved for clozapine, the first atypical, and to date the most effective medication for positive, negative, and disorganization symptoms of Schizophrenia. In the United States, clozapine is administered as a third-line agent, due to serious adverse effects, many of which can be minimized by careful clinical and laboratory monitoring. Encouraged by its effectiveness for non-FDA approved indications, an increasing number of clinicians are using clozapine off label, for indications such as refractory depression, atypical depression, bipolar disorder, anorexia, severe anxiety disorders, and personality disorder, among others. The complex pharmacodynamic profile of clozapine may in part explain such wide spectrum efficacy, which is related to either specific or combined mechanisms. In addition to serotonergic (5-HT2A, 5-HT1A) and dopaminergic antagonism (mostly at D4 receptors), clozapine is also a histone deacetylase (HDAC) inhibitor, thereby mediating epigenetic increase in GABA production and GABA modulation of cortical pyramidal neurons, an effect believed to improve cognitive processing and top-down cortical control of subcortical functions, which is beneficial for a number of psychiatric syndromes. Also, clozapine is believed to stimulate the synthesis of GABAergic neurosteroids, an effect that may explain its efficacy not only in psychosis but also in chronic anxiety and vulnerability to stress. By yet another mechanism, clozapine blocks glycine transport, an effect that may enhance NMDA neurotransmission (Javitt et al., 2005) and perhaps facilitate neuroplasticity and new learning. Clozapine can be combined with lithium, antidepressants, and anticonvulsants, notably valproate, the latter also a HDAC inhibitor with similar epigenetic effects on GABA production. If combined with antidepressants, fluvoxamine is the preferred partner (reviewed in Lu and Lane, 2003). We support proposals to use clozapine as a first- and second-line medication in adults with Schizophrenia (e.g., as in Great Britain and China, respectively).

Aripiprazole, originally marketed as an antipsychotic, is now more frequently used for other indications, such as bipolar disorder, major depression, dysthymia, impulsive aggression, and trait anxiety in individuals with and without personality disorder, either as monotherapy or as an augmentation strategy. As discussed, aripiprazole is frequently referred to as a "third-generation" psychotropic to illustrate its unique action profile which has been dubbed a "biased ligand" or "smart"[19] pharmacological

19. Due to the "smart" mode of action, aripiprazole may prevent the development of dopamine-related neurochemical adaptations that may possibly affect long-term response to antipsychotics (de Bartolomeis et al., 2015).

agent working at D2 and possibly D3 dopaminergic receptors. Aripiprazole is also a partial 5-HT1A agonist and a full 5-HT2A antagonist, and it has NMDA, histaminic, and adrenergic activity. The action profile also includes multiple cellular pathways and several cortical and subcortical neurotransmitter circuitries as well as modulation of gene expression distinct from other antipsychotics (reviewed in de Bartolomeis et al., 2015). Given its superb efficacy in depression, four- and six-week injectable aripiprazole can be thought of as the first long-acting injectable antidepressant.

Despite relative safety, caution is advised. The decision to use SGPs long term requires consideration of potential undesired effects and should be made with the informed consent of the patient. Body weight and blood sugar must be closely monitored, so that early signs of metabolic and other adverse effects are recognized and prevented. Following Lerner et al. (2007), we (DMS) have had success in treating parkinsonian side effects, including tardive dyskinesia, with high doses of pyridoxine (vitamin B6). Many clinicians combine pyridoxine with high-dose ascorbic acid (vitamin C), tocopherol (vitamin E), and zinc sulfate intravenously daily. The mechanisms of antiparkinsonian efficacy of antioxidants is unknown, although oxidative stress contributes to multiple neuropsychiatric conditions.

IS A PERSONALIZED BUT EVIDENCE-BASED APPROACH THE ULTIMATE ART AND SCIENCE OF HEALING?

Despite progress in efficacy/effectiveness, tolerability, and safety, prescribing psychoactive medications is still viewed by many as guesswork at best which may cause more harm than good. Reflecting on the explosion in the use of psychoactive drugs in the recent decades (dubbed "pharmageddon"),[20] concerns have been raised about the "medicalization of life," when normal but emotional life phases, such as bereavement or divorce, are treated with medication. The recent initiative to integrate an evidence-based or "average patient" approach (the science) and personalized or "unique patient" approach (the art) may help gain public trust in the pharmacotherapy of personality and non-psychotic syndromes. There is only a finite variation in the psychobiological organization of human beings notwithstanding, in all practicality, unique phenotypes. Personalized pharmacotherapy could be achieved by stratification of mechanistic-based

20. Sales of sertraline (Zoloft) outperformed the sales of Tide detergent in 2005 in the United States.

hypotheses developed by RCTs into fine-grained strata of averages for small groups of neuropsychologically close individuals (de Leon, 2012).

Some proponents of personalized medicine would not see unique patient approaches as "art" but rather as the ultimate science of a treatment based on individual genetics. This would be true if only somatic but not mental issues were considered. Personalized approach means not only the complete DNA sequence of individuals but also a detailed understanding to their unique intimate psychological reactions to illness, their coping and adjustment abilities, and their philosophy of life. These emerging properties within autonoetic consciousness ("meta-representations") are not readily, if at all, reducible to one's DNA sequence. The complex interactive triad of gene × brain/mind × environment, with many-to-many feedback and feedforward interactions, allow the same (different) conditions to lead to different (same) outcomes (the mentioned "multifinality" and "equifinality," respectively). Perhaps we are just naive, but we simply do not believe that a human being shall ever be completely understood by knowing his or her DNA sequence or by performing MRI scans, serum analysis, or by digitizing their mind output via smartphone-generated data, no matter how sophisticated these may become. In other words, phenotype, not technology, is the problem because at some point, beyond a certain level of cognitive abstraction, mental phenomena simply become too personal to be classified into averages. Even if a method becomes capable of reducing cognitive meta-representations to their network or protein substrates, the networks appear to be unique to the individual (Gratton et al., 2018) and may lose this uniqueness if averaged out across individuals, limiting the utility in evidence-based medicine but highlighting the benefit for precision and personalized medicine. Finally, epistasis and protein interactions may not necessarily account for functional mind interactions resulting in emerging cognitive abstractions which are the essence of the human mind. Yet, even the most esoteric mental conditions, such as one's philosophical standing about psychiatry, can and do significantly affect treatment effects in somatic therapies. The fact that therapists use countertransference proper and spontaneous emotional reactions (diagnostic countertransference) to understand the patient's dynamisms advocates strongly for the artistic component in diagnosis and treatment of personality disorder.

In a recent interview, Thomas Insel stated that "one surprise in recent years was the idea that you could talk to an avatar or a machine, and you would actually feel more at ease revealing your innermost secrets than if you had talked to another human" (Medscape, February 2018). Given the current fragmentation of traditional human relationships, Insel's point about non-human, blank-screen confidants seems valid. After all the concept of a neutral therapist was originally introduced by Freud who thought of neutrality as optimal for the patient's projections. However, personal information gathered by the machine will ultimately have to be interpreted by a therapist, who has the intangible tools (intuition, imagination, own nonconscious and conscious reactions) to "translate" the connection between the innermost secrets and the manifest struggles of the individual. As an analogy, computer translations into a different language do not lack the knowledge of words but lack the intuitive finesse necessary to produce acceptable outcomes. With this in mind, treatment of personality disorder will most likely have to remain face-to-face ("analog") in order to provide a natural stage for the corrective emotional experience, that is, to provide the opportunity for the mind to heal the way it naturally develops, through interactive experience. On the other hand, teletherapy and virtual communication seem quite appropriate for syndromes that develop later in the process of mental development, after the separation-individuation phase is mastered without deficits.

The new concept of "personalized evidence-based medicine" corresponds to what has been called the art and science of clinical work. With syndromes driven mainly by biogenetic factors (e.g., autism, Schizophrenia), the balance between art and science is skewed toward evidence-based treatments. Here, a clinician's insistence on his or her personal or intuitive style of treatment may be harmful. With nonpsychotic psychopathology, including personality disorder, loaded with intangible experiential factors, personalized and evidence-based approaches must remain evenly balanced. Only such a balanced, art-and-science approach can match the unique neurobiological context of the patient (the "neurobiological fingerprint") with his or her unique environmental and psychological contexts (the "psychosocial fingerprint") in order to help guide personalized treatments. Biomarkers have been elusive in psychiatry, partly because pathways involved in complex psychiatric syndromes have not been fully defined. Consequently, psychiatric diagnostics is built upon mostly subjective reports and consensus by master clinicians. In summary, the art and science of healing personality disorder is here to stay. Here, not only the talent but also the personal life experience of the clinician interpreting the nature of the patient's psychological problems (the art) is combined with a stratified evidence-based approach (the science) to find the treatment most likely to help the unique needs of any particular patient (personalized-and evidence based). This includes the important decision *not to treat at all,* as not every human problem requires psychotherapy or Prozac.

SUMMARY . . . AND WHAT LIES AHEAD FOR HUMAN PERSONALITY?

Heritable temperament trait vulnerabilities, inferior caregiving or psychological trauma, persisting fragmentation of early experiences, and a homeostatic maneuver of the mind to organize and survive through fantasy and deviance are the central concepts used in this book to explain the phenomenon of personality disorder. The neocortical engrams with episodic memory coupled with their respective engramized amygdala affects become the main source of self-related information pulled into nonconscious working memory (as nonconscious higher order representation), which is a function of the PFCx. Here, they operate as internalized object relations, as both the infrastructure and the function of the mind, and thus the basic units of all experience. We call them the elementary particles of the mind, each containing a percept, the related self-reflection, and the related connecting affect and are thus not divisible to lower order units of mental experience. From nonconscious working memory, internalized object relations are rerepresented by the general network of cognition, and amalgamated with other relevant neural information, all of which will be then integrated into the mental faculties (thought, conscious emotion, motivation). The faculties, highly personalized by the biases of early experiences, are interactively self-organized by punctuated homeostasis into the semi-stable subsystems of the mind: from the subcortical-cortical hybrid of temperament to the sense of self, character, moral values, and identity. Each of these partially overlapping but discernible subsystems or modules provides a specific adaptive advantage to the mind as a whole, in its personalized adaptation to the internal or the external environment.

Personality disorder follows the same developmental dynamics as normal personality but does so in the context of excessive affects and/or bad environment, rendering the elementary particles of experience polarized ("faulty") and the early mind both fragile and vulnerable to disintegration. We contend that such fragmented personality underlies all true cases of personality disorder. The mind resorts to omnipotent fantasies as a means to psychological survival. These fantasies, each a defensive ideal specific for individual variants of personality disorder, organize the fragmented core into an unrealistic but more stable self-image, dominant enough to compensate for mental fragility but further pathologizes personality by steering it into deviance. The process accounts for the duality of the self-subsystem in personality disorder, as the dominant compensatory self coexists with the weaker and split-off real self. The patients are thinly but unmistakably aware of the falsity of their own dictatorial self-ideal, which is merely a precarious pretense of a solution to fragility, hence the profound disintegration and existential anxieties that follow. Such fragmented personality and its subsystems are adaptively dysfunctional and continue to need sources of organization, both internally (through fantasy) and interpersonally (through selfobjects who are expected, frequently demanded, to define and maintain the unrealistic compensatory self). Interpersonal conflicts are actively sought to change others' reactions to one's own misconduct (alloplastic adaptation) or to coerce them into following the expected exposition supplied by the supporting cast. All of these together make a personality disorder, a syndrome arising from a homeostatic attempt of the mind to heal itself through the power of fantasy and the resulting unrealistic self-image.

In this book, we pioneer the concept of *dynamic nosology* of mental health and disorders. Our model of dimensional diagnostics defines a tridimensional diagnostic space, in which each individual is uniquely positioned. The coordinates cross-match the person's common level of functioning (vertical diagnosis) with his or her adaptive behavior style (horizontal diagnosis) at a point in space and for a given unit of time. Our model provides a highly individualized assessment (personalized diagnosis) that is always flexible, contextual, and time specific. Such dynamic nosology is inherently sensitive to fluctuations in mental functioning over time, in contrast to the static classifications of the DSM, the International Classification of Diseases, or other concepts of psychopathology.

Drawing from our model of personality disorder, we outline mechanism-based treatments: in-depth, reconstructive interpersonal psychotherapy (an integrative, trans-theoretical approach that relies on psychoanalytic and humanist traditions with elements of transactional-analytic and existential therapy) and mechanism-based pharmacotherapy of subcortical neurobiological vulnerabilities associated with excessive temperament traits (these overinfluence the mind relative to cognitive control and perpetuate personality fragmentation).

So what does lie ahead for human personality? On the basis of what was covered in this book, one is tempted to extrapolate our main points into the future for the sake of completeness, with all the usual risks involved in making such predictions. What follows is our best guess, not to be taken as the final word by any means.

Adaptive character traits and internalized moral values are a relatively recent phenomenon in the psychological evolution of humans, retrospectively traceable no earlier than the agricultural revolution (about 10,000 years ago) and the first civilizations in Egypt and Mesopotamia (modern-day Iran and Iraq). This may imply that personality as we know it is not the final word in human mental evolution but is still in its developing phase. Its future characteristics, especially if combined with technology-boosted brain processes and mental functions, are impossible to foresee with reasonable accuracy. The upcoming generations are expected, although not guaranteed, to find a way to adapt to such mega-changes, as has been the case throughout human history. Moving forward, adaptive priorities of the posthuman culture are hard to predict, but they shall heavily depend upon who holds the rein, humans or artificial intelligence. The goal is to integrate technology into our lives without being defeated by the very innovations we created. We contend that intuition (understanding without conscious reasoning) will become an extremely important aspect of future mental functioning, perhaps critical in order to master and maintain control over self-improving and independently learning technology. As a pocket of traditional humanity, intuition could become the bridge to maintain continuity with future hybrid (biological-technological) forms of human mental life, and perhaps its nonbiological forms as well.

It is important to keep in mind that both uncritical tolerance and unfettered intolerance are equally destructive to society, each in its own peculiar way. Both modern and postmodern culture were suppressive—one of tolerance, the other of intolerance. The postmodern mandate for policital correctness has brought us to the verge of democratic totalitarism, in which no one dares to express, perhaps even feel their real feelings or opinions about people and events lest their views be labeled of "stereotyping" or even "hatred." We are not advocating against political correctness but rather against its abuse, which blurs its own original noble intention: to protect individuals and groups against baseless villainization but not against criticism. Echoing Bloom (1987), we argue that the social mandate for political correctness may suppress common sense, which, in the changing world, might be the very last fortress of wisdom with a human touch to it.

The current liquid modernity period and swarm-like society—in which life considers highly what is transitory rather than what is permanent, the immediate rather than the long term, and regards utility as prior to any other value (Palese, 2013)—has a potential to become truly tolerant and democratic, but at the cost of dissolution of firm individuality. The swarm-like society of individuals weakly connected in the real world but cyber-represented via their depersonified choices, as momenty units of a trend, with ever-alternating leaders and followers, may be simply too ephemeral for sustained intolerance. This of course provided that no new methods of control of the cyber-masses become available, perhaps with technologies that combine microchips with brains and could be abused to control the cyborg's mind. The current trend to concretize and compress language (e.g., emoji, emoticons) in order to expedite communication reduces the world of abstract ideas into concrete images, akin to cave art. Such impoverished language could make dissent impossible because there may be no words not only to express it but also to even think of it (humans think thoughts in language), eerily reminiscent of George Orwell's *1984*. In other words, it is certainly possible that the increasing fragmentation of life in the real world and its organization in the virtual space may lead to hitherto unknown forms of radical, evil, or deviance. We, however, remain optimistic that the future holds more potentials than perils.

Cyber networks (social media) require regular identity updates in order to be included in the global world, defining internal direction from the outside and reducing the need for peersonalized identity. If people lose "solidity" and "personal" from personality, they are also likely to lose personality disorder as we know it. We in fact predict that the incidence of personality disorder shall decrease in the future. This prediction is not as audacious as it may sound. We believe that the focus of natural selection has moved away from individuals toward larger organized groups (societies), perhaps human race as a whole. As noted, the process of globalization does not in fact involve people, who are actually desocialized and depersonified by it, but the human mind, organized around collective choices floating in cyberspace as digitized clouds of databases. We understand the latter as the common selfobject for the collective mind of the human race. If this were the case, individual personality (the mind) of the past could be transformed into a collective personality (the mind) of the future, a form of eusociality of cognitive processes of humans. If this were the case, either no one or everyone will have a personality disorder, depending on one's point of view (as noted, we prefer the former view). Notwithstanding, one can envision the time when the famous phrase "Gens una sumus" ("we are one kind") by the Roman poet Claudian shall be finally materialized, although revised as "Mens una sumus" ("we are one mind"). In the meantime, however, in order to maintain our sensitivity to individual mental life in the rapidly changing world, clinical assessment should be very flexible, and time and context sensitive, in differentiating normalcy from pathology.

APPENDIX

Inventory of Mechanisms of Defense

The Inventory of Defense Mechanisms (iMOD), a 95-item self-report, represents an attempt to improve conceptualization and operationalization of defense mechanisms through a variety of behavioral and emotional manifestations, personal attitudes and beliefs, patterns of interpersonal relationships, and interpersonal feedback (the latter is a unique feature). The items are empirically derived, based on the authors' rich clinical experience in psychotherapy and available literature, and finalized through a series of clinical testing. The iMOD is, we believe, a modern, valid, and up-to-date test of defense mechanisms, a welcome addition to the available psychometric tests of personality in health and disorder.

The psychometric characteristics of iMOD: The questionnaire has 95 items assessed on a 4-point Likert scale and takes about 40 minutes to complete. It evaluates 19 defense mechanisms, that is, five to six items per mechanism, which we found was optimal to achieve good internal consistency and validity of the scales. Shorter versions of similar inventories have proven insufficiently reliable for a reliable diagnosis. We first tested the iMOD in a sample of university students of both sexes (N = 128), mean age 22 years (M = 22.29; SD = 4.65). The results showed a solid internal consistency (Cronbach's alpha ranging from 0.60 to 0.82), supporting the reliability of the scales. As the next step, in a sample of 58 nonpsychotic outpatients, the questionnaire successfully differentiated clinical from non-clinical subjects and functional from nonfunctional adaptation, supporting the discriminative validity of the iMOD. Similar to Mulder et al. (1996), low character scores as defined by Cloninger et al. (1993), were correlated with immature defense mechanisms and vice versa, supporting the concurrent validity of the iMOD. Together, the studies support the overall validity and reliability of the iMOD. The scoring and detailed interpretation are available upon request from Dr Dzamonja Ignjatovic (tamara.dzamonja@gmail.com)

INSTRUCTIONS

This inventory contains 95 statements describing common behaviors, opinions, attitudes, and feelings. Try to rate each statement to the degree it applies to your usual, typical behaviors, attitudes, and feelings, not the way you feel at the moment of completing this inventory. Please read each statement carefully but do not spend too much time looking for a perfect answer. Those answers that first come to mind are usually the right answers. It is important to rate every statement even if you are not completely certain in your ratings.

Circle one number for each statement on the scale from 1 to 4:

1- If you strongly disagree the statement applies to you
2- If you mostly disagree the statement applies to you
3- If you mostly agree the statement applies to you
4- If you strongly agree the statement applies to you

Please keep in mind that there are no right or wrong items in this inventory; you are asked to simply describe your own typical behaviors or feelings.

Your answers will be kept completely anonymous and the results are used solely in research.

Before you begin, please specify your:

Gender M F

Age (in years) ________________

Occupation ________________

LET'S START!

	Scoring: 1 – strongly disagree 2 – mostly disagree 3 –mostly agree 4 – strongly agree
1	I can easily laugh at my weaknesses or when I make a mistake.
2	When I have to face a difficult situation, I imagine it in advance in order to get better prepared.

3	When I have a problem, I am able to push it aside so it does not disturb me while I am doing other things.
4	I can handle anxiety or stress by starting to work on something interesting.
5	I feel satisfied when helping people, and I feel bad when I am unable to do so.
6	I often find myself being kind to people at whom I should be angry or unhappy with.
7	After I openly confront someone, I feel that I have to "iron things out" by explaining myself to him/her.
8	I possess special abilities that enable me to have a problem-free life.
9	Many people are so inferior that they deserve to be despised.
10	Fantasy and imagination give me more satisfaction than real life.
11	I am often disappointed in people when I uncover their real intentions.
12	It happens that I get physically sick when I have problems.
13	I always find a good reason or explanation for my failures.
14	Others often complain that I do not express my feelings.
15	I react impulsively when something irritates me or makes me nervous.
16	People tell me that I tend to ignore unpleasant facts.
17	I am said to be stubborn and difficult to satisfy.
18	I tend to see things and people as "black-or-white" (good or bad) rather than something in between.
19	No matter how frustrated I am, I never feel the urge to yell, curse, or hit something.
20	I am usually able to see the funny side of my troubles or problems.
	Scoring reminder: 1 – strongly disagree 2 – mostly disagree 3 –mostly agree 4 – strongly agree
21	I usually prepare in advance in my mind for possible unpleasant situations.
22	I can control my feelings when their expression might disturb me or other people.
23	I have passionate interests and hobbies that make me feel fulfilled.
24	I try to help others to solve their problems, even when they don't ask me for help.
25	I practice the saying "turn the other cheek" in real life.
26	When I do something inappropriate, it is important for me to "undo" it somehow later on.
27	I believe that I deserve special recognition or appreciation.
28	I am often disappointed by people whom, at first, I expected more from.
29	I deal with my problems more through fantasy and/or imagination than in a real life.
30	I am often cautious with people in order not to be used or get hurt.
31	I have headaches quite often.
32	I usually find some excuse when things are not unfolding as planned.
33	Frequently I do not feel anything in situations that provoke strong feelings in others.
34	I can't help "exploding" when somebody threatens me.
35	Problems that concern other people do not seem big or important to me.

36	It frequently appears to me that I irritate others.
37	I can completely reverse my opinions and/or feelings about somebody in a short period.
38	Often I don't know why am I anxious, tense, or moody.
39	I tend to defuse an unpleasant situation by making a joke.
40	When I am about to meet a person I have a conflict with, I think about it in advance in order to control my behavior more successfully.
	Scoring reminder: 1 – strongly disagree 2 – mostly disagree 3 –mostly agree 4 – strongly agree
41	I manage not to show my feelings or emotions if their expression would be inappropriate.
42	When I am engaged in work or other activities, I tend to forget my needs or worries.
43	If somebody does not accept my help, it hurts my feelings.
44	I am occasionally rude to or reserved with someone I actually care about.
45	If I criticize someone, I have the need to also praise or somehow comfort them later on.
46	All emotional relationships I have had so far were very special.
47	I often realize that others are worth much less than I originally thought.
48	I develop "scenarios" in my mind in which I successfully solve my problems that I don't attend to in reality.
49	I often wonder if I can trust my friends or acquaintances.
50	I often get physically ill when I worry about something for long.
51	Many things or goals I didn't accomplish were not worth my efforts anyway.
52	In my opinion, showing strong emotion is a sign of weakness.
53	I am very hasty and ill-advised in my reactions.
54	Others tell me that I don't recognize danger.
55	I typically make more mistakes if somebody is directly supervising me.
56	My relationships with people go through numerous major ups and downs.
57	I don't remember that I ever lied my way out of problems and/or trouble.
58	I can make a joke when I feel uncomfortable.
59	Prior to important events I usually "play the tape" of these situations in my mind.
60	I manage to calm down my anger when it might only aggravate the situation.
	Scoring reminder: 1 – strongly disagree 2 – mostly disagree 3 –mostly agree 4 – strongly agree
61	Admiring art is often completely absorbing and/or fulfilling to me.
62	I feel guilty if I am not helping somebody, even if I know realistically that I cannot help them or should not be doing so.
63	I am often particularly kind to someone who, in fact, irritates me or makes me nervous.

64	When I say something bad about someone, I feel compelled to add something positive about that person.
65	I notice that I especially like people who are similar to me.
66	The way I see it, there are only a handful of people who really deserve my time and attention.
67	When I wish for something, I fantasize about it more than I take concrete steps to make it happen.
68	The way I see it, it is best not to let people know much about me.
69	I usually have problems with my stomach when I am tense, anxious, or upset.
70	I think that I am too honest to be successful in today's world.
71	I am never overwhelmed by intense, dramatic feelings.
72	In a heated moment I don't "count to ten" but react immediately, regardless of the consequences.
73	Nothing can hurt my feelings.
74	When I don't want to do something, I tend to simply "forget" to do it.
75	I tend to suddenly change opinions about myself into almost completely the opposite.
76	I don't have any thoughts or needs that I could be ashamed about.
77	I usually make jokes in situations when there is a possibility that something will be disturbing to me.
78	When I have a problem, I usually make a plan of what should be done to resolve it.
79	I try not to think about unpleasant topics, and I am usually effective in doing so.
80	I spend a lot of time in work and different activities so I don't have idle time.
	Scoring reminder: 1 – strongly disagree 2 – mostly disagree 3 –mostly agree 4 – strongly agree
81	I am dealing with other peoples' problems more than anyone else I know.
82	I tend to express the opposite of what I really feel toward someone.
83	When I "blast" someone, I later try to compensate for that by being kind or offering help.
84	The vast majority of people I have met in my lifetime have been delighted with me.
85	In fact, nobody can really understand me.
86	I get more pleasure by fantasizing about ideal love than from actual close relationships.
87	Others often envy me.
88	I have physical problems so frequently that nobody takes them seriously anymore.
89	When I fail, I say to myself that "participation is more important than winning."
90	People say that I am a reserved and/or cold person.
91	Sometimes I punch, kick, or throw something when I am angry (doing the same to a person also counts).

92	Others sometimes tell me that I have a blind spot for my problems.
93	I often procrastinate when something is expected of me.
94	I've had numerous sudden changes in my goals and plans in my lifetime.
95	Others tell me their impressions about me which I do not recognize as my characteristics.

REFERENCES

aan het Rot M, Zarate Jr CA, Charney DS et al. (2012). Ketamine for depression: Where do we go from here? *Biological Psychiatry* 72(7):537–547.

Abbass AA, Kisely SR, Town JM et al. (2014). Short-term psychodynamic psychotherapies for common mental disorders. *Cochrane Database of Systematic Reviews* 1(7):CD004687.

Agrawal HR, Gunderson J, Holmes BM et al. (2004). Attachment studies with borderline patients: A review. *Harvard Review of Psychiatry* 12(2):94–104.

Alexander F, French TM (1946). *Psychoanalytic therapy: Principles and application.* University of Nebraska Press, Lincoln and London.

Allan K (1997). The postmodern self: A theoretical consideration. *Quarterly Journal of Ideology* 20:3–24.

Almaas AH (2001). *The point of existence: Transformations of narcissism in self-realization.* Shambala, Boston and London.

Aman MG, Smith T, Arnold LE et al. (2014). A review of atomoxetine effects in young people with developmental disabilities. *Research in Developmental Disabilities* 35(6):1412–1424.

American Psychological Association, Board of Scientific Affairs (1996). Intelligence: Knowns and unknowns. *American Psychologist* 51:77–101.

American Psychiatric Association (1952). *Diagnostic and statistical manual of mental disorders.* American Psychiatric Association, Washington, DC.

American Psychiatric Association (1980). *Diagnostic and statistical manual of mental disorders.* 3rd ed. American Psychiatric Association, Washington, DC.

American Psychiatric Association (1987). *Diagnostic and statistical manual of mental disorders.* 3rd ed. rev. American Psychiatric Association, Washington, DC.

American Psychiatric Association (1994). *Diagnostic and statistical manual of mental disorders.* 4th ed. American Psychiatric Association, Washington, DC.

American Psychiatric Association (2000). *Diagnostic and statistical manual of mental disorders.* 4th ed., text revision. American Psychiatric Association, Washington, DC.

American Psychiatric Association (2013). *Diagnostic and statistical manual of mental disorders.* 5th ed. American Psychiatric Association, Washington, DC.

Anacker C, Zunszain PA, Cattaneo A et al. (2011a). Antidepressants increase human hippocampal neurogenesis by activating the glucocorticoid receptor. *Molecular Psychiatry* 16(7):738–750.

Anacker C, Zunszain PA, Carvalho LA et al. (2011b). The glucocorticoid receptor: Pivot of depression and of antidepressant treatment? *Psychoneuroendocrinology* 36(3):415–425.

Andrews PW, Bharwania A, Leea KR et al. (2015). Is serotonin an upper or a downer? The evolution of the serotonergic system and its role in depression and the antidepressant response. *Neuroscience and Biobehavioral Reviews* 51:164–188.

Andrews-Hanna JR (2012). The Brain's Default Network and its Adaptive Role in Internal Mentation, *Neuroscientist* 18(3):251–270.

Arnsten AFT (2006). Fundamentals of attention-deficit/hyperactivity disorder: Circuits and pathways. *Journal of Clinical Psychiatry* 67(Suppl. 8):7–12.

Arnsten AFT, Rubia K (2012). Neurobiological circuits regulating attention, cognitive control, motivation, and emotion: Disruptions in neurodevelopmental psychiatric disorders. *Journal of the American Academy of Child and Adolescent Psychiatry* 51(4):356–367.

Ashley J, Cordy B, Lucia D et al. (2018). Retrovirus-like Gag protein Arc1 binds RNA and traffics across synaptic boutons. *Cell* 172(1–2):262–274.

Auchincloss E, Samberg, E (2012). *Psychoanalytic terms and concepts*. American Psychoanalytic Association and Yale University Press, New Haven and London.

Bakermans-Kranenburg MJ, van IJzendoorn MH (2013). Sniffing around oxytocin: Review and meta-analyses of trials in healthy and clinical groups with implications for pharmacotherapy. *Translational Psychiatry* 3:e258.

Barron F, Harrington DM (1981). Creativity, intelligence, and personality. *Annual Review of Psychology* 32:439–476.

Bartz J, Simeon D, Hamilton H et al. (2011a). Oxytocin can hinder trust and cooperation in borderline personality disorder. *Social Cognitive and Affective Neuroscience* 6:556–563.

Bartz, JA, Zaki J, Bolger N, Ochsner KN (2011b). Social effects of oxytocin in humans: Context and person matter. *Trends in Cognitive Sciences* 15(7): 301–309.

Bateman AW, Fonagy P (1999). Effectiveness of partial hospitalization in the treatment of borderline personality disorder: A randomized controlled trial. *American Journal of Psychiatry* 156:1563–1569.

Bateman AW, Fonagy P (2001). Treatment of borderline personality disorder with psychoanalytically-oriented partial hospitalization, an 18-month follow-up. *American Journal of Psychiatry* 158:36–42.

Bateman AW, Fonagy P (2004). *Psychotherapy for borderline personality disorder: Mentalization based treatment*. Oxford University Press, Oxford.

Bateman AW, Fonagy P (2008). 8-year follow-up of patients treated for borderline personality disorder: Mentalization-based treatment versus treatment as usual. *American Journal of Psychiatry* 165:631–638.

Bate C, Boduszek D, Dhingra K et al. (2014). Psychopathy, intelligence and emotional responding in a non-forensic sample: An experimental investigation. *The Journal of Forensic Psychiatry and Psychology* 25(5):600–612.

Bauman Z (2000). *Liquid modernity*. Blackwell, Oxford.

Beatson JA, Rao S (2102). Depression and borderline personality disorder. *The Medical Journal of Australia* 1(Suppl. 4):24–27.

Beaulieu JM, Caron MG (2008). Looking at lithium: Molecular moods and complex behavior. *Molecular Interventions* 8:230–241.

Beck A, Freeman A, Davis D et al. (2004). *Cognitive therapy and personality disorders*. 2nd ed. Guilford Press, New York.

Bedi G, Luan Phan K, Angstadt M, de Wit H (2009). Effects of MDMA on sociability and neural response to social threat and social reward. *Psychopharmacology* 207:73.

Bell CJ, Nicholson H, Mulder RT et al. (2006). Plasma oxytocin levels in depression and their correlation with the temperament dimension of reward dependence. *Journal of Psychopharmacology* 20(5):656–660.

Berger J (1980). *Treći roditelj: Novi pravci grupne psihoterapije*. Nolit, Beograd.

Berne E (1972). *What do you say after you say hello?* Bantam Books, New York.

Berridge KC, Kringelbach ML (2015). Pleasure systems in the brain. *Neuron* 86(3):646–664.

Bertsch K, Schmidinger I, Neumann GI et al. (2013). Reduced plasma oxytocin levels in female patients with borderline personality disorder. *Hormones and Behavior* 63:424–429.

Bess M (2015). *Our grandchildren redesigned*. Beacon Press, Boston.

Beutler LE, Clarkin JF (1990). *Systematic treatment selection: Towards targeted therapeutic interventions*. Brunner/Mazel, New York.

Beutel ME, Stark R, Pan H et al. (2010). Changes of brain activation pre- post short-term psychodynamic inpatient psychotherapy: An fMRI study of panic disorder patients. *Psychiatry Research* 184:96–104.

Bicks LK, Koike H, Akbarian S et al. (2015). Prefrontal cortex and social cognition in mouse and man. *Frontiers in Psychology* 6:1–15.

Bion W (1959). Attacks on linking. *International Journal of Psychoanalysis* 40:308–315.

Blais MA, Smallwood P, Groves JE et al. (2016). Personality and personality disorders. In Stern T, Fava M, Wilens TE, Rosenbaum (eds.), *Massachusetts General Hospital comprehensive clinical psychiatry*, pp. 433–444. Elsevier, New York.

Bloom A (1987). *The closing of the American mind*. Simon & Schuster, New York.

Bond M, Perry JC (2004). Long-term changes in defense styles with psychodynamic psychotherapy for depressive, anxiety, and personality disorders. *American Journal of Psychiatry* 161:1665–1671.

Bortolato M, Godar SC, Melis M et al. (2012). NMDARs mediate the role of monoamine oxidase A in pathological aggression. *Journal of Neuroscience* 32(25):8574–8582.

Bouret S, Sara SJ (2004). Reward expectation, orientation of attention and locus coeruleus-medial frontal cortex interplay during learning. *European Journal of Neuroscience* 20:791–802.

Bozukluklarının K, ve Ergenlerde C, Bulguları O (2015). Precursors of personality disorders in children and adolescents. *Current Approaches in Psychiatry* 7(4):368–381.

Caldwell HK, Albers HE (2016). Oxytocin, vasopressin, and the motivational forces that drive social behaviors. *Current Topics in Behavioral Neuroscience* 27:51–103.

Campbell A (2013). The evolutionary psychology of women's aggression. *Philosophical Transactions of the Royal Society B* 368:20130078.

Carruthers P (2006). *The architecture of the mind*. Oxford University Press, Oxford.

Champagne FA (2008). Epigenetic mechanisms and the transgenerational effects of maternal care. *Frontiers in Neuroendocrinology* 29:386–397.

Champagne FA, Curley JP (2009). Epigenetic mechanisms mediating the long-term effects of maternal care on development. *Neuroscience & Biobehavioral Reviews* 33:593–600.

Chen B, Gu T, Ma B et al. (2014). The CRHR1 gene contributes to genetic susceptibility of aggressive behavior towards others in Chinese Southwest Han population. *Journal of Molecular Neuroscience* 52:481–486.

Chomsky N (2000). On humanism and morality. Interviewed by Tor Wennerberg. Montreal Serai 13(3) [conducted in November 1998].

Chopra KK, Bagby M, Dickens S et al. (2005). A dimensional approach to personality in atypical depression. *Psychiatry Research* 134:161–167.

Clarkin J, Caligor E, Stern B et al. (2007a). Structured Interview of Personality Organization (STIPO). Personality Disorders Institute, Cornell University.

Clarkin JF, Levi KN, Lenzenweger MF et al. (2007). Evaluating three treatments for borderline personality disorder: A multiwave study. *American Journal of Psychiatry* 164:922–928.

Clarkin JF, Yeomans FE, Kernberg OF (2006). *Psychotherapy for borderline personality: Focusing on object relations.* American Psychiatric Publishing, Washington, DC.

Cloninger CR (1987). A systematic method for clinical description and classification of personality variants: A proposal. *Archives of General Psychiatry* 44: 573–588.

Cloninger CR, Svrakic DM (2017). Personality disorders. In Sadock B, Sadock V, Ruiz P. (eds.), *Kaplan & Sadock's comprehensive textbook of psychiatry.* 10th ed. Lipppincott, Williams & Wilkins, Philadelphia and Baltimore.

Cloninger CR, Svrakic DM, Przybeck TR, (1993). A psychobiological model of temperament and character. *Archives of General Psychiatry* 50:975–990.

Cloninger CR, Svrakic NM, Svrakic DM (1997). Role of personality in the development of mental order and disorder. *Development and Psychopathology* 9:881–906.

Cole MW, Bassett DS, Power JD et al. (2014). Intrinsic and task-evoked architectures of the human brain. *Neuron* 83(1):238–251.

Comai S, Tau M, Gobbi G et al. (2012a). The psychopharmacology of aggressive behavior: a translational approach part 1: Neurobiology. *Journal of Clinical Psychopharmacology* 32(1):83–94.

Comai S, Tau M, Pavlovic Z et al. (2012b). The psychopharmacology of aggressive behavior: A translational approach part 2: Clinical studies using atypical antipsychotics, anticonvulsants, and lithium. *Journal of Clinical Psychopharmacology* 32(2):237–260.

Conway MA (2005). Memory and the self. *Journal of Memory and Language* 53:594–628. doi:10.1016/j.jml.2005.08.005

Conway MA, Pleydell-Pearce CW (2000). The construction of autobiographical memories in the self-memory system. *Psychological Review* 107(2):261–288.

Conway MA, Pleydell-Pearce CW, Whitecross S.E (2001). The neuroanatomy of autobiographical memory: A slow cortical potential study of autobiographicamemory retrieval. *Journal of Memory and Language* 45:493–524.

Corbetta M, Patel G, Shulman GL (2008). The reorienting system of the human brain: From environment to theory of mind. *Neuron* 58(3):306–324.

Cyrulnik B (2008). *Autobiographie d'un épouvantail.* Odile Jacob, Paris.

Dadds MR, Moul C, Cauchi A et al. (2014a). Methylation of the oxytocin receptor gene and oxytocin blood levels in the development of psychopathy. *Development and Psychopathology* 26:33–40.

Dadds MR, Moul C, Cauchi A et al. (2014b). Polymorphisms in the oxytocin receptor gene are associated with the development of psychopathy. *Development and Psychopathology* 26:21–31.

Davidson RJ, Putnam KM, Larson CL (2000). Dysfunction in the neural circuitry of emotion regulation—a possible prelude to violence. *Science* 289:591–594.

de Bartolomeis A, Tomasetti C, Iasevoli F (2015). Update on the mechanism of action of aripiprazole: Translational insights into antipsychotic strategies beyond dopamine receptor antagonism. *CNS Drugs* 29:773–799.

de Boer SF, Koolhaas JM (2005). 5-HT1A and 5-HT1B receptor agonists and aggression: A pharmacological challenge of the serotonin deficiency hypothesis. *European Journal of Pharmacology* 526:125–139.

de Leon J (2012). Evidence-based medicine versus personalized medicine: Are they enemies? *Journal of Clinical Psychopharmacology* 32(2):153–164.

de Manzano Ö, Cervenka S, Karabanov A et al. (2010). Thinking outside a less intact box: Thalamic dopamine D2 receptor densities are negatively related to psychometric creativity in healthy individuals. *PLoS One* 5(5):e10670.

De Martino B, Strange BA, Dolan RJ (2008). Noradrenergic neuromodulation of human attention for emotional and neutral stimuli. *Psychopharmacology* 197:127–136.

Diedrich A, Voderholzer U (2015). Obsessive–compulsive personality disorder: A current review. *Current Psychiatry Report* 17:2.

Dimitrijevic A (2011). Pregled načela tretmana zasnovanog na mentalizovanju. *Psihijatrija danas* 43(1):5–20.

Divac-Jovanovic M (1979). Granična stanja na Roršahu. *Psihologija* 3–4:165–177.

Divac-Jovanovic M (1986). Rekonstrukcija referentnog okvira—Transakciono-analitički model psihoterapije graničnih poremećaja. *Psihijatrija danas* 2–3:291–303.

Divac-Jovanovic M, Čalovska Hercog N, Stojanovic D et al. (2005). Peer supervision across different psychotherapeutic modalities. In *European Identity and Psychotherapy*. 12th Congress of the European Association for Psychotherapy, pp. 99–104. Belgrade, Serbia.

Divac-Jovanovic M, Svrakic DM (2016). *Granicna lincost i njena razalicita lica*. Clio, Beograd, Srbija.

Divac-Jovanovic M, Svrakic DM, Lecic-Tosevski D (1993). Personality disorders: model for conceptual approach and classification, part I: General model. *American Journal of Psychotherapy* 47:558–571.

Divac-Jovanovic M, Tatar-Radojkovic S (1987). Treating borderline phenomena across diagnostic categories. *Transactional Analysis Journal* 17:4–10.

Dryden W (Ed.). (1996). *Developments in psychotherapy: Historical perspectives*. SAGE, Thousand Oaks, CA.

Džamonja Ignjatović T (1999). *Psihodijagnostika i savremeni modeli ličnosti*. Zadužbina Andrejević, Beograd.

Džamonja Ignjatović T, Divac-Jovanovic M, Milanović M et al. (2014). Konstrukcija i karakteristike upitnika za procenu mehanizama odbrane–MOD. *Psihijatrija danas* 2:155–173.

Faraone SV, Perlis RH, Doyle AE et al. (2005). Molecular genetics of attention-deficit/hyperactivity disorder. *Biological Psychiatry* 57(11):1313–1323.

Fiore D, Dimaggio G, Nicolo G et al. (2008). Metacognitive interpersonal therapy in a case of obsessive–compulsive and avoidant personality disorders. *Journal of Clinical Psychology* 64 (2):168–180.

Fodor JA (1983). *The modularity of mind*. MIT Press, Cambridge, MA.

Freud S (1930). *Unbehagen in der Kultur* [The uneasiness in civilization]. Translated by J. Strachey.

Frick A, Åhs F, Engman J et al. (2015). Serotonin synthesis and reuptake in social anxiety disorder: A positron emission tomography study. *JAMA Psychiatry* 72(8):794–802.

Garvey MJ, Noyes Jr R, Cook B et al. (1996). Preliminary confirmation of the proposed link between reward-dependence and norepinephrine. *Psychiatry Research* 65:61–64

Generoso MB, Trevizola AP, Kasper S et al. (2017): Pregabalin for generalized anxiety disorder: An updated systematic review and meta-analysis. *International Clinical Psychopharmacology* 32:49–55.

Gergen KJ (1991). *The saturated self: Dilemmas of identity in contemporary life*. Basic Books, New York.

Giesen-Bloo J, van Dyck R, Spinhoven P et al. (2006). Outpatient psychotherapy for borderline personality disorder: Randomized trial of schema-focused therapy vs transference-focused psychotherapy. *Archives of General Psychiatry* 63:649–658.

Goldman-Rakic PS (1995). Cellular basis of working memory. *Neuron* 14:477–485.

Goldman-Rakic PS (1996). The prefrontal landscape: Implications of functional architecture for understanding human mentation and the central executive. *Philosophical Transactions of the Royal Society of London. Series B, Biological Sciences* 351(1346):1445–1453.

Goldman-Rakic P, Lidow MS, Gallager DW (1990). Overlap of dopaminergic, adrenergic, and serotoninergic receptors and complementarity of their subtypes in primate prefrontal cortex. *Journal of Neuroscience* 10(7):2125–2138.

Goleman D (1995). *Emotional intelligence: Why it can matter more than IQ*. Bantam Books, New York.

Gottfredson LS (1997). Mainstream science on intelligence. *Intelligence* 24: 13–23

Gratton C, Laumann TO, Nielsen AN et al. (2018). Functional brain networks are dominated by stable group and individual factors, not cognitive or daily variation. *Neuron* 98(2):439–452.

Gregoire C, Kaufman SB (2016). Creative people's brains really do work differently [Blog].

Greenaway M, Elbe D (2009). Focus on aripiprazole: A review of its use in child and adolescent psychiatry. *Journal of the Canadian Academy of Child and Adolescent Psychiatry* 18(3):250–260.

Grilo C, Sanislow C, Gunderson J et al. (2004). Two-year stability and change of schizotypal, borderline, avoidant and obsessive-compulsive personality disorders. *Journal of Consulting and Clinical Psychology* 72:767–775.

Gusnard DA, Ollinger JM, Shulman GL et al. (2003). Persistence and brain circuitry, *PNAS* 100(6):3479–3484.

Hahn CG, Gyulai L, Baldassano CF et al. (2004). The current understanding of lamotrigine as a mood stabilizer. *Journal of Clinical Psychiatry* 65:791–804.

Haller J, Mikics E, Halász J et al. (2005a). Mechanisms differentiating normal from abnormal aggression: Glucocorticoids and serotonin. *European Journal of Pharmacology* 526:89–100.

Haller J, Toth M, Halasz J et al. (2005b). The activation of raphe serotonergic neurons in normal and hypoarousal-driven aggression: A double labeling study in rats. *Behavioral Brain Research* 161:88–94.

Hamilton WD (1964). The genetical evolution of social behaviour I and II. *Journal of Theoretical Biology* 7:1–52.

Hammock EAD (2015). Developmental perspectives on oxytocin and vasopressin. *Neuropsychopharmacology Reviews* 40:24–42.

Hankin BL, Abela JRZ (Eds.). (2005). *Development of psychopathology: A vulnerability-stress perspective*. SAGE, Thousand Oaks, CA.

Hare RD (1996). Psychopathy: A clinical construct whose time has come. *Criminal Justice and Behavior* 23:25–54.

Hebert MA, Potegal M, Moore T et al. (1996). Diazepam enhances conditioned defeat in hamsters (mesocricetus auratus). *Pharmacology Biochemistry and Behavior* 55:405–413.

Heinrichs M, Domes G (2008). Neuropeptides and social behavior: Effects of oxytocin and vasopressin in humans. *Progress in Brain Research* 170:337–350.

Heinz A, Grace AA, Beck A (2009). The intricacies of dopamine neuron modulation. *Biological Psychiatry* 65(2):101–102.

Heller J (1961). *Catch 22*. Simon & Schuster, New York.

Hirvonen J, Hietala J, Kajander J et al. (2011). Effects of antidepressant drug treatment and psychotherapy on striatal and thalamic dopamine D2/3 receptors in major depressive disorder studied with [11C]raclopride PET. *Journal of Psychopharmacology* 25:1329–1336.

Holland AC, Kensinger EA (2010). Emotion and autobiographical memory. *Physics of Life Reviews* 7(1):88–131.

Horney K (1937). *The neurotic personality of our time*. W.W. Norton, New York.

Horvarth AO, Symonds DB (1991). Relationship between working alliance and outcome in psychotherapy: a meta-analysis. *Journal of Counseling Psychology* 38:139–149.

Hunt RD, Arnsten ARF, Asbell D (1995). An open trial of guanfacine in the treatment of attention deficit hyperactivity disorder. *Journal of the American Child and Adolescent Psychiatry* 34:50–54.

Ishikawa SS, Raine A, Lencz T et al. (2001). Autonomic stress reactivity and executive functions in successful and unsuccessful criminal psychopaths from the community. *Journal of Abnormal Psychology* 110(3):423–432.

Jacobs BL, Azmitia EC (1992). Structure and function of the brain serotonin system. *Psychological Reviews* 72(1):165–205.

Jacobs BL, Fornal CA (1999). Activity of brain serotonergic neurons in the behaving animal. *Neuropsychopharmacology* 2(Suppl.):9–14.

Jacobson E (1964). *The self and the object world*. New York: International Universities Press.

James W (1992). *Writings 1878–1899*. Library of America, New York.

Javitt DC, Duncan L, Balla A et al. (2005). Inhibition of system A-mediated glycine transport in cortical synaptosomes by therapeutic concentrations of clozapine: implications for mechanisms of action. *Molecular Psychiatry* 10:276–286.

Jiang R, Calhoun VD, Zuo N, et al. (n.d.). Connectome-based Individualized Prediction of Temperament Traits scores [Unpublished data].

Johannessen CU, Johannessen SI (2003). Valproate: Past, present, and future. *CNS Drug Reviews* 9(2):199–216.

Joines V, Stewart I (2002). *Personality adaptation: A new guide to human understanding in psychotherapy and counselling*. Lifespace, Nottingham and Chapel Hill.

Jovanović Divac M, Svrakic DM (2017). Integrative treatment of personality disorder. Part I: Psychotherapy. *Psychiatria Danubina* 29(1):2–13.

Kaiser S, Lyne J, Agartz I et al. (2016). Individual negative symptoms and domains—relevance for assessment, pathomechanisms and treatment. *Schizophrenia Research* 186:39–45.

Karlsson H., Hirvonen J, Kajander J et al. (2010). Research letter: Psychotherapy increases brain serotonin 5-HT1A receptors in patients with major depressive disorder. *Psychological Medicine* 40:523–528.

Kazdin AE (2008). Evidence-based treatment and practice: New opportunities to bridge clinical research and practice, enhance the knowledge base, and improve patient care. *American Psychologist* 63:146–159.

Kendler KS (2009). An historical framework for psychiatric nosology. *Psychological Medicine* 39(12):1935–1941.

Kernberg OF (1975). *Borderline conditions and pathological narcissism.* Jason Aronson, New York.

Kernberg OF (1984). *Severe personality disorders.* Yale University Press, New Haven and London.

Kernberg OF (2015). Neurobiological correlates of object relations theory: The relationship between neurobiological and psychodynamic development. *International Forum of Psychoanalysis* 24(1):38–46.

Kernberg OF (2016). What is personality? *Journal of Personality Disorders* 30(2):145–156.

Kernberg OF, Selzer MA, Koenigsberg HW et al. (1989). *Psychodynamic psychotherapy of borderline patients.* Basic Books, New York.

Kernberg OF, Yeomans F, Clarkin J et al. (2008). Transference focused psychotherapy: Overview and update. *International Journal of Psychoanalysis* 89:601–620.

Kessler H, Stasch M, Cierpka M (2013). Operationalized psychodynamic diagnosis as an instrument to transfer psychodynamic constructs into neuroscience. *Frontiers in Human Neuroscience* 7:718.

Kitamura T, Ogawa SK, Roy DS et al. (2017). Engrams and circuits crucial for systems consolidation of a memory. *Science* 356(6333):73–78.

Klein M (1952). *Some theoretical conclusions regarding the emotional life of the infant. Envy and gratitude and other works 1946–1963*. Hogarth Press and the Institute of Psycho-Analysis, New York.

Klein M (1975). Love, Guilt and Reparation and Other Works 1921–1945. Karnac Books, London.

Klein SB (2013). Making the case that episodic recollection is attributable to operations occurring at retrieval rather than to content stored in a dedicated subsystem of 1ong-term memory. *Frontiers in Behavioral Neuroscience* 7(3):1–14.

Kohut H (1971). *The analysis of the self.* International Universities Press, Madison, CT.

Kohut H (1977). *The restoration of the self.* International Universities Press. New York.

Kohut H (1984). *How does analysis cure*? University of Chicago Press, Chicago.

Kohut H, Wolf ES (1978). The disorders of the self and their treatment: An outline. *International Journal of Psychoanalysis* 59:413–425.

Kreisman JJ, Strauss H (1991). *I hate you—don't leave me: Understanding the borderline personality*. William Morrow, New York.

Kyaga S, Lichtenstein P, Boman M et al. (2011). Creativity and mental disorder: Family study of 300,000 people with severe mental disorder. *British Journal of Psychiatry* 199(5):373–379.

Lang PJ, Bradley MM, Cuthbert BN (1998). Emotion, motivation, and anxiety: Brain mechanisms and psychophysiology. *Biological Psychiatry* 44:1248–1263.

Langley K, Fowler T, Ford T et al. (2010). Adolescent clinical outcomes for young people with attention-deficit hyperactivity disorder. *The British Journal of Psychiatry* 196:235–240.

Krebs RM, Schott BH, Duezel E (2009). Personality traits are differentially associated with patterns of reward and novelty processing in the human substantia nigra/ventral tegmental area. *Biological Psychiatry* 6(2):103–110.

Lai C, Daini S, Calcagni ML et al. (2007). Neural correlates of psychodynamic psychotherapy in borderline disorders—a pilot investigation. *Psychotherapy and Psychosomatics* 76:403–405.

Laing RD (1969). *Self and others*. Penguin, London.

Lečić-Toševski D, Divac-Jovanovic M (1989). Granična dekompenzacija afektivnog poremećaja. *Psihijatrija danas* 21:325–330.

LeDoux JE (2003). *Synaptic self*. Penguin, New York.

LeDoux JE, Brown R (2017). A higher-order theory of emotional consciousness. *PNAS* 114(10):E2016–E2025.

Leichsenring F, Leibing E (2003). The effectiveness of psychodynamic therapy and cognitive behavior therapy in the treatment of personality disorders: A meta-analysis. *American Journal of Psychiatry* 160:1223–1232.

Leichsenring F, Leibing E (2007). Psychodynamic psychotherapy: A systematic review of techniques, indications and empirical evidence. *Psychology and Psychotherapy: Theory, Research and Practice* 80:217–228.

Leichsenring F, Rabung S (2008). Effectiveness of long-term psychodynamic psychotherapy: A meta-analysis. *JAMA* 300:1551–1565.

Leichsenring F, Rabung S (2009). In response to Thombs et al. *JAMA* 301(9):931.

Lehto SM, Tolmunen T, Joensuu M et al. (2008). Changes in midbrain serotonin transporter availability in atypically depressed subjects after one year of psychotherapy. *Progress in Neuropsychopharmacology and Biological Psychiatry* 32:229–237.

Lerner V, Miodownik C, Kaptsan A et al. (2007). Vitamin B6 treatment for tardive dyskinesia: A randomized, double-blind, placebo-controlled, crossover study. *Journal of Clinical Psychiatry* 68(11):1648–1654.

Levy KN, Clarkin JF, Yeomans FE et al. (2006). The mechanisms of change in the treatment of borderline personality disorder with transference focused psychotherapy. *Journal of Clinical Psychology* 62(4): 481–501.

Lieb K, Zanarini MC, Schmahl C et al. (2004). Borderline personality disorder. *The Lancet* 364:453–461.

Lieb K, Völlm B, Gerta Rücker G et al. (2010). Pharmacotherapy for borderline personality disorder: Cochrane systematic review of randomized trials. *The British Journal of Psychiatry* 196:4–12.

Linehan MM (1993). *Cognitive-behavioral treatment of borderline personality disorder*. Guilford Press, New York.

Linehan MM, Heard HL (1999). Borderline personality disorder: Costs, course and treatment outcomes. In Miller N, Marguder KM (eds.), *Cost-effectiveness of psychotherapy: A guide for practitioners, researchers and policymakers*, pp. 291–305. New York: Oxford University Press.

Livesley J (2007). A framework for integrating dimensional and categorical classifications of personality disorders. *Journal of Personality Disorders* 21:199–224.

Livesley WJ, Jang KL, Vernon PA (1998). The phenotypic and genetic structure of traits delineating personality disorder. *Archives of General Psychiatry* 55:941–948.

Lu ML, Lane HY (2003). Adjunctive fluvoxamine with clozapine. *The British Journal of Psychiatry* 182 (1):81.

Luby J, Belden A, Botteron K et al. (2013). The effects of poverty on childhood brain development: The mediating effect of caregiving and stressful life events. *JAMA Pediatrics* 167(12):1135–1142.

Luby JL, Svrakic DM, McCallum K et al. (1999). The Junior Temperament and Character Inventory: Preliminary validation of a child self-report measure. *Psychological Reports* 84(3 Pt 2):1127–1138.

Lydiard BR (2003). The role of GABA in anxiety disorders. *Journal of Clinical Psychiatry* 64(Suppl. 3):21–27.

Lyoo IK, Kwon JS, Lee SJ et al. (2002). Decrease in genu of the corpus callosum in medication-naive, early-onset dysthymia and depressive personality disorder. *Biological Psychiatry* 52:1134–1143.

MacKinnon DW (1962). The nature and nurture of creative talent. *American Psychologist* 17:484–495.

Maffei C (Ed.). (1993). *Il disturbo borderline di personalita. Prospettive sulla diagnosi.* Bollati Boringhieri, Torino, Italy.

Mahler M, Pine F, Bergman A (1975). *The psychological birth of a human infant*. Basic Books, New York.

Maier W, Lichtermann D, Minges J, et al. (1994). Personality disorders among the relatives of schizophrenia patients. *Schizophrenia Bulletin* 20(3):481–493.

McAdams DP (2017). Self and identity. In Biswas-Diener R, Diener E (eds.), *Noba textbook series: Psychology*. Champaign, IL: DEF Publishers.

McClure Gulding M, Gulding R (1979). *Changing lives through redecision therapy*. Brunner/Mazel, New York.

McCracken JT, Smalley SL, McGough JJ (2000). Evidence for linkage of a tandem duplication polymorphism upstream of the dopamine D4 receptor gene (DRD4) with attention deficit hyperactivity disorder (ADHD). *Molecular Psychiatry* 5:531–536.

McGlashan T, Grilo C, Sanislow C et al. (2005). Two-year prevalence and stability of individual DSM-IV criteria for schizotypal, borderline, avoidant, and obsessive-compulsive personality disorders: Toward a hybrid model of axis II disorders. *American Journal of Psychiatry* 162:883–889.

McGowan PO, Sasaki A, D'Alessio AC et al. (2009): Epigenetic regulation of the glucocorticoid receptor in human brain associates with childhood abuse. *Nature Neursocience* 12(3):342–348.

McPherson M, Smith-Lovin L, Brashears ME (2006). Social isolation in America: Changes in core discussion networks over two decades. *American Sociological Review* 71:353–375.

Mead GH (1934). *Mind, self and society from the standpoint of a social behaviorist*. Edited by Charles W. Morris. University of Chicago Press, Chicago.

Messerly JG (2017). Reason and meaning. Review of Michael Bess', *Our Grandchildren Redesigned*. https://ieet.org/index.php/IEET/more/Messerly20160323

Miczek KA, Almeida RMM, Kravitz EA et al. (2007). Neurobiology of escalated aggression and violence. *Journal of Neuroscience* 27(44):11803–11806.

Miczek KA, de Almeida RMM (2012). The case for basic research on the psychopharmacology of aggression. *Journal of Clinical Psychopharmacology* 32(1):1–2.

Miczek KA, Faccidomo S, De Almeida RMM et al. (2004). Escalated aggressive behavior: New pharmacotherapeutic approaches and opportunities. *Annals of the New York Academy of Sciences* 1036:336–355.

Miczek KA, Fish EW (2005). Dopamine, glutamate and aggression. In Schmidt WJ, Reith MEA (eds.), *Dopamine and glutamate in psychiatric disorders*, pp. 237–263. Humana Press, Totowa, NJ.

Miczek KA, Fish EW, de Bold JF et al. (2002). Social and neural determinants of aggressive behavior: Pharmacotherapeutic targets at serotonin, dopamine and gamma-aminobutyric acid systems. *Psychopharmacology* 163:434–458.

Miczek KA, Takahashi A, Gobrogge KL et al. (2015). Escalated aggression in animal models: Shedding new light on mesocorticolimbic circuits. *Current Opinions in Behavioral Sciences* 3:90–95.

Miettunen J, Kantojarvi L, Veijola J et al. (2006). International comparison of Cloninger's temperament dimensions. *Personality and Individual Differences* 41:1515–1526.

Millon T (2000). Personality disorders in modern life. John Wiley, New York.

Millon T, Millon C, Davis R, Grossman S (2009). *MCMI-III manual.* 4th ed. Pearson Education, Minneapolis, MN.

Mitchell J (1986). *The selected Melanie Klein.* Penguin Books, London.

Mitra A, Snyder AZ, Blazey T et al. (2015). Lag threads organize the brain's intrinsic activity. *PNAS* 112(52):E7307.

Mitra A, Kraft A, Wright P et al. (2018). Spontaneous infra-slow brain activity has unique spatiotemporal dynamics and laminar structure. *Neuron* 98:1–9.

Mollon P (n.d.). Releasing the unknown self [website version] www.selfpsychologypsychoanalysis.org

Monasterio E, Mei-Dan O, Hackney AC et al. (2016). Stress reactivity and personality in extreme sport athletes: The psychobiology of BASE jumpers. *Physiology and Behavior* 167:289–297.

Mulder RT, Joyce PR, Sellman JD et al. (1996). Towards an understanding of defense style in terms of temperament and character. *Acta Psychiatrica Scandinavica* 93:99–104.

Munafo MR, Yalcin B, Willis-Owen SA et al. (2008). Association of the DAD4 receptor (DRD4) gene and approach-related personality traits: Meta-analysis and new data. *Biological Psychiatry* 63(2):197–206.

Naslund J, Studer E, Pettersson R et al. (2015). Differences in anxiety-like behavior within a batch of Wistar rats are associated with differences in serotonergic transmission, enhanced by acute SRI administration, and abolished by serotonin depletion. *International Journal of Neuropsychopharmacology* 18(8):1–9.

Neppe V (1999). The serotonin 1A modulation of aggression: Bimodal buspirone dosage as a prototype anti-irritability agent in adults. *Australian Journal of Psychopharmacology* 9:8–25.

Nestler EJ, Hyman SE, Holtzman DM, Malenka RC (2015). *Molecular neuropharmacology: A foundation for clinical neuroscience*. 3rd ed. McGraw-Hill, New York.

New AS, Goodman M, Triebwasser J et al. (2008). Recent advances in the biological study of personality disorders. *Psychiatric Clinics of North America* 31:441–461.

Newman SW (1999). The medial extended amygdala in male reproductive behavior: A node in the mammalian social behavior network. *Annals of the New York Academy of Sciences* 877:242–257.

Novellino M (1984). Self-analysis of countertransference in integrative transactional analysis. *Transactional Analysis Journal* 14:63–75.

Nowak MA, Tarnita CE, Wilson EO (2010). The evolution of eusociality. *Nature* 466(7310):1057–1062.

Ogden TH (1979). On projective identification. *International Journal of Psychoanalysis* 60:357–373.

OPD Task Force (2008). *Operationalized Psychodynamic Diagnosis (OPD-2) manual of diagnosis and treatment planning.* Hogrefe, Cambridge, MA.

Oyserman D, Elmore K, Smith G (2012). Self, self-concept, and identity. In M. R. Leary, J. P. Tangeney (eds.), *Handbook of self and identity*, pp. 69–104. Guilford Press, New York and London.

Palese E (2013). Individual and society in the liquid modernity. *SpringerPlus* 2:191. http://www.springerplus.com/content/2/1/191

Panksepp J (1998). *Affective neuroscience: The foundations of human and animal emotions*. Oxford University Press, New York.

Pariante CM, Mako A, Lovestone S et al. (2001). Antidepressants enhance glucocorticoid receptor function in vitro by modulating the membrane steroid transporters. *British Journal of Pharmacology* 134:1335–1343.

Parker G (2014). Is borderline personality disorder a mood disorder? *The British Journal of Psychiatry* 204:252–253.

Pascual L, Rodrigues P, Gallardo-Pujol D (2013). How does morality work in the brain? A functional and structural perspective of moral behavior. *Frontiers in Neuroscience* 7:1–8.

Pasquali L, Busceti CL, Fulceri F et al. (2010). Intracellular pathways underlying the effects of lithium. *Behavior Pharmacology* 21:473–492.

Pastuzyn ED, Day CE, Kearns RB et al (2018). The neuronal gene arc encodes repurposed retrotransposon gag protein that mediates intercellular RNA transfer. *Cell* 172(1–2):275–288.

Pazzagli A, Monti MR (2000). Dysphoria and aloneness in borderline personality disorder. *Psychopathology* 33(4):220–226.

PDM Task Force (2006). *Psychodynamic diagnostic manual*. Alliance of Psychoanalysis Organizations, Silver Spring, MD.

Phelps EA (2004). Human emotion and memory: Interactions of the amygdala and hippocampal complex. *Current Opinion in Neurobiology* 14:198–202.

Posner M, Rothbarth M (2006). Temperament, attention, and developmental psychopathology. In D Cicchetti & DJ Cohen (Eds.), *Handbook of developmental psychopathology*. John Wiley, New York.

Posternak MA, Zimmerman M (2005). Dual reuptake inhibitors incur lower rates of tachyphylaxis than selective serotonin reuptake inhibitors: A retrospective study. *Journal of Clinical Psychiatry* 66(6):705–707.

Power RA, Steinberg S, Bjornsdottir G et al. (2015). Polygenic risk scores for schizophrenia and bipolar disorder predict creativity. *Nature Neuroscience* 18: 953–955.

Preston SD, de Waal FBM (2002). Empathy: Its ultimate and proximate bases. *Behavioral and Brain Sciences* 25:1–72.

Prochaska JO, Norcross JC (2003). *Systems of psychotherapy. A transtheoretical analysis*. Thompson, Brooks/Cole, Stamford, CN.

Proust M (1913). *À la recherche du temps perdu* (In Search of Lost Time). Grasset and Gallimard, Paris.

Proust J (2009). What is a mental function? In Brenner A, Gayon J (eds.), *Philosophy of science contemporary research in France*. Springer, New York.

Puig VM, Gulledge AT (2011). Serotonin and prefrontal cortex function: Neurons, networks, and circuits. *Molecular Neurobiology* 44(3):449–464.

Quadros IM, Hwa LS, Shimamoto A et al. (2014). Prevention of alcohol-heightened aggression by CRF-R1 antagonists in mice: Critical role for DRN-PFC serotonin pathway. *Neuropsychopharmacology* 39:2874–2883.

Raine A, Yang Y (2006). The anatomical bases of psychopathy: A review of brain imaging findings. In Patrick, CJ (ed.), *Handbook of psychopathy*, pp. 278–295. Guilford Press, New York.

Robbins P (2017). Modularity of mind. In *Stanford encyclopedia of philosophy* (Winter 2017 edition), Edward N. Zalta (ed.). https://plato.stanford.edu/archives/win2017/entries/modularity-mind

Robins, CJ, Rosenthal MZ, Cuper PF (2010). Dialectical behavior therapy. In Magnavita J (ed.), *Evidence based treatment of personality dysfunction*, pp. 49–78. American Psychological Association, Washington, DC.

Roy Byrne PP (2005). The GABA–benzodiazepine receptor complex: Structure, function, and role in anxiety. *Journal of Clinical Psychiatry* 66(Suppl. 2):14–20.

Salovey P, Mayer J, Caruso D (2004). Emotional intelligence: Theory, findings, and implications. *Psychological Inquiry* 15(3):197–215.

Savin-Williams RC, Demo DH (1983). Situational and transituational determinants of adolescent self-feelings. *Journal of Personality and Social Psychology* 44:824–833.

Schreckenberger M, Klega A, Grunder G et al. (2008). Opioid receptor PET reveals the psychobiologic correlates of reward processing. *Journal of Nuclear Medicine* 49:1257–1261.

Schiff J, Schiff A, Mellor K et al. (1975). *Cathexis reader: Transactional analysis treatment of psychosis.* Harper & Row, New York.

Schnell K, Herpertz SC (2007). Effects of dialectic-behavioral-therapy on the neural correlates of affective hyperarousal in borderline personality disorder. *Journal of Psychiatric Research* 41:837–847.

Schosser A, Fuchs K, Scharl T et al. (2010). Interaction between serotonin 5-HT2A receptor gene and dopamine transporter (DAT1) gene polymorphisms influences personality trait of persistence in Austrian Caucasians. *The World Journal of Biological Psychiatry* 11(2):417–424.

Schwartz F (1981). Psychic structure. *International Journal of Psychoanalysis* 62(1):61–72.

Scully JL (2004). What is a disease? Disease, disability and their definitions. *EMBO Reports* 5(7):650–653.

Searls HF (1986). *My work with borderline patients*. Aronson, New York.

Shedler J (2010). The efficacy of psychodynamic psychotherapy. *American Psychologist* 65(2):98–109.

Siddiqui SV, Chatterjee U, Kumar D et al. (2008). Neuropsychology of prefrontal cortex *Indian Journal of Psychiatry* 50(3):202–208.

Siegel A, Roeling TAP, Gregg TR et al. (1999). Neuropharmacology of brain-stimulation-evoked aggression. *Neuroscience and Biobehavioral Reviews* 23:359–389.

Siegel A, Victoroff J (2009). Understanding human aggression: New insights from neuroscience. *International Journal of Law and Psychiatry* 32:209–215.

Siever LJ, Weinstein LN (2009). The neurobiology of personality disorders: Implications for psychoanalysis. *Journal of the American Psychoanalytic Association* 57(2):361–398.

Simeon D (2004). Depersonalisation disorder: A contemporary overview. *CNS Drugs* 18(6):343–54.

Skodol AE, Stout RL, McGlashan TH et al. (1999). Co-occurrence of mood and personality disorders: A report from the Collaborative Longitudinal Personality Disorders Study (CLPS). *Depression and Anxiety* 10:175–182.

Sporns O, Betzel RF (2016). Modular brain networks. *Annual Review of Psychology* 4(67):613–640.

Sporns O, Kötter R (2004). Motifs in brain networks. *PLoS Biology* 2(11):e369.

Starcevic V, Uhlenhuth EH, Stephanie Fallon S et al. (1996). Personality dimensions in panic disorder and generalized anxiety disorder. *Journal of Affective Disorders* 37:75–79.

Stevens GW, Deuling JK, Armenakis AA (2012). Successful psychopaths: Are they unethical decision-makers and why? *Journal of Business Ethics* 105(2):139–149

Stewart I, Joines V (1987). TA today: A new introduction to transactional analysis. Lifespace, Nottingham; Chapel Hill.

Stone I (1934). *Lust for life*. Longmans, Green, NY.

Sui J, Humphreys GW (2015). The integrative self: How self-reference integrates perception and memory. *Trends in Cognitive Sciences* 19(12):719–728.

Suzuki H, Luby J, Botteron KN et al. (2014). Early life stress and trauma and enhanced limbic activation to emotionally valenced faces in depressed and healthy children. *Journal of the American Academy for Child and Adolescent Psychiatry* 53(7):800–813.

Svoboda E, McKinnon MC, Levine B (2006). The functional neuroanatomy of autobiographical memory: A meta-analysis. *Neuropsychologia* 44(12): 2189–2208.

Svrakic DM (1990). The functional dynamics of narcissistic personality. *American Journal of Psychotherapy* 44(2):189–203.

Svrakic DM, Whitehead CA, Przybeck TR et al. (1993). Differential diagnosis of personality disorders by the seven-factor Temperament and Character Inventory. *Archives of General Psychiatry* 50:991–999.

Svrakic DM, Draganic S, Hill K et al. (2002). Temperament, character, and personality disorders: Etiologic, diagnostic, treatment issues. *Acta Psychiatrica Scandinavica* 106:189–195.

Svrakic DM, Lečić-Toševski D, Divac-Jovanovic M (2009). DSM Axis II: Personality disorders or adaptation disorders? *Current Opinion in Psychiatry* 29:111–117.

Svrakic DM, Zorumski CF, Svrakic N et al. (2013). Risk architecture of schizophrenia: The role of epigenetics. *Current Opinion in Psychiatry* 26:1–8.

Švrakić M (1962). *Šta su neuroze?* Kultura, Beograd.

Svrakic NM, Svrakic DM, Cloninger CR (1996). A general quantitative theory of personality development: Fundamentals of a self-organizing psychobiological complex. *Development and Psychopathology* 8:247–272.

Takahashi A, Lee RX, Iwasato TI et al. (2015). Glutamate input in the dorsal raphe nucleus as a determinant of escalated aggression in male mice. *Journal of Neuroscience* 35(16):6452–6463.

Takahashi A, Quadros IM, de Almeida RMM et al. (2011). Brain serotonin receptors and transporters: Initiation vs. termination of escalated aggression. *Psychopharmacology* 213:183–212.

Talvik M, Nordström A-L, Olsson H et al. (2003). Decreased thalamic D2/D3 receptor binding in drug-naive patients with schizophrenia:A PET study with [11C]FLB 457. *International Journal of Neuropsychopharmacology* 6:361–370.

Thase ME (2008). Are SNRIs more effective than SSRIs? A review of the current state of the controversy. *Psychopharmacology Bulletin* 41(2):58–85.

Thomas A, Chess S (1984). Genesis and evolution of behavioral disorders: From infancy to early adult life. *American Journal of Psychiatry* 141:1–9.

Thombs BD, Bassel M, Jewett LR (2009). Analyzing effectiveness of long-term psychodynamic psychotherapy. *JAMA* 301:930–933.

Tienari P, Wynne LC, Sorri A et al. (2004). Genotype-environment interaction in schizophrenia-spectrum disorder: Long-term follow-up study of Finnish adoptees. *The British Journal of Psychiatry* 184:216–222.

Todd RD, Neuman RJ (2007). Gene-environment interactions in the development of combined type ADHD: Evidence for a synapse-based model. *American Journal of Medical Genetics B: Neuropsychiatric Genetics* 144B(8):971–975.

Tolstoy L (2010). *My life* (Serbian translation). LOM, Belgrade, Serbia.

Town JE, Abbass A, Hardy G (2011). Short-term psychodynamic psychotherapy for personality disorders: A critical review of randomized controlled trials. *Journal of Personality Disorders* 25:723–740.

Trull TJ, Durrett CA (2005). Categorical and dimensional models of personality disorder. *Annual Review of Clinical Psychology* 1:355–380.

Tseelon E (1992). Is the presented self sincere? Goffman, impression management and the postmodern self. *Theory, Culture & Society* 9:115–128.

Turkle S (2010). *Alone together: Why we expect more from technology and less form each other*. Basic Books, New York.

Tyrer P, Crawford M, Mulder R (2011). Reclassifying personality disorders. *The Lancet* 377:1814–1815.

Vaillant G (1992). Ego Mechanisms of Defense: A Guide for Clinicans and Researchers, American Psychiatric Press, Inc., Washington DC, London England.

Van Tol HHM, Bunzow JR, Guan H-C et al. (1991). Cloning of the gene for the human dopamine D4 receptor with high affinity for the antipsychotic clozapine. *Nature* 350:610–614.

Victoroff J (2017). The neurpopsychiatry of human aggression. In Sadock BJ, Sadock VA, Ruiz P (eds.), *Kaplan and Sadock's comprehensive textbook of psychiatry*, 10th ed., pp. 2471–2504. Wolters Kluwer, New York.

Vitiello B, Stoff DM (1997). Subtypes of aggression and their relevance to child psychiatry. *Journal of American Academy of Child and Adolescent Psychiatry* 36:307–315.

Warneken F, Tomasello M (2009). The roots of human altruism. *British Journal of Psychology* 100:455–471.

Williams HL, Conway MA, Cohen G (2008). Autobiographical memory. In Cohen G and Conway MA (Eds.), *Memory in the real world*. 3rd ed., pp. 21–90. Psychology Press, Hove, UK.

Wilkinson-Ryan, Westen D (2000). Identity disturbance in borderline personality disorder: An empirical investigation. *American Journal of Psychiatry* 157(4):528–541.

Willick MS (1983). On the concept of primitive defences. *Journal of the American Psychoanalytic Association* 31(Suppl.):175–200.

Wilson S, Stroud CB, Emily DC (2017). Interpersonal dysfunction in personality disorders: A meta-analytic review. *Psychological Bulletin* 143(7):677–734.

World Health Organization (1994). *International classification of diseases*, 10th revision. World Health Organization, Geneva.

World Health Organization (2018). *International classification of diseases*, 11th revision. World Health Organization, Geneva (coming into effect in 2022).

Wright R (1999). *Non zero: The logic of human destiny*. Pantheon Books, New York.

Wright AGC, Hallquist MN, Morse JQ et al. (2013). Clarifying interpersonal heterogeneity in borderline personality disorder using latent mixture modeling. *Journal of Personality Disorders* 27(2):125–143.

Wynn K (2009). Constraints on natural altruism. *British Journal of Psychology* 100:481–485.

Wynn K (2013). Born good? Babies help unlock the origins of morality. *60 Minutes*, July 28.

Yalom ID (2009). *The gift of therapy*. HarperCollins, New York.

Yang M, Coid J, Tyrer P (2010). Personality pathology recorded by severity: National survey. *The British Journal of Psychiatry* 197:193–199.

Young JE, Klosko J, Weishaar ME (2003). *Schema therapy. A practitioner's guide*. Guilford Press, New York.

Zald DH, Cowan RL, Riccardi P et al. (2008). Midbrain DA receptor availability is inversely associated with novelty-seeking traits in humans. *Journal of Neuroscience* 28(53):14372–14378.

Zhou Y, Liang M, Tian L et al. (2007). Functional disintegration in paranoid Schizophrenia using resting-state fMR. *Schizophrenia Research* 97(1–3):194–205.

Zimmerman M, Chelminski I, Young D et al. (2011). Does DSM-IV already capture the dimensional nature of personality disorders? *Journal of Clinical Psychiatry* 72(10):1333–1339.

Zorumski CF, Conway CR (2017). Use of ketamine in clinical practice: A time for optimism and caution. *JAMA Psychiatry* 74(4):405–406.

Zorumski CF, Rubin E (2011). *Psychiatry and clinical neuroscience: A primer*. Oxford University Press, New York.

INDEX

Made in the USA
Coppell, TX
13 December 2025

65609077R00201